T0329855

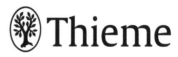

Fractures of the Hand and Carpus

FESSH 2018 Instructional Course Book

Michel E. H. Boeckstyns, MD, PhD
Consultant Hand Surgeon
Capio-CFR Hospital
Hellerup, Denmark

Martin Richter, MD
Director
Department of Hand Surgery
Malteser Hospital Seliger Gerhard
Bonn, Germany

629 illustrations

Thieme
Stuttgart • New York • Delhi • Rio de Janeiro

Library of Congress Cataloging-in-Publication Data is available from the publisher.

© 2018 by Georg Thieme Verlag KG

Thieme Publishers Stuttgart
Rüdigerstrasse 14, 70469 Stuttgart, Germany
+49 [0]711 8931 421, customerservice@thieme.de

Thieme Publishers New York
333 Seventh Avenue, New York, NY 10001 USA
+1 800 782 3488, customerservice@thieme.com

Thieme Publishers Delhi
A-12, Second Floor, Sector-2, Noida-201301
Uttar Pradesh, India
+91 120 45 566 00, customerservice@thieme.in

Thieme Publishers Rio, Thieme Publicações Ltda.
Edifício Rodolpho de Paoli, 25º andar
Av. Nilo Peçanha, 50 - Sala 2508
Rio de Janeiro 20020-906 Brasil
+55 21 3172 2297 / +55 21 3172 1896

Cover design: Thieme Publishing Group
Typesetting by Ditech Process Solutions, India

Printed in Germany by CPI Books GmbH   5 4 3 2 1

ISBN 978-3-13-241720-5

Also available as an e-book:
eISBN 978-3-13-241721-2

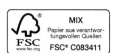

Contents

Preface ix

Contributors x

Section I General Chapters 1

1   Epidemiology and Specific Challenges 3
Kevin C. Chung, Sandra V. Kotsis

1.1   Incidence of Hand and Carpal Fractures   3

2   Evidence in the Treatment of Hand Fractures 11
János Rupnik

2.1   Introduction   11   2.3   Results................................... 12
2.2   Quality and Distribution of the Studies   11   2.4   Discussion 13

3   Nonoperative Management of Hand Fractures 15
Grey Giddins

3.1   Introduction   15   3.3   Results................................... 15
3.2   Methods and Materials....................   15   3.4   Discussion 25

4   K-wire Fixation, Intraosseous Wiring, Tension Band Wiring 29
Lindsay Muir, Anuj Mishra, Zafar Naqui

4.1   Intraosseous and Cerclage Wiring..........   29   4.2   K-wire Fixation........................... 31

5   Intramedullary Screw Fixation of the Metacarpals and Phalanges of the Hand 41
Maurizio Calcagni, Lisa Reissner, Christoph Erling, Thomas Giesen

5.1   Introduction   41   5.4   Results................................... 46
5.2   Indications..............................   42   5.5   Complications 46
5.3   Surgical Technique.......................   42   5.6   Conclusions 46

6   Plate and Screw Fixation of Hand and Carpal Fractures 47
Philippe Cuénod

6.1   Introduction and Historical Perspective   47   6.4   Specific Indications and Procedures 52
6.2   Implants and Technical Principles..........   47   6.5   Complications 61
6.3   General Considerations and Indications   51

7   External Minifixation 65
Frédéric Schuind, Fabian Moungondo, Wissam El Kazzi

7.1   Introduction   65   7.4   Results................................... 69
7.2   Surgical Technique.......................   65   7.5   Discussion 69
7.3   Indications..............................   68

8   Role of Arthroscopy in the Treatment of Carpal Fractures and Nonunion 73
Peter Jørgsholm

8.1   Introduction   73   8.3   Method 75
8.2   Indications..............................   73   8.4   Conclusion 79

9   **Strategies in Compound Hand Injuries**.. 81
         Thomas Giesen, Olga Politikou, Maurizio Calcagni

9.1   Introduction 81   9.5   Classification............................. 82
9.2   Patient Expectation 81   9.6   Timing.................................... 82
9.3   Clinical Examination 81   9.7   Surgery 83
9.4   Imaging.................................. 81   9.8   Surgical Steps 83

10   **Pediatric Hand Fractures**.. 91
         Pernille Leicht

10.1   Introduction 91   10.2   Special Children Fractures 92

11   **Fractures in the Paralytic Extremity** 101
         Gürsel Leblebicioğlu, Egemen Ayhan, Tüzün Fırat

11.1   Introduction 101   11.5   Diagnosis 105
11.2   Basic Science 101   11.6   Management of Fractures 105
11.3   Epidemiology 104   11.7   Evidence 105
11.4   Prevention 104   11.8   Future 105

12   **Hand Injuries in the Athlete** 109
         William Geissler, David Alvarez

12.1   Metacarpal and Phalangeal Fractures....... 109   12.3   Scapholunate Injuries 118
12.2   Carpal Fractures 113

13   **Special Aspects in Musicians** 123
         Philippe Cuénod

13.1   Introduction and Historical Perspective 123   13.3   General Principles and Clinical Examples ... 128
13.2   Instruments and Movements Required to   13.4   Conclusions 133
       Play Them.............................. 124

14   **Fractures of the Hand and Carpus: Complications and Their Treatment** 135
         Adnan Prsic, Jing Chen, Jin Bo Tang

14.1   Infection/Osteomyelitis 135   14.6   Summary of Clinical Points to Aid in
14.2   Malunion 136   Prevention of Complications.............. 141
14.3   Nonunion.............................. 139   14.7   Special Clinical Points in Judgment and
14.4   Bone Necrosis 140   Surgical Treatment....................... 142
14.5   Complications of Intra-articular Fracture:
       Osteoarthritis and Stiffness of Ligaments ... 141

15   **Rehabilitation of Hand and Finger Fractures** 145
         Jürgen Mack

15.1   Challenges in Rehabilitation of Hand and   15.3   Techniques Used in Rehabilitation.......... 146
       Wrist Fractures 145   15.4   Extension and Traction.................... 150
15.2   Patient Evaluation before Therapy......... 145   15.5   Summary 155

Section II Phalangeal Fractures 157

16   **Fractures at the Base of the Proximal Phalanx** 159
         Lars S. Vadstrup

16.1   Trauma Mechanism...................... 159   16.3   Clinical Signs and Tests.................... 159
16.2   Classification........................... 159   16.4   Investigatory Examinations................ 160

16.5	Possible Concurrent Lesions of Bone and Soft Tissue 160	16.8	Alternative Treatment Options. 161
16.6	Evidence. 160	16.9	Prognosis 161
16.7	Author's Favored Treatment Option 160		

17   Extra-articular Fractures of the Phalanges. 163
David J. Shewring

17.1	Trauma Mechanism. 163	17.7	Author's Favored Treatment Options 165
17.2	Classification. 163	17.8	Alternative Treatment Options. 167
17.3	Clinical Signs and Tests. 164	17.9	Treatment of Specific Fracture Configurations. 169
17.4	Investigatory Examinations. 164		
17.5	Concurrent Soft Tissue Lesions. 164	17.10	Prognosis 173
17.6	Evidence. 165	17.11	Tips and Tricks 173

18   Intra-articular Fractures of the Proximal Interphalangeal Joint 175
David J. Shewring

18.1	Trauma Mechanism. 175	18.5	Evidence. 176
18.2	Classification. 175	18.6	Author's Favored Treatment Options 180
18.3	Clinical Signs and Tests. 175	18.7	Alternative Treatment Options. 182
18.4	Investigatory Examinations. 175	18.8	Prognosis 183

19   Avulsion Fractures of the Flexor and Extensor Tendons 185
Michael Solomons

19.1	Extensor Avulsion Fractures 185	19.2	Flexor Avulsion Fractures. 190

Section III Metacarpal Fractures 193

20   Intra-articular Fractures and Dislocations at the Base of Metacarpals 2 to 5. 195
Michael Schädel-Höpfner

20.1	Introduction 195	20.6	Treatment. 197
20.2	Trauma Mechanism and Anatomy. 195	20.7	Evidence. 201
20.3	Classification. 195	20.8	Author's Favored Treatment Option 201
20.4	Clinical Signs and Tests. 196	20.9	Tips and Tricks 203
20.5	Investigatory Examinations. 197	20.10	Prognosis 203

21   Intra-articular Fractures at the Base of the First Metacarpal. 205
Yuka Igeta, Sybille Facca, Philippe A. Liverneaux

21.1	Trauma Mechanism. 205	21.6	Evidence. 206
21.2	Classification. 205	21.7	Authors' Favored Treatment Option 206
21.3	Clinical Signs and Tests. 206	21.8	Alternative Treatment Options. 207
21.4	Investigatory Examinations. 206	21.9	Prognosis 210
21.5	Possible Concurrent Lesions of Bone and Soft Tissue 206	21.10	Tips and Tricks 210

22   Diaphyseal Fractures of the Metacarpals. 213
Pierluigi Tos, Simona Odella, Ugo Dacatra, Jane Messina, Emilio Pedrini

22.1	Trauma Mechanism. 213	22.5	Possible Concurrent Lesions of Bone and Soft Tissue 214
22.2	Classification. 213		
22.3	Clinical Signs 213	22.6	Evidence and Anatomical Considerations . . . 214
22.4	Investigatory Examination. 213	22.7	Indications for Surgery. 214

22.8 Authors' Favored Treatment Option 215
22.9 Alternative Treatment Options............. 220

22.10 Prognosis 220
22.11 Tips and Tricks 220

23   Metacarpal Neck Fractures 223
Hebe Désirée Kvernmo

23.1 Trauma Mechanism....................... 223
23.2 Classification............................. 223
23.3 Clinical Signs and Tests.................... 223
23.4 Radiographs............................. 225
23.5 Possible Concurrent Lesions of Bone and
     Soft Tissue 226

23.6 Evidence.................................. 226
23.7 Author's Favored Treatment Option 227
23.8 Alternative Treatment Options............. 230
23.9 Prognosis 230
23.10 Tips and Tricks 230

24   Correction of Malunion in Metacarpal and Phalangeal Fractures 233
Hermann Krimmer

24.1 Trauma Mechanism....................... 233
24.2 Classification............................. 233
24.3 Clinical Signs and Tests.................... 233
24.4 Evidence 233

24.5 Author's Favored Treatment Options 233
24.6 Clinical Results 235
24.7 Tips and Tricks 235

Section IV Carpal Fractures 237

25   Acute Scaphoid Fractures 239
Joseph J. Dias, Lambros Athanatos

25.1 Introduction 239
25.2 Trauma Mechanism....................... 239
25.3 Clinical Signs and Tests.................... 239
25.4 Investigatory Examinations................ 241

25.5 Alternative Treatment Options............. 242
25.6 Prognosis 244
25.7 Conclusion 246

26   Nonunion of the Scaphoid 249
Susanne Roberts, Scott W. Wolfe

26.1 Trauma Mechanism....................... 249
26.2 Diagnostic Techniques and Criteria......... 251
26.3 Treatment Options....................... 251

26.4 Evidence and Prognosis 258
26.5 Salvage Procedures 258

27   Other Carpal Fractures 261
Martin Richter

27.1 General Considerations 261
27.2 Fracture of Triquetrum.................... 262
27.3 Fracture of the Pisiform 264
27.4 Fracture of the Lunate.................... 265

27.5 Fracture of the Trapezium 266
27.6 Fracture of Capitate...................... 269
27.7 Fracture of Hamate 271

Index 275

Preface

This year's Instructional Course "Fractures of the Hand and Carpus" for the XXIII congress of the FESSH is possible thanks to the contributions of a number of prominent experts, to whom we are deeply indebted. The accompanying book is a comprehensive summary of the current state of the art of the management of hand fractures.

The book consists of a number of chapters, which include anatomy and general principles as well as a variety of techniques for the management of specific fractures. It will become evident that more than one approach may be applicable for any given situation. This may range from nonoperative methods such as splint or cast immobilization to percutaneous pin fixation, external and internal fixation. The most appropriate method for any given case will depend on the available evidence and the surgeon's personal experience as well as individual patient considerations. The emphasis in each case is on regaining anatomical alignment and a functional finger range of motion. In some cases, a less than perfect alignment may be sacrificed at the expense of optimizing hand function. An early and aggressive postoperative hand therapy program is often integral to the final outcome in many cases and cannot be overemphasized.

Although any opinions expressed in this book should not be considered as the official guidelines of the FESSH, we are certain that this book will be useful for both the entry level surgeon and the experienced operator. We hope you will enjoy reading this book as much as we enjoyed producing it.

Michel E. H. Boeckstyns, MD, PhD
Martin Richter, MD

Contributors

David Alvarez, MD
Hand and Upper Extremity Surgery Fellow
Department of Orthopaedic Surgery
University of Mississippi Medical Center
Jackson, MS, USA

Lambros Athanatos, MRCS (Ed)
Specialist Trainee in Trauma and Orthopaedic Surgery
University Hospitals of Leicester
Leicester General Hospital
Leicester, UK

Egemen Ayhan, MD
Hand Surgeon
Department of Orthopaedics and Traumatology
University of Health Sciences
Diskapi Yildirim Beyazit Training and Research Hospital
Ankara, Turkey

Maurizio Calcagni, MD
Vice Chairman
Division of Plastic Surgery and Hand Surgery
University Hospital Zurich
Zurich, Switzerland

Jing Chen, MD
Attending Surgeon
Department of Hand Surgery
Affiliated Hospital of Nantong University
Jiangsu, China

Kevin C. Chung, MD, MS
Professor of Surgery
Section of Plastic Surgery
Department of Surgery
Assistant Dean for Faculty Affairs
University of Michigan Medical School
Ann Arbor, MI, USA

Philippe Cuénod, MD
Specialist for Hand Surgery FMH
CH8 - Center for Hand Surgery and Therapy
Geneva, Switzerland

Ugo Dacatra, MD
Head of Clinic
Division of Hand Surgery
Gaetano Pini Orthopaedic Institute
Milan, Italy

Joseph J. Dias, MD, FRCS
Professor of Hand and Orthopaedic Surgery
University Hospitals of Leicester
Leicester General Hospital
Leicester, UK

Christoph Erling, MD
Senior Physician
Department of Plastic Surgery and Hand Surgery
University Hospital Zurich
Zurich, Switzerland

Sybille Facca, MD, PhD
Surgeon
Department of Hand Surgery
University Hospital of Strasbourg, FMTS
CNRS, University of Strasbourg
Strasbourg, France

Tüzün Fırat, PT, PhD
Associate Professor
Department of Physiotherapy and Rehabilitation
Faculty of Health Sciences
University of Hacettepe
Ankara, Turkey

William Geissler, MD
Alan E Freeland Chair of Hand Surgery
Professor and Chief
Division of Hand and Upper Extremity Surgery
Chief, Section of Arthroscopic Surgery and Sports Medicine
Director, Hand and Upper Extremity Fellowship
Department of Orthopaedic Surgery
University of Mississippi Medical Center
Jackson, MS, USA

Grey Giddins, FRCS (Orth), Dip Hand Surg (Eur)
Professor
Orthopaedic Department
Royal United Hospital
Bath, UK

Thomas Giesen, MD
Consultant Hand Surgeon
Free Lecturer of the University of Zurich
Swissparc AG
Zurich, Switzerland
Centro Manoegomito
Clinica Ars Medica
Lugano, Switzerland

Yuka Igeta, MD
Hand Surgeon
Department of Orthopaedic Surgery
Juntendo University Tokyo
Tokyo, Japan
Department of Hand Surgery
University Hospital of Strasbourg, FMTS
University of Strasbourg
Strasbourg, France

Peter Jørgsholm, MD, PhD
Head of Clinic, Hand Surgeon
Private Hospital Mølholm
Vejle, Denmark

Wissam El Kazzi, MD
Head
Hand Surgery Clinic
Erasme University Hospital
Brussels, Belgium

Sandra V. Kotsis, MPH
Research Associate
Section of Plastic Surgery
Department of Surgery
University of Michigan Medical School
Ann Arbor, MI, USA

Hermann Krimmer, MD
Hand Surgeon
Hand Center Ravensburg
Clinic St. Elisabeth Ravensburg
Ravensburg, Germany

Hebe Désirée Kvernmo, MD, PhD
Professor
Hand Unit, Orthopaedic Department
University Hospital of North Norway
Senior Consultant
Institute of Clinical Medicine
University of Tromsø - The Arctic University of Norway
Tromsø, Norway

Gürsel Leblebicioğlu, MD
Professor of Orthopaedic Surgery and Traumatology
Hand Surgeon
Division of Hand Surgery
Department of Orthopaedic Surgery and Traumatology
University of Hacettepe Medical School
Ankara, Turkey

Pernille Leicht, MD
Consultant
Orthopaedic Clinic, Hand Surgery Section
Copenhagen University
Rigshospitalet
Copenhagen, Denmark

Philippe A. Liverneaux, MD, PhD
Chairman
Department of Hand Surgery
University Hospital of Strasbourg, FMTS
University of Strasbourg
Strasbourg, France

Jürgen Mack
Physiotherapist, Hand and Manual Therapist
Private practice
Institute for Physiotherapy and Hand Therapy
Ulm, Germany

Jane Messina, MD
Specialist in Orthopaedics and Traumatology
Operative Surgery Unit
Hand Institute Gaetano Pini
Milan, Italy

Anuj Mishra, MD
Consultant Plastic, Reconstructive and Hand Surgeon
Manchester Hand Centre
University Hospital of South Manchester
NHS Foundation Trust
Manchester, UK

Fabian Moungondo, MD
Hand Surgeon
Erasme University Hospital
Brussels, Belgium

Lindsay Muir, MB, MCh Orth, FRCS (Orth)
Consultant Hand Surgeon
Manchester Hand Institute
Salford Royal NHS Foundation Trust
University of Manchester
Manchester, UK

Zafar Naqui, BDHS, EBHD, MSc Hand Surg.
Consultant Hand and Wrist Surgeon
Manchester Hand Centre
Salford Royal FT
University of Manchester
Manchester, UK

Simona Odella, MD
Hand Surgeon
Hand Surgery and Reconstructive Microsurgery Unit
ASST Orthopaedic and Trauma Center Pini-CTO
Milan, Italy

Emilio Pedrini, MD
Hand Surgeon
Hand Surgery and Reconstructive Microsurgery Unit
Orthopaedic Institute G. Pini-CTO
Milan, Italy

Olga Politikou, MD
Assistant Hand Surgeon
Department of Plastic and Hand Surgery
University of Zurich
Zurich, Switzerland

Adnan Prsic, MD
Hand and Microsurgery Fellow
Department of Orthopaedics and Sports Medicine
University of Washington
Seattle, WA, USA

Lisa Reissner, MD
Consultant
Department of Plastic Surgery and Hand Surgery
University Hospital Zurich
Zurich, Switzerland

Martin Richter, MD
Director
Department of Hand Surgery
Malteser Hospital Seliger Gerhard
Bonn, Germany

Susanne Roberts, MD
Assistant Professor
Department of Orthopaedic Surgery
Columbia University Medical Center
New York, NY, USA

János Rupnik, MD
Head
Department of Hand Surgery
Péterfy Hospital National Institute of Traumatology
Budapest, Hungary

Michael Schädel-Höpfner, MD
Head
Department of Orthopaedic and Hand Surgery
Lukas Hospital
Neuss, Germany

Frédéric Schuind, MD, PhD
Full Professor
Université libre de Bruxelles
Head
Department of Orthopaedics and Traumatology
Erasme University Hospital
Brussels, Belgium

David J. Shewring, MB BCh, FRCS(Orth), Dip Hand Surg (Eur)
Consultant Hand Surgeon
Department of Hand Surgery
University Hospital of Wales
Cardiff, Wales

Michael Solomons, MD, FCS (SA) Orth
Associate Professor
Department of Orthopaedics
University of Cape Town
Cape Town, South Africa

Jin Bo Tang, MD
Professor and Chair
Department of Hand Surgery
The Hand Surgery Research Center
Affiliated Hospital of Nantong University
Jiangsu, China

Pierluigi Tos, MD, PhD
Chief
Hand Surgery and Reconstructive Microsurgery Unit,
Orthopaedic Institute G. Pini-CTO
Milan, Italy

Lars S. Vadstrup, MD
Head
Hand Surgery Clinic
Gentofte Hospital
Copenhagen, Denmark

Scott W. Wolfe, MD
Professor
Department of Orthopaedic Surgery
Hospital for Special Surgery
Weill Medical College of Cornell University
New York, NY, USA

Section I
General Chapters

1 Epidemiology and Specific
Challenges 3

2 Evidence in the Treatment of
Hand Fractures 11

3 Nonoperative Management
of Hand Fractures 15

4 K-wire Fixation, Intraosseous
Wiring, Tension Band Wiring 29

5 Intramedullary Screw Fixation
of the Metacarpals and
Phalanxes of the Hand 41

6 Plate and Screw Fixation of
Hand and Carpal Fractures 47

7 External Minifixation 65

8 Role of Arthroscopy in the
Treatment of Carpal Fractures
and Nonunion 73

9 Strategies in Compound Hand
Injuries 81

10 Pediatric Hand Fractures 91

11 Fractures in the Paralytic
Extremity 101

12 Hand Injuries in the Athlete 109

13 Special Aspects in Musicians 123

14 Fractures of the Hand and Carpus:
Complications and Their
Treatmentment 135

15 Rehabilitation of Hand and
Finger Fractures 145

1 Epidemiology and Specific Challenges

Kevin C. Chung, Sandra V. Kotsis

Abstract

Knowing the epidemiology of hand fractures can aid in clinical care by recognizing the types of fractures and the mechanisms of injury that commonly affect each age group. The incidence of hand and wrist fractures continues to rise, particularly in adolescents, owing to increased participation in competitive sports. Metacarpal fractures have the highest incidence in 10- to 20-year-olds and phalangeal fractures have the highest incidence in 11- to 15-year-olds. In phalangeal fractures, for most age groups, the thumb is the second most commonly fractured digit after the small finger. However, in individuals older than 65 years, excluding metacarpal fractures, the thumb is the most commonly injured digit. Children of age 5 to 14 years represent the age group most commonly seen with a carpal fracture and the scaphoid has the highest fracture rate of all the carpal bones. Future research collaborations aiming to reduce the incidence of sports-related hand fractures are needed as well as increased emphasis on safety measures at work to prevent fall-related fractures.

Keywords: epidemiology, incidence, etiology, pediatric, metacarpal, phalangeal, thumb, carpal, scaphoid, Salter-Harris

1.1 Incidence of Hand and Carpal Fractures

The incidence of hand and wrist fractures has increased and continues to do so, mainly because of the competitive nature of sports at the high school and college levels and the increased participation in sports for all ages of the general population.[1] In 2010, 15% of all emergency department visits for children aged 19 years or younger were fracture related and the three most common fracture locations were in the upper extremities (forearm, finger, and wrist).[2] Approximately 46% of high school students in the United States participated in a sport in the 2009 to 2010 academic year.[3] Using the National High School Sports-Related Injury Surveillance System, it was found that the hand/finger was the most commonly fractured body site (32%). This was true for football, boys' soccer, volleyball, boys' and girls' basketball, wrestling, baseball, and softball.[4] Additionally, a large number of children and adolescents participate in non-school–related activities that result in hand injuries, such as skateboarding and scooter-riding.[5] Although sports are the most common cause of hand fracture in school-aged children, a study of pediatric hand fractures found that children between the ages of 1 and 3 years are most affected by crush injuries.[6] Thus, biphasic peaks in fracture incidence are seen in 1- to 3-year-olds and again in 10- to 12-year-olds.[6]

Knowing the epidemiology of hand fractures can aid in clinical care by recognizing the types of fractures that commonly affect each age group and the mechanisms of injury that cause different fractures.

1.1.1 Metacarpal Fractures

Metacarpal fractures comprise 33% of all hand fractures reported in a national injury database during a 5-year period[7] and 18% of all hand and/or forearm fractures in U.S. emergency departments.[8] The most common location for fracture was at home.[7] Metacarpal fractures have been reported to have the highest incidence in 10- to 19-year-olds,[7] 15- to 24-year-olds,[8] and 16- to 20-year-olds[9] (▶ Fig. 1.1). In a study of pediatric hand fractures, the metacarpals of the small digit had the second highest incidence of fractures and most fractures were concentrated around the metacarpophalangeal joint of the small finger.[10] Similarly, a study in Norway consisting of patients of all ages presenting with fracture found that the two most common sites of fractures were around the small finger metacarpophalangeal joint and the small finger metacarpal as a whole.[11]

Males are more likely to incur a metacarpal fracture compared to females.[7,8] An interaction between age and sex has been shown to be significant; younger men are at the greatest risk of having a metacarpal fracture.[7] Males also show peaks of hand, wrist, and forearm fracture occurrence in May and September, which is thought to be associated with participation in sports.[9]

Metacarpal fractures can be divided into base, shaft, head, and neck fractures (▶ Fig. 1.2).[12] Metacarpal neck fractures are the most common metacarpal fractures due to the weakness of the bone in this region. The cause of injury is usually punching a firm object which results in fracture of the metacarpal neck of the small finger, and is inappropriately termed a "boxer's fracture." In a national database, the most common mechanism of non-sports–related injury for a metacarpal fracture was "contact with a wall."[7] One case-control study found that patients with a boxer's fracture had significantly higher mean scores than controls for self-defeating, borderline, and antisocial personality disorders.[13]

1.1.2 Phalangeal Fractures

After radius and ulna fractures, phalangeal fractures have the highest incidence of upper extremity fractures followed by metacarpal fractures (▶ Table 1.1).[8,14] Chung and Spilson reported that 5- to 14-year-olds have the highest incidence of phalangeal fractures[8] (▶ Fig. 1.3), and Immerman et al similarly reported that 11- to 15-year-olds had the highest rate of phalangeal fractures.[9] A 23-year retrospective review of patients in the Netherlands found

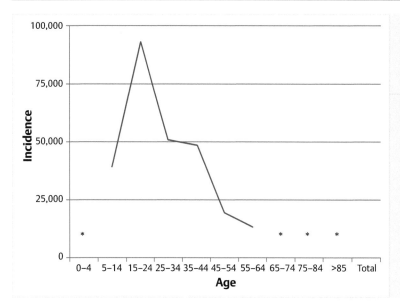

Fig. 1.1 Incidence of metacarpal fractures by age treated in U.S. emergency departments.
* Age groups 0–4, 65–74, 75–84, and > 85 had unreliable estimates and thus are lacking data. (Data from Chung KC, Spilson SV. The frequency and epidemiology of hand and forearm fractures in the United States. J Hand Surg 2001;26A:908–915.)

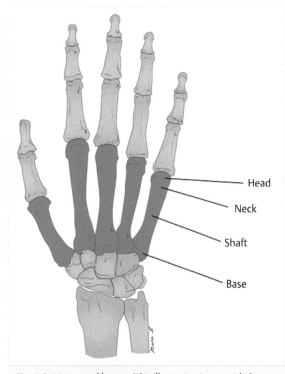

Fig. 1.2 Metacarpal bones. (This illustration is a provided courtesy of Dr. Nasa Fujihara.)

Table 1.1 Fracture incidence by anatomical site in U.S. emergency departments

Anatomical site	Number of fractures	%	95% confidence interval
Radius and/or ulna	643,087	44	584,712–701,462
Phalanx/phalanges	341,305	23	310,254–372,356
Metacarpal(s)	264,642	18	240,533–288,751
Carpal	207,880	14	188,910–226,850
Multiple hand bones	8,960	1	8,012–9,908
Total	1,465,874	100	1,333,002–1,598,746

Used with permission from Chung KC, Spilson SV. The frequency and epidemiology of hand and forearm fractures in the United States. J Hand Surg 2001;26A:908–915.

that men in the ages 10 to 29 years had the greatest proportion of phalangeal fractures.[15] In this study, most phalangeal fractures in both men and women were caused by sports (22 and 30%, respectively). However, machinery was the leading cause of injury in men in the ages of 40 to 69. Another study found that the odds of incurring a phalangeal fracture were four times higher (odds ratio [OR] 4.04 [3.04, 5.36]) in college field hockey players (who do not wear gloves) compared to gloved athletes in stick-handling sports (women's lacrosse, men's ice hockey, and men's lacrosse). Gloves are not currently required nor recommended in women's field hockey. Young children, ages 0 to 5 years, are susceptible to phalangeal fractures due to crush injuries,[16] such as getting fingers stuck in a door. Distal tuft fractures of the phalanges are most common in this age group.[17,18]

Phalangeal fractures can be divided into base, shaft, and condylar fractures[12] (►Fig. 1.4) and fractures more commonly occur at the base.[10] In studies of pediatric hand fractures, the proximal phalanx of the small finger[6,16,19] or the thumb[10] had the highest incidence of fractures. Fractures involving the physis (growth plate) are described by the Salter-Harris classification system, types I to V (►Fig. 1.5). Phalangeal and metacarpal epiphyseal plates in the hand remain open until approximately 14½ years in girls and 16½ years in boys.[20] One retrospective review over a 2-year period consisted of 354 metacarpal or phalangeal fractures in children aged 18 years or younger in a single emergency room and hand clinic.[19] The authors found that 34% of

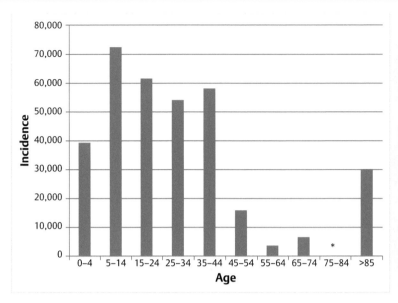

Fig. 1.3 Incidence of phalangeal fractures by age treated in U.S. emergency departments.
* Age group 75–84 had unreliable estimate and thus is lacking data. (Data from Chung KC, Spilson SV. The frequency and epidemiology of hand and forearm fractures in the United States. J Hand Surg 2001;26A:908–915.)

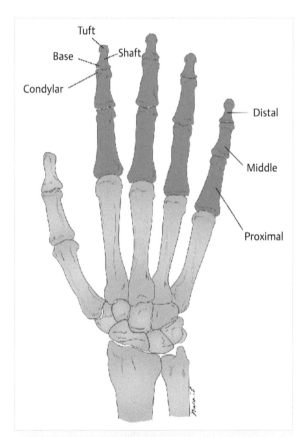

Fig. 1.4 Phalangeal bones. (This illustration is a provided courtesy of Dr. Nasa Fujihara.)

all fractures involved an epiphyseal plate. Of these injuries, 7.4% were Salter I, 78.7% were Salter II, 13.1% were Salter III, and 1.8% were Salter IV. A similar distribution of Salter-Harris fractures in the phalanges was observed in another study of children aged 21 years or younger.[21] The majority (37%) of Salter II fractures occurred in the small finger and 69% of Salter II fractures occurred in the proximal phalanx.[19]

Thumb Fractures

In phalangeal fractures, for most age groups, the thumb is the second most commonly fractured digit after the small finger. However, in individuals older than 65 years of age, excluding metacarpal fractures, the thumb was the most commonly injured digit (33% of hand fractures in this age group).[22] Fractures involving the metacarpal shaft of the thumb are uncommon because force directed to the shaft is often transferred to the base resulting in a fracture through the metacarpal base.[23] Salter-Harris type II fractures were found to be the most common fracture (72%) of the base of the proximal phalanx of the thumb in children aged 10 years or younger.[24] A review of 823 hand and carpal fractures from patients aged 16 years or younger found an incidence of 1.3% for Salter-Harris type III fractures. Four out of eleven of these fractures involved the thumb and 91% (10/11) were caused by an athletic injury.[25] A Bennett fracture is an intra-articular fracture separating the volar–ulnar aspect of the metacarpal base from the remaining thumb metacarpal[26] (▶Fig. 1.6). It is classified into three types: type 1 is a fracture with a large single ulnar fragment and subluxation of the metacarpal base, type 2 is an impaction fracture without subluxation of the thumb metacarpal, and type 3 is an injury with a small ulnar avulsion fragment in association with metacarpal dislocation.[27] In a record review of 71 fractures at the base of the thumb, Bennett's fracture represented 63% of fractures (45/71). The majority of these fractures (96%) were incurred by men. The remaining 37% of fractures in this study were oblique comminuted basal fractures that were also incurred mainly by men.[28] A Rolando fracture describes

5

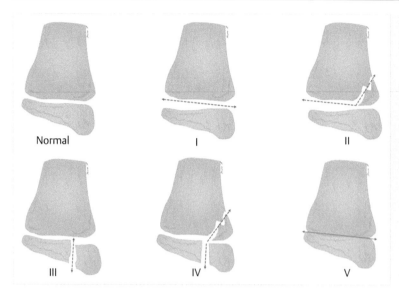

Fig. 1.5 Salter-Harris classification. (This illustration is a provided courtesy of Dr. Nasa Fujihara.)

Normal I II III IV V

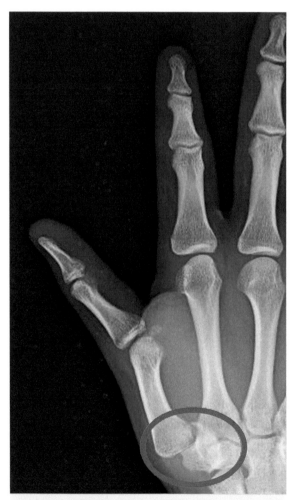

Fig. 1.6 Radiograph of Bennett's fracture.

review of 17 cases of Rolando fracture, the majority (71%) occurred in men and the cause of injury was a fall on the hand (53%), a blow to the thumb (35%), or the hand being jammed (12%).

1.1.3 Carpal Fractures

Carpal fractures are reported to comprise 14% of all hand and/or forearm fractures treated in U.S. emergency departments. Children of age 5 to 14 represent the age group most commonly seen with a carpal fracture, followed closely by those of age 15 to 24 (▶ Fig. 1.7).[8] Females have more carpal fractures (67%) compared to males (33%). Most carpal fractures are the result of a fall on an outstretched hand.[29]

Some studies have found increases in the incidence of carpal fracture over time in the pediatric population, particularly in relation to sports. One study analyzed the National Electronic Injury Surveillance System (NEISS) database for pediatric wrist fractures over a 16-year timespan. This database collects data from a sample of U.S. emergency room visits involving an injury and designates the products or activities that were involved at the time of injury. This study showed that the fewest pediatric wrist fractures occurred in the winter months and the top three causes of injury were bicycles, football, and playground equipment. Over the 16-year period, there was a decline in bicycle- and basketball-related wrist fractures and a rise in soccer-related wrist fractures.[30] A retrospective study analyzing inpatient and outpatient data from children and adolescents with wrist fractures in the Netherlands from 1997 to 2009 found an increase in the incidence over time in 5- to 9-year-olds and 10- to 14-year-olds. Wrist fractures in 5- to 9-year-olds were mainly caused by home accidents whereas most fractures in 10- to 14-year-olds were sports-related. In boys, most sports-related fractures were due to soccer. In girls, most sports-related fractures were due to soccer and school gymnastics.[31]

comminuted fractures of the base of the thumb but should, ideally, be reserved for Y- or T-pattern fractures that include the volar–ulnar Bennett's fragment in addition to a dorsal radial fragment.[23] In a retrospective

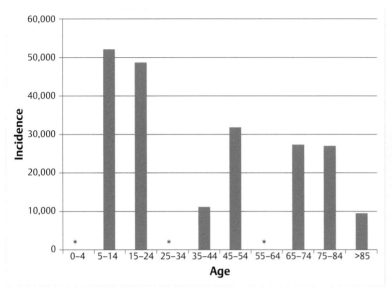

Fig. 1.7 Incidence of carpal fractures by age treated in U.S. emergency departments.
* Age groups 0–4, 25–34, and 55–64 had unreliable estimates and thus are lacking data. (Data from Chung KC, Spilson SV. The frequency and epidemiology of hand and forearm fractures in the United States. J Hand Surg 2001;26A:908–915.)

Scaphoid Fractures

Studies agree that the scaphoid has the highest fracture rate of all the carpal bones, comprising 58 to 66% of all carpal fractures[11,32,33] (▶Fig. 1.8). Scaphoid fractures are divided into the waist, proximal pole, distal pole, and tubercle. The majority of fractures occur at the scaphoid waist.[33,34] The incidence of scaphoid fractures is variable depending on the study sample. In the United States, using the NEISS database, the incidence rate was 1.5 fractures per 100,000 person-years. This rate, obtained from a weighted estimate of all injuries presenting to U.S. emergency departments, appears to be on the low end, only representing 2% of all wrist fractures.[35] In a trauma unit located in the United Kingdom, the incidence rate was 29 fractures per 100,000 person-years.[34] In a U.S. military population, the incidence rate was 121 fractures per 100,000 person-years,[36] but military personnel are more likely to have a scaphoid fracture.[11] A retrospective study in Singapore found a significant association between the incidence of isolated scaphoid and other carpal fractures and age (20–29 years) and an association with male gender.[33] Other studies have similarly found that scaphoid fractures are most common in men of age 15 to 30 years.[34,37]

Scaphoid fractures are most commonly caused by a fall on an outstretched hand, but other common mechanisms of injury include sports such as soccer,[34,38] basketball, bicycling, and skateboarding.[35] One study found an increasing incidence of scaphoid fractures associated with "test your strength" punching bag machines.[38] Another estimate places the incidence of scaphoid fractures in college football players as 1 in 100.[39]

Triquetral Fractures

Triquetral fractures are cited to comprise as little as 3 to 5%[40–43] to as many as 15 to 18%[29,42,44,45] of all carpal fractures (▶Fig. 1.8). Fractures of the triquetrum are generally observed as a dorsal chip (cortical fracture) or a body fracture. The dorsal chip fracture is reported to comprise approximately 93% of all triquetral fractures.[42] The most common clinical presentation is a fall onto an ulnarly-deviated wrist that is flexed in a dorsal direction.[46]

Trapezium Fractures

Trapezium fractures comprise 3 to 5% of all carpal fractures (▶Fig. 1.8).[29,47–51] Fractures of the trapezium body are described as horizontal and sagittal split, transarticular, dorsoradial tuberosity, and comminuted.[52] Sagittal split is the most common fracture.[46] Many trapezium fractures are the result of high-energy injuries such as motor vehicle accidents.[53] Fractures also occur due to a fall on an outstretched hand where there is axial compression force from the thumb metacarpal.[54,55] This fracture type frequently accompanies a Bennett fracture.[54]

Hamate Fractures

Hamate fractures are reported to comprise 2% of all carpal fractures,[29] but the true incidence may be higher because the diagnosis is easily missed[46,56] (▶Fig. 1.8). The hamate hook is at risk of fracture from "compressive forces when the palm is struck and shear forces from the adjacent flexor tendons arise during forceful torque of the wrist."[57] Such forces arise in the dominant hand of sports such as tennis or other racquet sports when only one hand receives the force of impact. The nondominant hand is usually at risk when playing a sport that requires a two-handed swing, such as baseball or golf.[29] Hook fractures have also been reported in hockey players, who sustain the injury from a direct blow from the puck, repetitive trauma, or from falling onto the hockey stick.[58] The hamate body is less commonly fractured than the hook. The mechanism of injury is variable and includes shearing, direct blow, high-energy trauma, and axial loading.[54]

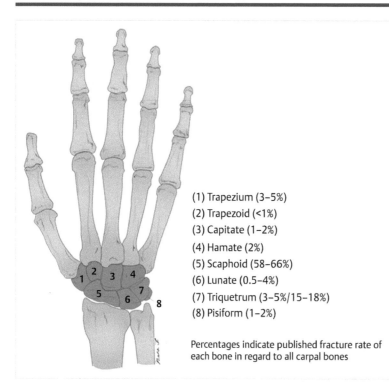

Fig. 1.8 Carpal bones. (This illustration is a provided courtesy of Dr. Nasa Fujihara.)

(1) Trapezium (3–5%)
(2) Trapezoid (<1%)
(3) Capitate (1–2%)
(4) Hamate (2%)
(5) Scaphoid (58–66%)
(6) Lunate (0.5–4%)
(7) Triquetrum (3–5%/15–18%)
(8) Pisiform (1–2%)

Percentages indicate published fracture rate of each bone in regard to all carpal bones

Capitate Fractures

Capitate fractures comprise 1 to 2% of all carpal fractures[29] (►Fig. 1.8). Isolated capitate fractures are rare, representing less than 0.5% of all carpal injuries,[59] and are more common with a perilunate injury.[11,56,59–61] The mechanism of injury of isolated capitate fractures is debated. Some say the fracture results from a direct blow or by an axial load through the third metacarpal with a flexed wrist.[62] Others say that they commonly occur through a fall onto an extended wrist that is ulnarly deviated.[54] The fracture patterns are transverse body (most common), transverse pole, verticofrontal, and parasagittal.[54]

Pisiform Fractures

Pisiform fractures comprise approximately 1 to 2% of all carpal fractures[47] (►Fig. 1.8). They are described as transverse, parasagittal, comminuted, and pisiform-triquetral impaction fractures.[47] They generally result from a direct blow, commonly in racquet sports[63] or from a baseball bat.[46] They may also result from the force transmitted when firing a handgun.[55]

Lunate Fractures

Lunate fractures are rare, constituting 0.5 to 4% of all carpal fractures[11,64–66] (►Fig. 1.8). Lunate fractures are classified into five subtypes: volar pole, dorsal pole, transverse body, sagittal body, and osteochondral chip fractures. Volar pole fractures are the most common subtype.[64] The mechanism of injury generally is a fall on

an outstretched hand.[46] In sports, a blow to the hand by a ball in line with the forearm has also been reported.[67] At-risk athletes include gymnasts and weight lifters, who both require extreme weight-bearing through an extended wrist.[68]

Trapezoid Fractures

Trapezoid fracture is a rare occurrence[11,32,33] accounting for less than 1% of all carpal fractures[29] (►Fig. 1.8). A case series over 10 years at a single institution found only 11 cases.[69] Fractures typically result from high-energy injuries to the hand.[46] Trapezoid fractures are classified as either dorsal rim or body types.[47] Both are often found in conjunction with other fractures or carpometacarpal dislocations.[54]

1.1.4 Implications

The majority of hand fractures affect adolescents who are participating in athletics. The use of safety gear, such as gloves in field hockey, is recommended. The University of Michigan has created the Exercise & Sport Science Initiative which "draws on expertise from a wide range of faculty across the University of Michigan campus, Michigan Athletics and industry partners to optimize physical performance and health for people of all ages and abilities."[70] Through this initiative, a professor in mechanical engineering developed a specialized batting glove to assist a college baseball player with a broken bone in his hand. The glove helped to reduce force and dissipate energy, allowing the player to return to play after having surgery.[71] Similar research collaborations can aid in reducing the occurrence of future sports-related injuries.

In adults, falls and work injuries are common causes of hand and carpal fractures. In 2015, fractures (all types) accounted for 9% of occupational injuries and illnesses resulting in days away from work. A hand or wrist injury resulted in a median time of 6 and 13 days, respectively, away from work.[72] Safety at work must be emphasized to avoid injuries due to machinery and/or falls. Additionally, the use of safety items, such as door hinge guards, by parents and in public facilities is recommended to prevent finger crush injuries in young children.

References

[1] Geissler WB, Burkett JL. Ligamentous sports injuries of the hand and wrist. Sports Med Arthrosc Rev. 2014; 22(1):39–44

[2] Naranje SM, Erali RA, Warner WC, Jr, Sawyer JR, Kelly DM. Epidemiology of pediatric fractures presenting to emergency departments in the United States. J Pediatr Orthop. 2016; 36(4):e45–e48

[3] Swenson DM, Henke NM, Collins CL, Fields SK, Comstock RD. Epidemiology of United States high school sports-related fractures, 2008–09 to 2010–11. Am J Sports Med. 2012; 40(9):2078–2084

[4] Swenson DM, Yard EE, Collins CL, Fields SK, Comstock RD. Epidemiology of US high school sports-related fractures, 2005–2009. Clin J Sport Med. 2010; 20(4):293–299

[5] Zalavras C, Nikolopoulou G, Essin D, Manjra N, Zionts LE. Pediatric fractures during skateboarding, roller skating, and scooter riding. Am J Sports Med. 2005; 33(4):568–573

[6] Liu EH, Alqahtani S, Alsaaran RN, Ho ES, Zuker RM, Borschel GH. A prospective study of pediatric hand fractures and review of the literature. Pediatr Emerg Care. 2014; 30(5):299–304

[7] Nakashian MN, Pointer L, Owens BD, Wolf JM. Incidence of metacarpal fractures in the US population. Hand (NY). 2012; 7(4):426–430

[8] Chung KC, Spilson SV. The frequency and epidemiology of hand and forearm fractures in the United States. J Hand Surg Am. 2001; 26(5):908–915

[9] Immerman I, Livermore MS, Szabo RM. Use of emergency department services for hand, wrist, and forearm fractures in the United States in 2008. J Surg Orthop Adv. 2014; 23(2):98–104

[10] Mahabir RC, Kazemi AR, Cannon WG, Courtemanche DJ. Pediatric hand fractures: a review. Pediatr Emerg Care. 2001; 17(3):153–156

[11] Hove LM. Fractures of the hand. Distribution and relative incidence. Scand J Plast Reconstr Surg Hand Surg. 1993; 27(4):317–319

[12] Cotterell IH, Richard MJ. Metacarpal and phalangeal fractures in athletes. Clin Sports Med. 2015; 34(1):69–98

[13] Mercan S, Uzun M, Ertugrul A, Ozturk I, Demir B, Sulun T. Psychopathology and personality features in orthopedic patients with boxer's fractures. Gen Hosp Psychiatry. 2005; 27(1):13–17

[14] Karl JW, Olson PR, Rosenwasser MP. The epidemiology of upper extremity fractures in the United States, 2009. J Orthop Trauma. 2015; 29(8):e242–e244

[15] De Jonge JJ, Kingma J, van der Lei B, Klasen HJ. Phalangeal fractures of the hand. An analysis of gender and age-related incidence and aetiology. J Hand Surg [Br]. 1994; 19(2):168–170

[16] Chew EM, Chong AK. Hand fractures in children: epidemiology and misdiagnosis in a tertiary referral hospital. J Hand Surg Am. 2012; 37(8):1684–1688

[17] Lankachandra M, Wells CR, Cheng CJ, Hutchison RL. Complications of distal phalanx fractures in children. J Hand Surg Am. 2017; 42(7):574.e1–574.e6

[18] Rajesh A, Basu AK, Vaidhyanath R, Finlay D. Hand fractures: a study of their site and type in childhood. Clin Radiol. 2001; 56(8):667–669

[19] Hastings H, II, Simmons BP. Hand fractures in children. A statistical analysis. Clin Orthop Relat Res. 1984(188):120–130

[20] Greulich W, Pyle P. Radiographic Atlas of Skeletal Development of the Hand and Wrist. 2nd ed. Stanford, CA: Stanford University Press; 1959

[21] Peterson HA, Madhok R, Benson JT, Ilstrup DM, Melton LJ, III. Physeal fractures: part 1. Epidemiology in Olmsted County, Minnesota, 1979–1988. J Pediatr Orthop. 1994; 14(4):423–430

[22] Stanton JS, Dias JJ, Burke FD. Fractures of the tubular bones of the hand. J Hand Surg Eur Vol. 2007; 32(6):626–636

[23] Carlsen BT, Moran SL. Thumb trauma: Bennett fractures, Rolando fractures, and ulnar collateral ligament injuries. J Hand Surg Am. 2009; 34(5):945–952

[24] Al-Qattan MM, Al-Zahrani K, Al-Boukai AA. The relative incidence of fractures at the base of the proximal phalanx of the thumb in children. J Hand Surg Eur Vol. 2009; 34(1):110–114

[25] Crick JC, Lemel MS. Salter-Harris type III epiphyseal fractures of the proximal phalanx. J South Orthop Assoc. 1998; 7(4):259–263

[26] Edmunds JO. Traumatic dislocations and instability of the trapeziometacarpal joint of the thumb. Hand Clin. 2006; 22(3):365–392

[27] Gedda KO. Studies on Bennett's fracture; anatomy, roentgenology, and therapy. Acta Chir Scand Suppl. 1954; 193:1–114

[28] Griffiths JC. Fractures at the base of the first metacarpal bone. J Bone Joint Surg Br. 1964; 46:712–719

[29] Garcia-Elias M. Carpal bone fractures (excluding scaphoid fractures). In: Watson HK, ed. The Wrist. Philadelphia, PA: Lippincott Williams & Wilkins; 2001:174–181

[30] Shah NS, Buzas D, Zinberg EM. Epidemiologic dynamics contributing to pediatric wrist fractures in the United States. Hand (NY). 2015; 10(2):266–271

[31] de Putter CE, van Beeck EF, Looman CW, Toet H, Hovius SE, Selles RW. Trends in wrist fractures in children and adolescents, 1997–2009. J Hand Surg Am. 2011; 36(11):1810–1815.e2

[32] van Onselen EB, Karim RB, Hage JJ, Ritt MJ. Prevalence and distribution of hand fractures. J Hand Surg [Br]. 2003; 28(5):491–495

[33] Hey HW, Chong AK, Murphy D. Prevalence of carpal fracture in Singapore. J Hand Surg Am. 2011; 36(2):278–283

[34] Duckworth AD, Jenkins PJ, Aitken SA, Clement ND, Court-Brown CM, McQueen MM. Scaphoid fracture epidemiology. J Trauma Acute Care Surg. 2012; 72(2):E41–E45

[35] Van Tassel DC, Owens BD, Wolf JM. Incidence estimates and demographics of scaphoid fracture in the U.S. population. J Hand Surg Am. 2010; 35(8):1242–1245

[36] Wolf JM, Dawson L, Mountcastle SB, Owens BD. The incidence of scaphoid fracture in a military population. Injury. 2009; 40(12):1316–1319

[37] van der Molen AB, Groothoff JW, Visser GJ, Robinson PH, Eisma WH. Time off work due to scaphoid fractures and other carpal injuries in The Netherlands in the period 1990 to 1993. J Hand Surg [Br]. 1999; 24(2):193–198

[38] Sutton PA, Clifford O, Davis TR. A new mechanism of injury for scaphoid fractures: 'test your strength' punch-bag machines. J Hand Surg Eur Vol. 2010; 35(5):419–420

[39] Rettig A, Ryan R, Stone J. Epidemiology of hand injuries in sports. In: Strickland J, Rettig A, eds. Hand Injuries in Athletes. Philadelphia, PA: WB Saunders; 1992:37–48

[40] Bartone NF, Grieco RV. Fractures of the triquetrum. J Bone Joint Surg Am. 1956; 38-A(2):353–356

[41] Bryan RS, Dobyns JH. Fractures of the carpal bones other than lunate and navicular. Clin Orthop Relat Res. 1980(149):107–111

[42] Höcker K, Menschik A. Chip fractures of the triquetrum. Mechanism, classification and results. J Hand Surg [Br]. 1994; 19(5):584–588

[43] Bonnin JG. Fractures of the triquetrum. Br J Surg. 1944; 31:278–283

[44] Garcia-Elias M. Dorsal fractures of the triquetrum-avulsion or compression fractures? J Hand Surg Am. 1987; 12(2):266–268

[45] Levy M, Fischel RE, Stern GM, Goldberg I. Chip fractures of the os triquetrum: the mechanism of injury. J Bone Joint Surg Br. 1979; 61-B(3):355–357

[46] Marchessault J, Conti M, Baratz ME. Carpal fractures in athletes excluding the scaphoid. Hand Clin. 2009; 25(3):371–388

[47] Putnam M, Meyer N. Carpal fractures excluding the scaphoid. In: Trumble T, ed. Hand Surgery Update 3: Hand, Elbow, and Shoulder. Rosemont, IL: American Society for Surgery of the Hand; 2003:175

[48] Garcia-Elias M, Henríquez-Lluch A, Rossignani P, Fernandez de Retana P, Orovio de Elízaga J. Bennett's fracture combined with fracture of the trapezium. A report of three cases. J Hand Surg [Br]. 1993; 18(4):523–526

[49] Cordrey LJ, Ferrer-Torells M. Management of fractures of the greater multangular. Report of five cases. J Bone Joint Surg Am. 1960; 42-A:1111–1118

[50] Palmer AK. Trapezial ridge fractures. J Hand Surg Am. 1981; 6(6):561–564

[51] Razemon J. Fractures of the carpal bones. In: R T, ed. The Hand. Philadelphia, PA: WB Saunders; 1985:821

[52] Walker JL, Greene TL, Lunseth PA. Fractures of the body of the trapezium. J Orthop Trauma. 1988; 2(1):22–28

[53] McGuigan FX, Culp RW. Surgical treatment of intra-articular fractures of the trapezium. J Hand Surg Am. 2002; 27(4):697–703

[54] Suh N, Ek ET, Wolfe SW. Carpal fractures. J Hand Surg Am. 2014; 39(4):785–791, quiz 791

[55] Geissler WB. Carpal fractures in athletes. Clin Sports Med. 2001; 20(1):167–188

[56] Papp S. Carpal bone fractures. Hand Clin. 2010; 26(1):119–127

[57] Walsh JJ, IV, Bishop AT. Diagnosis and management of hamate hook fractures. Hand Clin. 2000; 16(3):397–403, viii

[58] Husband JB. Hook of hamate and pisiform fractures in basketball and hockey players. Hand Clin. 2012; 28(3):303

[59] Rand JA, Linscheid RL, Dobyns JH. Capitate fractures: a long-term follow-up. Clin Orthop Relat Res. 1982(165):209–216

[60] Sabat D, Arora S, Dhal A. Isolated capitate fracture with dorsal dislocation of proximal pole: a case report. Hand (NY). 2011; 6(3):333–336

[61] Apostolides JG, Lifchez SD, Christy MR. Complex and rare fracture patterns in perilunate dislocations. Hand (NY). 2011; 6(3):287–294

[62] Vance RM, Gelberman RH, Evans EF. Scaphocapitate fractures. Patterns of dislocation, mechanisms of injury, and preliminary results of treatment. J Bone Joint Surg Am. 1980; 62(2): 271–276

[63] Helal B. Racquet player's pisiform. Hand. 1978; 10(1):87–90

[64] Teisen H, Hjarbaek J. Classification of fresh fractures of the lunate. J Hand Surg [Br]. 1988; 13(4):458–462

[65] Cetti R, Christensen SE, Reuther K. Fracture of the lunate bone. Hand. 1982; 14(1):80–84

[66] Kaewlai R, Avery LL, Asrani AV, Abujudeh HH, Sacknoff R, Novelline RA. Multidetector CT of carpal injuries: anatomy, fractures, and fracture-dislocations. Radiographics. 2008; 28(6):1771–1784

[67] Teisen H, Hjarbaek J, Jensen EK. Follow-up investigation of fresh lunate bone fracture. Handchir Mikrochir Plast Chir. 1990; 22(1):20–22

[68] Slade JF, III, Milewski MD. Management of carpal instability in athletes. Hand Clin. 2009; 25(3):395–408

[69] Kain N, Heras-Palou C. Trapezoid fractures: report of 11 cases. J Hand Surg Am. 2012; 37(6):1159–1162

[70] University of Michigan Exercise & Sport Science Initiative. http://essi.umich.edu/. Accessed June 22, 2017

[71] Science in Sport. http://research.umich.edu/news-issues/michigan-research/science-sport. Accessed June 22, 2017

[72] Bureau of Labor Statistics, US Department of Labor. Nonfatal Occupational Injuries and Illnesses Requiring Days Away from Work, 2015; https://www.bls.gov/news.release/pdf/osh2.pdf. Accessed June 22, 2017

2 Evidence in the Treatment of Hand Fractures

János Rupnik

Abstract

In this chapter, we reviewed the hand fracture management in relation with the concept of evidence and the recent literature from the following aspects: distribution of studies regarding anatomical localization on the hand, according to the research topic, the level of evidence of the study and from the point of view of practical effectiveness of the research. We do not make any conclusions about the treatment of fractures of different bones of the hand, since these are detailed in other chapters. Our inquiry focused on what questions can we get answer and whether this has a practical effect in the management of hand fractures.

Keywords: hand fractures, evidence level, role of evidence, fracture treatment

2.1 Introduction

Evidence-based medicine (EBM)—as an interdisciplinary science—has been a determining concept in medical science and research over the past two decades. The widespread expansion of medical knowledge, the multiplication of scientific articles led to the need to develop a method which helps to properly evaluate the unmanageable amount of data. Evaluating the quality of articles has become fundamental in scientific work. In addition to fully restructure the expectations of scientific publications, EBM became an independent science. We found 74,989 articles in the PubMed database by searching for "evidence-based medicine." In 1996, the number of articles containing the term was 241; in 2017, this number was 4,605. The increase in search results starts in 1996, and we can expect EBM to be introduced from that time. In relation to the EBM, it should also be mentioned that in addition to its clear positive effect, it may also have some potentially negative or real negative consequences, such as devaluating the basic knowledge and the accumulated clinical experience, and may not provide useful guidance in a specific case.[1]

The human hand consists of both long and short bones, which basically have different functions, biomechanical and healing properties. Partly because of this, there is a large number of conservative and operative treatment options and it is often difficult to find the best treatment method. There are management principles and guidelines, protocols that should be used. The question is how the scientific evidence relates to clinical practice. In a recent study, the level of evidence of hand surgery articles has been reviewed.[2] In the study, 993 original publications published between 1993 and 2013 were evaluated. The results show a continuous increase in the evidence level of articles, but, according to the authors, high level of evidence work is still uncommon. When developing a guideline, beyond the textbooks, we have to use the current studies with strongest recommendations. The grade A recommendations are directly based on level 1 evidence, grade B to level 2, and so on.[3] Nevertheless, in clinical use, we must pay attention to the fact, that not all randomized controlled trials are conducted properly and the results should be carefully evaluated.[4]

It does not occur in everyday practice that a treatment is based on a new prospective randomized trial. The decision making during the management of a fracture basically depends on the surgeon's knowledge, training, and experience. The basic principles of the fracture treatment provide a precise guideline. However, very often there are no scientifically proven answers to simple questions to decide, such as operative or conservative treatment, choice between different implants (K-wire, screw, compression screw, plate, fixateur externe), bone graft versus vascularized bone graft, and last but not least the question of cost benefit. The research was performed according to these considerations. The following terms were searched for in the Cochrane database: "phalangeal, metacarpal, thumb, carpal, scaphoid, and fracture, cost benefit, and treatment" in different combination. Only the articles from 2012 to 2016 were included. Through this sample, we tried to conclude the usefulness of the data obtained here in direct clinical practice.

2.2 Quality and Distribution of the Studies

2.2.1 Phalangeal Fractures

The search resulted 16 articles, among them there was no systemic review. In the period of 2012 to 2016, there were five articles, four were prospective randomized trials and one was biomechanical cadaver study. The topics of clinical studies were as follows: (1) Extra-articular fractures of the proximal phalanges of the fingers; comparison of functional, conservative treatment.[5] (2) Comparison of conservative and operative treatment, distal phalanx.[6] (3) Two different physiotherapeutic methods after proximal phalanx fracture fixation.[7] (4) The use of denatured cellulose barrier after plate osteosynthesis of the proximal phalanx.[8] (5) The stability of four different fixation methods was analyzed on a proximal phalanx distal intra-articular fracture cadaver model.[9]

2.2.2 Metacarpal Fractures

Only the articles published in the last 5 years have been studied. The search in the Cochrane database resulted in one systematic review and meta-analysis, six clinical trials and one biomechanical study. The systematic review investigated the outcomes of the antegrade intramedullary nailing compared to other surgical interventions in the treatment for fifth metacarpal neck fractures.[10] In five of the six clinical trials, the subject was the fractures of fifth metacarpal neck fracture. One prospective study compared the intramedullary nail and low-profile plate for unstable metacarpal neck fractures.[11] Two prospective studies analyzed the antegrade intramedullary technique.[12,13] Two compared the conventional conservative (plaster cast) treatment and splinting of the fifth metacarpal neck fracture.[14,15] One multicenter randomized control study focused on the conservative versus operative management of the fifth metacarpal neck fracture.[16] The biomechanical cadaver study compares plate fixation using mono and bicortical screws in transverse metacarpal fracture model.[17]

2.2.3 Scaphoid Fractures

The search for the carpal bones and scaphoid resulted in three systematic reviews and 10 prospective trials. Each of them dealt with the scaphoid. One of the reviews was a systematic review and meta-analysis of different randomized controlled trials comparing different operative and conservative treatments of acute scaphoid fractures.[18] The second review's goal was to determine and compare the usefulness of two different free vascularized bone grafts in the treatment of scaphoid nonunion, 245 cases have been included in the study through the articles.[19] The third review was a meta-analysis of comparative studies of the management of displaced scaphoid waist fractures.[20] Ten trials were found regarding scaphoid fracture treatment, one was a registered ongoing prospective randomized study of operative versus nonoperative treatment of minimally displaced fractures of adults. One study focused on the acute minimally or nondisplaced scaphoid fractures and compared the conservative treatment with the arthroscopic-assisted antegrade screw fixation.[21] It was a long-term study (6 years). Two clinical trials dealt with the question of the vascularized versus nonvascularized bone grafting for scaphoid nonunion.[22,23] In the next study, the comparison of the palmar and dorsal minimal invasive technique in the treatment of nondisplaced acute scaphoid fractures found the two methods as equivalent.[24] One biomechanical cadaveric study was found. In this paper, two percutaneous volar approaches were compared: the standard volar approach and the transtrapezial approach.[25] Regarding conservative treatment, two articles were investigated: one compared the thumb included and the other thumb excluded below elbow cast.[26] The effect of pulsed electromagnetic fields in the treatment of acute scaphoid fractures was investigated in a prospective randomized double-blind placebo-controlled study.[27] The results were evaluated by computed tomography (CT) scan. Two studies focused on the navigation during surgery, new techniques have been tested, a cadaver study for the computer-assisted navigation for dorsal percutaneous scaphoid placement,[28] and an in vitro model to evaluate the computer-assisted 3D navigation system.[29]

2.3 Results
2.3.1 Distribution

- Distal phalanges 1
- Proximal phalanges 4
- Metacarpals 8
- Carpal bones (scaphoid) 13

Four were systematic reviews; the others were prospective randomized studies. The grades of recommendations of the studies were "A" or "B" based on the levels of evidence.

2.3.2 Recommendations

In the conclusions, the following recommendations and evidences based on biomechanical studies are found.

Conservative Treatment

- Well reduced, minimally angulated or minimally displaced fractures of the proximal phalanges of the fingers can be effectively treated with functional casts without immobilizing the wrist.
- No statistically significant differences existed in pain, mobility of the metacarpophalangeal (MP) joint, satisfaction with the aesthetic appearance, and power grip between the groups of fifth metacarpal neck fractures treated with soft wrap/buddy taping or reduction and casting.
- Treatment of pediatric fifth metacarpal neck fracture with hand-based thermoplastic splints resulted in improved early range of motion (ROM) and grip strength, compared with conventional ulnar gutter splints.
- There is no advantage of an above-elbow cast over a below-elbow cast to treat acute scaphoid fractures.
- Immobilization of the thumb in the cast is not necessary in conservative treatment of nondisplaced or minimally displaced fractures of the waist of the scaphoid.
- The addition of pulsed electromagnetic field's bone growth stimulation to the conservative treatment of acute scaphoid fractures does not accelerate bone healing.

Conservative versus Operative Treatment

- Conservative treatment compared with bouquet pinning in fifth metacarpal neck fractures did not prove statistical differences between the groups in Quick DASH score, pain, and satisfaction, finger ROM, grip strength, or quality of life.
- The antegrade intramedullary K-wire fixation minimizes the functional loss and allows earlier return to daily activities compared to the conventional ulnar gutter splinting.

- Operative treatment of scaphoid does not result into a higher union rate in undisplaced fractures.
- Conservative treatment is more advantageous for non- and minimally displaced scaphoid waist fractures.
- Operative treatment of nondisplaced scaphoid fracture gives an improved functional outcome at 26 weeks, but after a median of 6 years' follow-up radiographic signs of arthritis in the radioscaphoid joint were more common compared with the conservative treatment.

Operative Treatment

- Implantation of a denaturized cellulose adhesion barrier after plate osteosynthesis of the proximal phalanx did not prove to be beneficial to the function.
- Antegrade intramedullary pinning (nailing) is more advantageous regarding the ROM and grip strengths during the early recovery period (at 3 months postoperatively) than percutaneous retrograde intramedullary pinning for treatment of displaced fifth metacarpal neck fractures.
- The comparison of antegrade intramedullary nailing versus low-profile plate for unstable metacarpal neck fractures showed that plate fixation provides earlier recovery of powerful hand function, and intramedullary nailing allows a wide range of finger motion.
- The palmar percutaneous approach is not more effective in the treatment of nondisplaced and minimally displaced scaphoid fractures than the dorsal limited approach.

Nonvascularized versus Vascularized Grafts

- There is no advantage of the iliac crest (free vascularized) graft over the distal radius (nonvascularized) graft in the treatment of scaphoid nonunion.
- The dorsal vascularized bone graft and the nonvascularized bone graft from the distal radius resulted in the same union rate in the treatment of scaphoid nonunions.

Biomechanical Results

- Biomechanical stability—examined on cadaveric model—did not differ among the fixation methods (1.1-mm K-wire, two 1.1-mm K-wires, headless compression screw, and lag screw) for proximal phalanx unicondylar fractures in a flexion–extension active ROM model.
- A biomechanical advantage was found when using bicortical screws versus monocortical screws in metacarpal fracture plating.
- In a cadaveric osteotomy-simulated scaphoid waist fracture model, the transtrapezial approach has advantage compared with the standard volar approach, regarding the central position of the screw in the distal pole.

Postoperative Treatment

- Exercises with the MP joint constrained in flexion and exercises with the MP joint unconstrained have similar effects after open reduction and internal fixation of proximal phalanx.

2.4 Discussion

With regard to conservative treatment, there is a tendency toward limited fixations and more mobilization. Comparing conservative and operative treatments, there is no benefit of operative treatment in the management of nondisplaced fractures even in the scaphoid nondisplaced waist fractures. The use of vascular graft does not appear to be better against nonvascular grafts for the treatment of scaphoid nonunions. For the treatment of the fifth metacarpal neck fractures, the antegrade intramedullary K-wiring is best in terms of functional and aesthetic aspects.

References

[1] Greenhalgh T, Howick J, Maskrey N; Evidence Based Medicine Renaissance Group. Evidence based medicine: a movement in crisis? BMJ. 2014; 348:g3725
[2] Sugrue CM, Joyce CW, Sugrue RM, Carroll SM. Trends in the level of evidence in clinical hand surgery research Hand (NY). 2016; 11(2):211–215
[3] Shekelle PG, Woolf SH, Eccles M, Grimshaw J. Developing clinical guidelines. West J Med. 1999; 170(6):348–351
[4] Burns PB, Rohrich RJ, Chung KC. The levels of evidence and their role in evidence-based medicine. Plast Reconstr Surg. 2011; 128(1):305–310
[5] Franz T, von Wartburg U, Schibli-Beer S, et al. Extra-articular fractures of the proximal phalanges of the fingers: a comparison of 2 methods of functional, conservative treatment. J Hand Surg Am. 2012; 37(5):889–898
[6] Apic G, Mentzel M, Röhm A, Schöll H, Gülke J. [Distal phalangeal fractures of the finger. Results of conservative and surgical treatment] Unfallchirurg. 2014; 117(6):533–538
[7] Miller L, Crosbie J, Wajon A, Ada L. No difference between two types of exercise after proximal phalangeal fracture fixation: a randomised trial. J Physiother. 2016; 62(1):12–19
[8] Kappos EA, Esenwein P, Meoli M, Meier R, Grünert J. Implantation of a denatured cellulose adhesion barrier after plate osteosynthesis of finger proximal phalangeal fractures: results of a randomized controlled trial. J Hand Surg Eur Vol. 2016; 41(4):413–420
[9] Sirota MA, Parks BG, Higgins JP, Means KR, Jr. Stability of fixation of proximal phalanx unicondylar fractures of the hand: a biomechanical cadaver study. J Hand Surg Am. 2013; 38(1):77–81
[10] Yammine K, Harvey A. Antegrade intramedullary nailing for fifth metacarpal neck fractures: a systematic review and meta-analysis. Eur J Orthop Surg Traumatol. 2014; 24(3):273–278
[11] Fujitani R, Omokawa S, Shigematsu K, Tanaka Y. Comparison of the intramedullary nail and low-profile plate for unstable metacarpal neck fractures. J Orthop Sci. 2012; 17(4):450–456
[12] Kim JK, Kim DJ. Antegrade intramedullary pinning versus retrograde intramedullary pinning for displaced fifth metacarpal neck fractures. Clin Orthop Relat Res. 2015; 473(5):1747–1754
[13] Cepni SK, Aykut S, Bekmezci T, Kilic A. A minimally invasive fixation technique for selected patients with fifth metacarpal neck fracture. Injury. 2016; 47(6):1270–1275
[14] Davison PG. . Boudreau N, Burrows R, Wilson KL, Bezuhly M. Forearm-based ulnar gutter versus hand-based thermoplastic splint for pediatric metacarpal neck fractures: a blinded, randomized trial. Plast Reconstr Surg. 2016; 137(3):908–916

[15] van Aaken J, Fusetti C, Luchina S, et al. Fifth metacarpal neck fractures treated with soft wrap/buddy taping compared to reduction and casting: results of a prospective, multicenter, randomized trial. Arch Orthop Trauma Surg. 2016; 136(1):135–142

[16] Sletten IN, Hellund JC, Olsen B, Clementsen S, Kvernmo HD, Nordsletten L. Conservative treatment has comparable outcome with bouquet pinning of little finger metacarpal neck fractures: a multicentre randomized controlled study of 85 patients. J Hand Surg Eur Vol. 2015; 40(1):76–83

[17] Afshar R, Fong TS, Latifi MH, Kanthan SR, Kamarul T. A biomechanical study comparing plate fixation using unicortical and bicortical screws in transverse metacarpal fracture models subjected to cyclic loading. J Hand Surg Eur Vol. 2012; 37(5):396–401

[18] Alshryda S, Shah A, Odak S, Al-Shryda J, Ilango B, Murali SR. Acute fractures of the scaphoid bone: systematic review and meta-analysis. Surgeon. 2012; 10(4):218–229

[19] Al-Jabri T, Mannan A, Giannoudis P. The use of the free vascularised bone graft for nonunion of the scaphoid: a systematic review. J Orthop Surg. 2014; 9:21

[20] Singh HP, Taub N, Dias JJ. Management of displaced fractures of the waist of the scaphoid: meta-analyses of comparative studies. Injury. 2012; 43(6):933–939

[21] Clementson M, Jørgsholm P, Besjakov J, Thomsen N, Björkman A. A conservative treatment versus arthroscopic-assisted screw fixation of scaphoid waist fractures—a randomized trial with minimum 4-year follow-up. J Hand Surg Am. 2015; 40(7):1341–1348

[22] Goyal T, Sankineani SR, Tripathy SK. Local distal radius bone graft versus iliac crest bone graft for scaphoid nonunion: a comparative study. Musculoskelet Surg. 2013; 97(2):109–114

[23] Caporrino FA, Dos Santos JB, Penteado FT, de Moraes VY, Belloti JC, Faloppa F. Dorsal vascularized grafting for scaphoid nonunion: a comparison of two surgical techniques. J Orthop Trauma. 2014; 28(3):e44–e48

[24] Drac P, Cizmar I, Manak P, et al. Comparison of the results and complications of palmar and dorsal miniinvasive approaches in the surgery of scaphoid fractures. A prospective randomized study. Biomed Pap Med Fac Univ Palacky Olomouc Czech Repub. 2014; 158(2):277–281

[25] Meermans G, Van Glabbeek F, Braem MJ, van Riet RP, Hubens G, Verstreken F. Comparison of two percutaneous volar approaches for screw fixation of scaphoid waist fractures: radiographic and biomechanical study of an osteotomy-simulated model. J Bone Joint Surg Am. 2014; 96(16):1369–1376

[26] Buijze GA, Goslings JC, Rhemrev SJ, et al; CAST Trial Collaboration. Cast immobilization with and without immobilization of the thumb for nondisplaced and minimally displaced scaphoid waist fractures: a multicenter, randomized, controlled trial. J Hand Surg Am. 2014; 39(4):621–627

[27] Hannemann PF, van Wezenbeek MR, Kolkman KA, et al. CT scan-evaluated outcome of pulsed electromagnetic fields in the treatment of acute scaphoid fractures: a randomised, multicentre, double-blind, placebo-controlled trial. Bone Joint J. 2014; 96-B(8):1070–1076

[28] Kam CC, Greenberg JA. Computer-assisted navigation for dorsal percutaneous scaphoid screw placement: a cadaveric study. J Hand Surg Am. 2014; 39(4):613–620

[29] Smith EJ, Al-Sanawi H, Gammon B, Pichora DR, Ellis RE. Volume rendering of three-dimensional fluoroscopic images for percutaneous scaphoid fixation: an in vitro study. Proc Inst Mech Eng H. 2013; 227(4):384–392

3 Nonoperative Management of Hand Fractures

Grey Giddins

Abstract

Historically most hand fractures were treated nonoperatively. While operative techniques have improved considerably, most fractures still do so well with nonoperative treatment that surgery is not warranted. There are strongly conflicting opinions in the published literature on the treatment of some hand fractures. This review aims to reconcile those and highlight subset bias, which may be skewing opinions.

A literature review was performed; spiral or long oblique metacarpal fractures and metacarpal neck fractures treated with mobilization, and transverse metacarpal shaft fracture treated with initial splintage or plaster support and then mobilization all do so well that currently surgery cannot reliably improve the outcomes, so the risks of surgery outweigh the likely benefits.

Thumb and finger metacarpophalangeal (MP) joint bony avulsion injuries would appear to need surgical stabilization to avoid instability. Many techniques have been described not least to prevent nonunion, but that does not seem to affect the outcome; the results of nonoperative treatment are so good that surgery is rarely required.

The treatment of bone mallet injuries and base of middle phalanx fractures appears not to be primarily to restore bone alignment but to restore gliding as opposed to pivoting. This is established for bony mallet injuries and suggested for proximal interphalangeal (PIP) joint injuries. Extension stress testing of bony mallet injuries and flexing PIP joint injuries appears reliable in predicting the outcome and so the need for surgery. For some of these injuries, there may be a small subset which would benefit from surgery. These need to be identified to improve treatment and to reconcile the strong and conflicting views of surgeons.

Keywords: hand fractures, metacarpal, spiral, transverse, avulsion, mallet, gliding, pivoting

3.1 Introduction

Historically, most hand fractures were treated nonoperatively (conservatively). More recently surgical treatment of many hand fractures has become popular. This involves closed or open reduction and stabilization with Kirschner (K) wires or internal fixation, the latter led by the AO group.[1] Although closed K-wiring or open reduction and internal fixation (ORIF) and their many variants can be used to treat almost any hand fracture, it does not mean they should. Clinicians and patients can easily be misled by the purported advantages of surgery. Case series reporting good results may be presented or published and surgeons may be persuaded to follow the new technique despite limited information about its efficacy and particularly the risks. Yet most hand fractures do well with nonoperative treatment.[2] Even relatively unsuccessful surgical treatment, for example, malunion following K-wiring or ORIF, may give good subjective and objective outcome despite the operation.

The choice to recommend surgery or not will depend on many factors not just objective medical evidence. Training, surgeon and patient beliefs about the efficacy of surgery, remuneration, targets, workload, ignorance, bias related to a recent case, and other factors will influence how clinicians guide patients and how they respond. Ideally, the advice we give should be fully informed and objective, but it is given by humans to humans, so biased by many factors; this is part of the art of medicine. Nonetheless, the advice should be supported by the best available evidence although that is usually suboptimal. Above all, I believe we should know how well a particular injury responds to nonoperative treatment before trying to improve that with surgery because of the increased risks and costs to society and the individual.

The aim of this review is to identify the fractures which can still be best treated nonoperatively. A secondary aim is to try to establish where there may be subgroups of those fractures which might benefit from different treatment such as surgery.

3.2 Methods and Materials

Multiple electronic and subsequent hand searches of published literature were performed in 2015 to identify fractures that do so well with nonoperative treatment that it is currently too difficult for surgery to provide significant further benefit. This review of the literature was updated in 2017. The inclusion criteria were all adult (ε 16 years of age) fractures of the hand, that is, excluding carpal injuries; papers which had a minimum of five cases; and papers with a minimum follow-up of 2 years. This proved impractical as so few had such adequate follow-up and so all papers with a minimum follow-up of 6 weeks were included. Even then reports often had patients younger than 16 years who could not be separated out. The exclusion criteria were fractures where surgery is plainly needed and proven to have been beneficial: many open fractures; replantations; many crush injuries (▶Fig. 3.1); displaced intra-articular fractures (excluding bony mallet injuries and ligament avulsion fractures); and pediatric fractures.

3.3 Results

Fingers

3.3.1 Spiral or Long Oblique Metacarpal Fractures

The spiral or long oblique fractures of the metacarpals are very common (▶Fig. 3.2). They can be treated surgically;

various techniques have been described and good results reported.[3-5] Similar good results have been reported with nonoperative treatment.[6] Khan and Giddins (2015)[7] showed that all spiral metacarpal fractures, even in the presence of initial malrotation, can be treated nonoperatively with excellent or very good outcomes and minimal morbidity (▶Table 3.1). This also applies to double spiral fractures and probably to triple spiral fractures, but they are rare, so the data are not robust. All the patients in their study were treated with early mobilization, without a splint or plaster. They were encouraged to "make a fist" at the first-hand clinic visit in order to correct any malrotation and ensure early mobilization. Twenty-five of 30 patients were reviewed at a minimum of 6 months following their injury. Objectively, they had full, painless movement, and grip strength of at least 90% of the other (uninjured) hand. The only adverse outcomes were minimal malrotation in one patient and mild discomfort in another.

Other authors have highlighted the risk of hand dysfunction caused by shortening of the metacarpals

following nonoperative treatment;[8-10] a biomechanical study in 2013 suggested that shortening up to 5 mm is not biomechanically significant.[11] This fits with the results of the study of Khan and Giddins. It is confirmed in humans and cadavers that the metacarpals derotate through tightening of the intermetacarpal ligaments. This limits shortening to 2 to 5 mm. Their results further confirm that shortening of 2 to 5 mm is not typically clinically relevant.

Malrotation following spiral metacarpal fractures almost always corrects with finger flexion. If it does not, then encouragement or (very rarely) manipulation under local anesthetic would be appropriate to avoid of rotational malunion. Nonoperative treatment gives such good results that recommending surgery seems unjustifiable in almost all patients.

Recently, I have given some patients wrist splints for comfort for the first 1 to 2 weeks from injury. My concern is in restricting full finger flexion, but I suspect that is not a problem and some patients are very sore for the first week or two following these fractures.

3.3.2 Finger Transverse Metacarpal Fractures—Shaft and Neck

In the past, virtually all patients with transverse metacarpal shaft (▶Fig. 3.3a, b) and particularly neck (boxer's) fractures were mobilized freely; the fractures healed with some deformity but almost always with good function. In the United Kingdom, Barton[2] showed the benefits of a small plaster or splint support to reduce and successfully maintain an improved angulation for transverse metacarpal shaft fractures with very good functional results. More recently the results of surgical treatments have been reported with equally good outcomes.

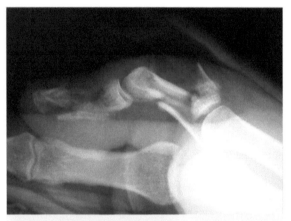

Fig. 3.1 Comminuted crush fracture of the thumb.

Fig. 3.2 (a, b) Spiral metacarpal fracture.

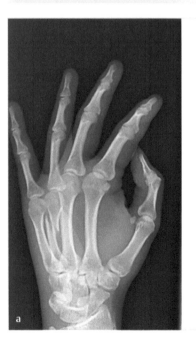
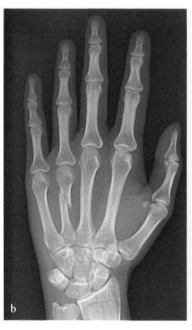

Table 3.1 The outcome of finger spiral or long oblique metacarpal fractures

Paper and year of publication	Treatments	Numbers of patients (fingers)	Mean follow-up (range) months	Mean age (range) years	Ranges of motion	Grip strength	Complications
Al-Qattan 2008 a	Cerclage wiring and interosseous loop wiring	24 (25)	2.5 (1.5–7)	32 (20–42)	Full in 23		CRPS in one
Al-Qattan 2008 b	Splint and mobilization	42 (54)	Min 1.5 Max 12	29 (20–48)		94% in those seen at 1 year	
Al-Qattan and Al-Lazzam 2007	Cerclage wire	19	2 (1.5 –3)	35 (18–45)	Full		Nil
Khan and Giddins 2015	Early mobilization	25 (28)	Min 6 (6–14)	27 (17–60)	Full	> 90% in all	Mild malrotation in one. Mild discomfort in a boxer

Abbreviation: CRPS, Complex regional pain syndrome.

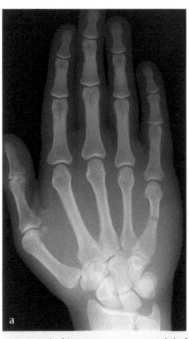
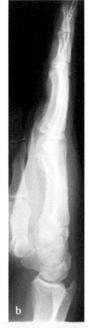

Fig. 3.3 (a, b) Transverse metacarpal shaft fracture.

A crucial question is what degree of metacarpal malunion is acceptable? The answer is not clear. For metacarpal neck (boxer's) fractures, it has been suggested by various authors as 50 to 60 degrees[12]; 30 degrees[13,14]; and 20 degrees of flexion[15,16]; of note, the amount of acceptable angulation has increased over time. For little finger metacarpal shaft fractures, 30 degrees[12,17] has been suggested as acceptable. These recommendations are only expert opinion.

The outcome of nonoperative treatment has been reported widely and apart from a mild cosmetic abnormality, there is typically an excellent functional outcome (Cochrane review 2005 [updated 2009]).[18] The Cochrane review also noted that there is no good evidence that more marked malunion reduces hand function or gives an unacceptable deformity.[18]

Many surgical techniques have been described including intramedullary nailing,[19] intra-medullary screw fixation,[20–22] K-wire (bouquet) fixation,[23–25] intraosseous loop wire fixation,[3] and external fixation.[26] The results of these techniques are not reliably better than nonoperative treatment and they introduce complications not seen with nonoperative treatment. Nonoperative treatment has complications but apart from malunion these are rare.

Comparative studies, particularly randomized controlled studies (RCTs) provide the best way to assess different treatments. Excellent RCTs in hand surgery are rare, but there are some useful comparative studies. Westbrook et al[27] compared the nonsurgical and surgical treatment of metacarpal neck and shaft fractures in a retrospective study. About 105 metacarpal neck fractures were treated nonoperatively, compared with 18 treated operatively (intramedullary K-wiring in 13 and plating in 5 cases); and 113 metacarpal shaft fractures were treated nonoperatively compared with 26 treated operatively (K-wiring in 4 and plating in 22 cases). At a minimum follow-up of 2 years, there were no differences in DASH score, grip strengths, or aesthetics between the nonoperative and operative groups. However, there was a significantly higher complication rate in the patients treated operatively compared to those treated nonoperatively. The follow-up rates were low (17% for nonoperative treatment and 54% for operative treatment); this is typical in these patient groups. A randomized study of metacarpal neck fractures by Strub et al[28] has suggested that surgery may give very slightly better outcomes than nonoperative treatment, primarily better cosmesis due to less malunion. They studied two groups each of 20 patients who were pseudo-randomized between nonoperative treatment and intramedullary (bouquet) wiring. The latter required a minimum of two operations each: one to insert and one to remove the wires. The only complications were in the operative group; they also had more dissatisfied as well as very satisfied patients. This study did not measure the inconvenience and costs to the patient or the health care system, so the cost of this possible small benefit is unknown. Of particular note in this and many other studies of surgery for hand fractures, it is not clear how many patients need to be improved from "satisfied" to "very satisfied" to compensate for one "dissatisfied" patient.

Overall, there may be a small cosmetic benefit from surgery for transverse metacarpal shaft and neck fractures of the ring and little fingers, but the costs and the risks are probably not worth the small potential benefit to most patients and in particular most health care systems. The index and middle fingers tolerate transverse metacarpal shaft and neck fracture malunion less well because of the stiffness of the carpometacarpal (CMC) joints, so the indications for surgery are greater. However, only so few studies have been reported that it is not possible to provide a reliable conclusion about their best treatment.

3.3.3 Finger Proximal Phalanx Collateral Ligament Avulsion Fractures

Bekler et al[29] stated that avulsion fractures of the bases of the phalanges of the fingers are challenging to treat (▶Fig. 3.4); they also stated that "Avulsion fractures (of the bases of the phalanges) are intra-articular according to their configuration and need anatomical reduction." There was no evidence to support this opinion.

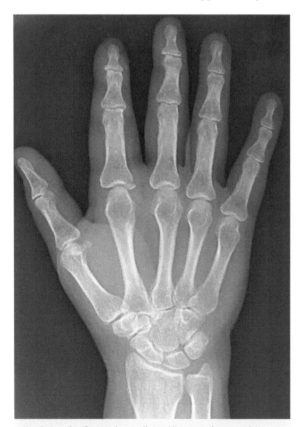

Fig. 3.4 Index finger ulnar collateral ligament bony avulsion injury.

Despite this assertion, finger proximal phalanx avulsion fractures attract a full range of "proven" treatment advice.

Many authors have recommended that all base of finger avulsion fractures should be treated surgically because of the high rate of symptomatic non- or delayed union.[30-35] In particular Shewring and Thomas[35] reported that of eight of their patients treated nonoperatively all had delayed union; seven were treated with ORIF and bone grafting. They report very good results at discharge from follow-up at 3 months following surgery. In contrast, Sawant et al[36] reported that finger proximal phalanx avulsion fractures of up to 25% of the articular surface on the posteroanterior (PA) radiograph achieve very good results with early protected mobilization, that is, with buddy strapping and avoidance of heavy activity for 4 to 6 weeks. Even that level of support may not be necessary or not for so long, but that has not yet been established. Overall, it appears that for avulsion fractures protected mobilization gives results that cannot easily be improved by surgery (▶Table 3.2). The data are, however, limited; these are small series or have limited follow-up. The dichotomy with the experience of Shewring and Thomas[35] who reported symptomatic delayed union in eight consecutive patients and the excellent results of Sawant et al[36] may be because many of these injuries do not unite with bone (as for thumb MP joint ulnar collateral ligament [UCL] avulsions[37]) but heal with sufficient stability that surgery is not required. This seems to be true for the central as much as for the border digits including the radial collateral ligament (RCL) insertion to the index finger.

As so often in the hand bone union appears much less important than elsewhere in the long bones, but it is such an obvious measure to assess that it can encourage treatment that is not functionally justified.

3.3.4 Bony Mallet Injuries

There are multiple papers reporting on a myriad of techniques for reducing and holding the dorsal avulsion fracture fragment in bony mallet injuries.[38-51] Yet, this is an operation with an acknowledged high risk of complications.[30,52,53] Authors of more recent techniques report fewer complications particularly skin breakdown.[38-51] In general, good results are reported for various surgical treatments of bony mallet injuries with a dorsal fracture fragment of one-third or more (▶Table 3.3). A number of authors, especially Stark et al,[54] have recommended surgery to treat fractures of one-third or more. These authors have been concerned about achieving "anatomical reduction" of the fracture and prevention of subluxation of the main distal phalanx fracture fragment.[39-51] How much subluxation needs to be treated is unproven, but it is known that some cases do progress to symptomatic dislocation. In one of the most widely cited papers, Wehbe and Schneider[53] reported that among patients with dorsal fracture fragments of over one-third followed up for a mean of 3.2 years, the 15 patients treated nonoperatively did as well as the six treated operatively. They concluded that operative treatment gave no better results than nonoperative treatment. Similarly,

Table 3.2 The outcome of finger proximal phalanx avulsion fractures (the data could not be extracted from many papers)

Paper	Treatment	Numbers of patients (fingers)	Mean follow-up (range) months	Mean age (range) years	Pain (VAS 0–10)	Function DASH scores	Ranges of motion	Grip strength
Sawant et al 2007	Early mobilization	7 (7)	57 (8–94)	39 (16–68)	0.6 (0–2)	1.3 (0–4.2)	Full	> 90%
Mikami et al 2011	K-wiring	4 (5)	43 (30–72)	21 (11–57)	NR	3.0 (0.8–10.8)	85	NR
Shewring and Thomas 2003	Open reduction and internal fixation	33	3	26 (15–44)	NR	NR	Full	NR

Abbreviation: NR, not recorded.

Table 3.3 Thumb MP joint ulnar collateral ligament bony avulsions

Paper and year	Treatment	Number of patients (thumbs)	Mean follow-up (range) months	Mean age (range) years	Ranges of MP joint movement	Grip strength	Notes
Kozin and Bishop 1994	Tension band wiring	9	26	20 (15–41)	77%	96%	
Kuz et al 1999	Plaster cast or splint for 4 weeks	30	3.1 (1–5.2)	30	The same	NR	No pain in 19 of 30. Unstable in 2/20. Nonunion 5/20
Landsman et al 1995	Thumb spica splint for 8–12 weeks	12	38 (12–60)	30 (17–48)	84 (60–100) %	92 (80–100) %	All healed but data on ROM and strength includes tendinous injuries, which overall did worse than the avulsion injuries
Sorene and Goodwin 2003	Plaster cast	28	30 (12–48)	34 (17–62)	NR	97%	No pain in 26. Nonunion 17

Abbreviations: MP, metacarpophalangeal; NR, not recorded; ROM, range of motion.
Kozin and Bishop's two cases were RCL injuries.

another series of cases with a 5-year follow-up has shown that both tendinous and bony mallet injuries treated nonoperatively achieve good objective and very good subjective outcomes.[55] Among the bony mallet injuries were some with fracture fragments greater than one-third, but they are not reported separately. They also reported some evidence of degeneration at the distal interphalangeal (DIP) joint in 10 of 11 patients with large fracture fragments within 5 years. Wehbe and Schneider[53] noted no difference in the rates of radiographic DIP joint osteoarthritis (OA) between operative and nonoperative treatment. Other authors have reported rates up to 50%, yet some reported 0% (▶Table 3.3). Almost certainly their criteria (which are reported rarely) differ, making comparison difficult. The risk of radiographic OA would be a potential concern except that long-term symptomatic degenerative arthritis in the DIP joints is not widely reported in patients who have had bony mallet injuries, that is, as hand surgeons we rarely see patients requiring treatment for symptomatic DIP joint arthritis who had bony mallet injuries decades earlier. It would appear that the majority of patients with bony mallet injuries do not require surgical treatment.

A Cochrane review of bony mallet injuries reported that there was a paucity of good studies and there was no evidence that surgery was better than nonoperative (typically splint) treatment for all types of mallet injury.[56] They did, however, acknowledge that there may be a subgroup of these injuries that would benefit from surgery.

The key concern is volar subluxation of the bulk of the distal phalanx (▶Fig. 3.5). Several recent papers have clarified further the risk of subluxation: Kim and Kim[57] showed that over 50% of patients with a fracture fragment involving greater than one-third of the base on the lateral radiograph did not progress to subluxation. They noted a cutoff of at a fracture fragment size of 48% of the base, above which subluxation was more likely. This is also similar to the findings in the study of Giddins[58] who noted that stable injuries had a mean fracture fragment size of 49%. Kim and Kim[57] also related subluxation to delay in application of a splint, particularly to a delay of longer than 12 days. Moradi et al[59] reviewed 392 bony mallet injuries. They showed that subluxation did not occur with a fracture fragment smaller than 39% on the lateral radiograph. The risk of subluxation increased

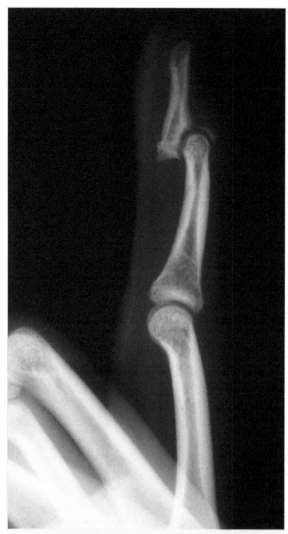

Fig. 3.5 Chronic distal interphalangeal joint (DIPJ) subluxation following a mallet injury.

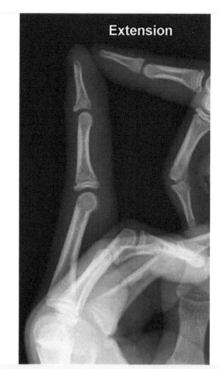

Fig. 3.6 Gliding of a bony mallet injury on extension stress testing.

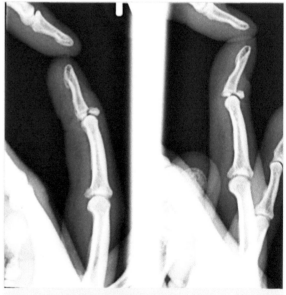

Fig. 3.7 Pivoting of a bony mallet injury on extension stress testing.

with increasing size of the fragment, increased displacement of the fragment, and time from injury to treatment. Nonetheless, most (68%) did not sublux even with a fracture fragment greater than 39%. Giddins[58] has shown that the risk of subluxation can be assessed by a lateral hyperextension radiograph performed within 1 to 2 weeks of injury. If there is gliding of the joint (▶Fig. 3.6), that is, it remains congruent as it rotates into extension, then this is a stable joint. The presumption is that there has not been so much volar plate and collateral ligament injury that subluxation will occur. If there is pivoting (▶Fig. 3.7), then subluxation will usually occur, although this may only be mild. A third subgroup occurs described as tilting (▶Fig. 3.8). This appears to be a variant on gliding and is not typically associated with subluxation. Exactly what level of subluxation requires treatment is unclear.

Together these recent papers establish that basing treatment on a fracture fragment greater than one-third of the base of the distal phalanx is unreliable in predicting subluxation. It will lead to substantial overtreatment and so

should be discarded. Rather a combination of a fracture fragment greater than 39%, displacement, and particularly the response to hyperextension testing should indicate the very small number of patients who require surgery to prevent appreciable, that is, long-term symptomatic, subluxation. The vast majority of patients with these injuries should do well with splintage for about 4 weeks (even that may be longer than is necessary). The recent work on

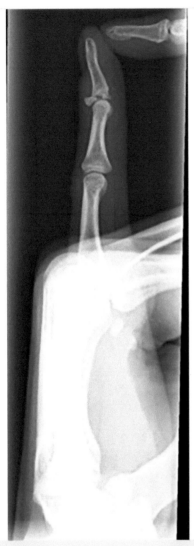

Fig. 3.8 Tilting of a bony mallet injury on extension stress testing.

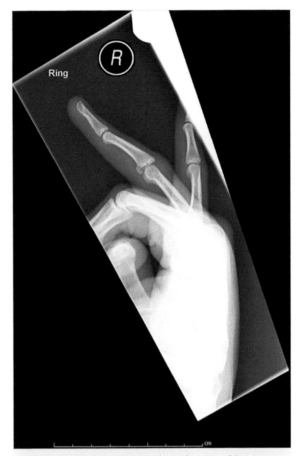

Fig. 3.9 Proximal interphalangeal joint fracture subluxation.

this injury is helping define treatment by highlighting the subgroups where surgery is indicated and helping exclude more patients from needing operations.

3.3.5 Base of Middle Phalanx Injuries

Fractures of the base of the middle phalanx are common but can be difficult to treat. The two common injuries are dorsal fracture subluxations/dislocations and pilon fractures. There are many recommended treatments: immobilization, early mobilization, manipulation and K-wire stabilization, static external fixation, dynamic external fixation, ORIF, and immediate hemihamate arthroplasty. Stable injuries, particularly fracture subluxations, with a fracture of the base of the middle phalanx of less than one-third on the lateral radiograph or pilon fractures without too much displacement appear to do well with nonoperative treatment. Typically, the

remainder are treated surgically. While many patients achieve good results with surgical treatment, there are some very poor results especially if a postoperative infection occurs. Recent work that I have done suggests that lateral flexion radiographs (comparable to the lateral extension radiographs in the assessment of stability in bony mallet injuries) can predict the injuries that need surgery and those that do not. Patients attending their first outpatient clinic appointment (within 10 days of injury) are encouraged to flex their injured PIP joint as much as possible, ideally at least 40 degrees at the PIP joint. A lateral flexion radiograph is performed. If this shows gliding (▶Fig. 3.9, ▶Fig. 3.10), specifically not pivoting, then the finger can be treated with early mobilization anticipating a very good outcome with little pain and a range of motion (ROM) of at least 10 to 90 degrees, that is, as good as reported surgical series. If the middle phalanx pivots about the volar margin of the bulk of the base of the middle phalanx (▶Fig. 3.11) as the finger flexes, then there is likely to be a poor outcome and surgery is recommended (these patients often struggle to flex > 20 degrees). I have not thought it "ethical" to treat the fingers that pivot, nonoperatively, in order to assess whether surgery would have been needed so I can only report on the fingers that glide. I have treated 10 fingers which glided with consistent results even when the fracture pattern includes

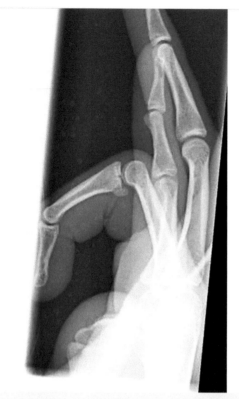

Fig. 3.10 Gliding on proximal interphalangeal joint flexion.

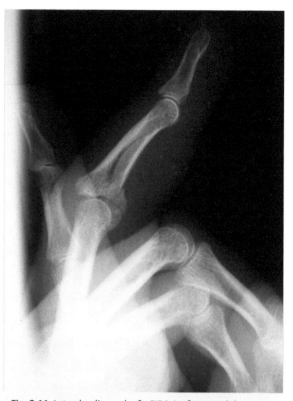

Fig. 3.11 Lateral radiograph of a PIP joint fracture dislocation pivoting with flexion.

an increased sagittal width of the base of the middle phalanx (▶Fig. 3.9) which has been suggested as an indication for surgery. I recommend careful and regular review for a minimum of 3 weeks from injury, with repeat radiographs to ensure there is no further late collapse of the fracture and to ensure that good early mobilization occurs. So far, I have not seen late collapse or any poor outcomes.

It is hardly surprising that maintenance/restoration of gliding gives good results in IP joints. I believe that the aim of treatment of intra-articular hand fractures is not primarily reduction of the fracture to a certain angle but restoration of gliding with acceptable alignment. I believe I have established that for bony mallet injuries and will sow it for PIP joint injuries. This fits with our clinical experience. Thus, condylar fractures at the IP joints do not need reduction to restore gliding as that is maintained as shown by angular malunions with good ROM; rather surgical reduction is needed to maintain the overall alignment of the injured digit.

Thumb

3.3.6 Metacarpophalangeal Joint Avulsion Fractures

Ulnar Collateral Ligament Injuries

The outcome of thumb MP joint avulsion fractures (▶Fig. 3.12) treated nonoperatively is also disputed.

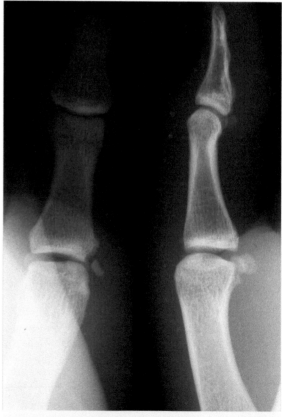

Fig. 3.12 Thumb metacarpophalangeal joint radial collateral ligament bony avulsion injury.

A Stener lesion, whether or not there is a bony avulsion, will almost always give a poor long-term outcome with nonoperative treatment.[60] For less displaced injuries without a Stener lesion, some authors have reported poor outcomes of avulsion fractures treated nonoperatively: Dinowitz et al[61] reported on nine cases with minimally displaced fractures (up to 2 mm) treated in plaster within 6 days. They reported that all had persistent pain, which largely resolved with surgical stabilization. Kuz et al[62] reported on 30 patients with thumb MP joint avulsion fractures treated nonoperatively: 30 were reviewed by questionnaire, and 20 were seen in person. Nineteen of the 30 patients who completed questionnaires reported no pain; all 30 reported being satisfied by their treatment and none had had to change their jobs. Of the 20 patients assessed in person, there were no statistically significant reductions in pinch or grip strength, but 2 patients had some instability on stress testing. The authors reviewed the radiographs of 20 patients; they reported a nonunion rate of ¼ (5 of 20). Sorene and Goodwin (2003)[37] reported on 28 patients who suffered thumb UCL avulsion fractures were stable at original assessment. The patients were treated with immobilization in plaster for 6 weeks and thereafter followed up for a mean of 2.5 (range 1–4) years. Twenty-six of the 28 patients had no pain at rest or on movement and all 28 patients had the same pinch and grip strength as their contralateral

uninjured side, yet 60% had radiological evidence of persistent nonunion of the avulsion fracture fragment. Comparable very good results have been reported in many surgical series.[30,63] Overall, it appears that stable thumb UCL bony avulsion injuries can be immobilized in plaster with the expectation of a very good clinical outcome even though radiological union may not be achieved (▶Table 3.4).

The treatment of unstable thumb MP joint UCL avulsion injuries is less clear; at present, surgery is probably the default position, but, as so often, the data are inadequate. There are many different types of thumb UCL avulsion injury from small bony avulsions, which seem primarily to be a soft tissue problem through to large rotated bone avulsion fragments. It is highly likely this is an injury with subtypes requiring different treatment; some of these injuries may do appreciably better treated surgically while the majority may not. This remains unproven, but it would in part explain the dichotomy between the advocates of nonoperative and operative treatment. An adequately powered (probably quite large study in order to identify the subtypes) multicenter RCT is needed. While nonoperative management should remain the treatment of choice for thumb MP joint, UCL bony avulsion fractures' surgeons need to be aware that there is a range of injuries and the best treatment for each subgroup is currently unclear.

Table 3.4 The outcome of treatment of bony mallet injuries with fracture fragments greater than or equal to one-third and a minimum follow-up of 12 months

Paper and year	Treatment	Numbers of patients (fingers)	Mean FU (range) months	Mean age (range) years	DIPJ ranges of motion (degrees)	% of bone involved on the lateral radiograph	Crawford (or other) score E = excellent, G = good, F = fair	Radiological evidence of osteoarthritis
Damron and Engber 1994	Pull-through suture and K-wire	18	97 (24–147)	23 (17–32)	1–69 (15 patients)	51 (38–67)	10 pain-free, 13 no functional limitation	7 of 15
Darder-Prats et al 1998	K-wire	22	25 (18–48)	23 (14–34)	NR	> 33	18 E, 3 G, 1 F	0
Fritz et al 2005	K-wire	24	Mean unclear (min 12 months)	31 (15–53)	1–72	> 33	19 no pain W and N criteria	
Okafor et al 1997	Splint for 7 (6–12) weeks	11	66 (but includes tendinous as well)	NK	9–51	NR	NR	10 of 11
Hofmeister et al 2003	Closed K-wiring	23 (24)	> 1 year	24	4–77	40	22 E/G, 2 F	
Takami et al 2000	Open reduction and K-wiring	33	29	32 (19–63)	4–67	> 33	NR	
Tetik and Gudemez 2002	Closed K-wiring	18	27	29 (22–47)	2–81	40	NR	

Abbreviation: NR, not recorded.

Radial Collateral Ligament Injuries

There are fewer reports on the management of RCL injuries of the thumb MP joint (▶ Fig. 3.13). As there is no adductor hood to give a Stener-type lesion, nonoperative treatment should give good results, that is, immobilization in plaster or a splint for 4 to 6 weeks. Despite this, surgical treatment of these injuries has been debated for a long time.[64–67] There are also rare reports of radial-sided "Stener" lesions.[68,69]

Köttstorfer et al[70] showed that mildly displaced RCL avulsion fractures treated nonoperatively usually achieve a very good outcome. The role of surgery for more widely displaced or unstable injuries is unclear. Köttstorfer et al[70] also noted that many surgeons believe that surgery is required for unstable injuries as "considerable displacement of torn ends can prevent the RCL from healing." Good results have been reported with surgical stabilization for more unstable injuries, but the original premise that the ligament will not heal with marked displacement or instability is unproven. In addition, it is well known that in the hand considerable ligament disruption can usually be repaired by the body's own mechanisms avoiding instability and there are many instances of considerable gaps between bone ends which heal with bone in the hand, for example, bony mallet injuries. One reason for the differences in treatment may be the lengthy recover from thumb MP joint RCL and UCL avulsion injuries. This may skew the clinical impression of treatment outcome in shorter-term reviews. RCL injuries should not be assumed to be a single problem requiring one type of treatment. The optimal treatment for each subgroup is not yet established, but again nonoperative treatment should be presumed to be the management of choice for the large majority of these injuries.

3.3.7 Bennetts's Fracture Subluxation

The treatment of Bennett's fracture subluxations (▶ Fig. 3.14) has moved from a strong preference for nonoperative treatment 30 or more years ago to an almost uniform preference for surgical stabilization in part based on publications stating that conservative treatment is less good than operative treatment. Whether this is proven by the published literature in not clear.

A recent systematic review (2016) looked at the evidence in the treatment of Bennett's fractures.[71] Thirty-eight different retrospective studies were reviewed; they were published from 1958 to 2015. There were 11 different types of treatment from immobilization for only 1 week to ORIF. The reporting of the data was not consistent preventing a meta-analysis. It was, nonetheless, possible to compare the outcomes for hundreds of patients. Pain was reported in 31 studies, return to work in 28 studies, and radiological evidence of OA in 31 studies (▶ Table 3.5). The long-term assessment of pain could be compared for 645 patients: 75 of 224 (33%) patients treated nonsurgically had pain at final review (mean time 12, range 6–26 years), compared with 73 of 421 (17%) treated surgically (mean time 5, range 2–11 years) ($p < 0.0001$). Data

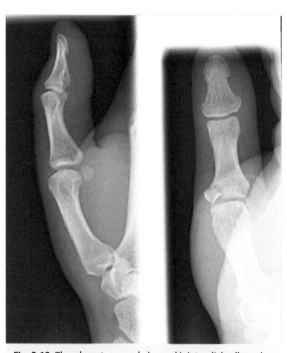

Fig. 3.13 Thumb metacarpophalangeal joint radial collateral ligament bony avulsion injury.

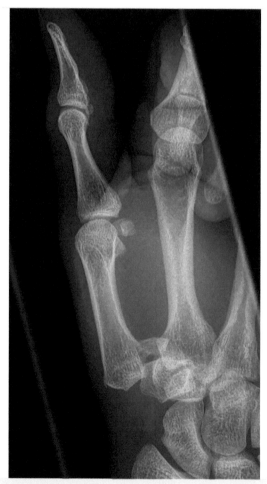

Fig. 3.14 Bennett's fracture subluxation.

Table 3.5 Outcomes of treatments of Bennett's fractures

Study	Numbers of patients available for review	Mean final assessment time (years)	Intervention	Intervention 2	Intervention 3
Blaskova 1958	48 (48)	2	MUA & POP (48)		
Spangberg 1963	34 (34)	4	Traction (34)		
Griffiths 1964	45 (21)	6.8	Unreduced & POP (8)	Partial reduction & POP (3)	Reduced & POP (10)
Ziffko 1980	100 (100)	2–22	MUA & POP (100)		
Wang 1981	40 (31)	2.8	Duck billed splint 40 (31)		
Livesley 1990	33 (17)	26.4	None 5 (2)	Traction 4 (4)	MUA & POP 1–6 weeks 24 (11)
Oosterbos 1995	22 (20)	13	MUA & POP 22 (20)		
Milosevic 2005	50 (50)	9	MUA & POP (50)		

on return to work could be compared for 474 patients. One hundred and twenty of 122 (98%) patients treated nonsurgically returned to their previous employment at a mean of 11 (range 2–26) years, compared with 351 of 352 (99%) of those treated surgically at a mean of 6 (range 1–12) years. Radiological evidence of osteoarthritis was reported in 839 patients: 99 of 299 (33%) patients treated nonsurgically had osteoarthritis at a mean of 8 (range 2–26) years, compared with 182 of 540 (33%) patients treated surgically at a mean of 4 (range 1–12) years. Data on complications of treatment were available for 956 patients; only 2 of 287 (< 1%) of patients treated nonsurgically had complications compared to 88 of 669 (13%) treated surgically; 56 patients treated surgically required a second operation for removal of metalwork, primarily prominent tension band wires ($p = 0.0001$).

The quality of the data is not high, nonetheless, it seems that patients are more likely to suffer long-term pain following nonsurgical treatment and much more likely to suffer complications with surgical treatment. Otherwise, the data for return to work and long-term OA are comparable.

The longest review (mean 26 years) is from Livesley.[72] It is cited frequently as evidence in favor of treating these injuries operatively rather than nonoperatively.[73] Yet in Livesley's cohort of 17 patients, no comment is made on the quality of the reduction at the beginning of treatment and three different methods of treatment were used: no immobilization in two cases, traction in four cases, and manipulation and plaster in 11 cases. The duration of treatment varied between 1 and 6 weeks. Despite this relatively poor treatment by current standards, 11 of the 17 had no or mild pain and 16 of the 17 had returned to their previous employment at the final review. Furthermore, although this paper has the longest follow-up, when degenerative changes may be expected to lead to symptoms, their results are not significantly different in terms of pain and function to similar conservative studies and perhaps more importantly to several of the operative studies.[74–77]

Overall, there is currently no high-quality evidence as to the optimal treatment method for a Bennett's fracture subluxation. Surgeons should aim to achieve and hold an adequate reduction of the fracture until bone union. This is harder to do nonoperatively but not impossible. In my experience, use of a modified Bennett's plaster holding the thumb MP joint flexed helps achieve and maintain reduction of the fracture in a plaster cast in most but not all cases. Thus, many of these injuries can be treated nonoperatively and an adequate reduction achieved and maintained. In theory, this should give as good an outcome as successful surgical treatment. Ultimately, one or more randomized controlled trials comparing nonsurgical or surgical treatments are required to advance the treatment of this common injury.

3.4 Discussion

The published literature in the treatment of common hand fractures is weak; there are few RCTs; there is bias in many of the studies: often incomplete data, outdated outcome reporting, and in particular, inadequate descriptions of the methods especially for nonoperative techniques. While we recognize that closed reduction and percutaneous K-wring is very different to ORIF, papers describing nonoperative treatment often do not differentiate clearly between uninhibited mobilization, supervised mobilization with regular follow-up, and immobilization and follow-up. In addition, the quality of postoperative care such as regular review of radiographs is rarely described despite its importance in assessing and maintaining fracture alignment in the first few weeks following injury.

The available data suggest that for the fractures described above surgery either does not reliably confer benefit over "good" nonoperative treatment or considering gliding/pivoting for certain IP joint injuries can further reduce those requiring surgery. For some injuries, surgery is rarely likely to be required, for example, spiral metacarpal fractures. For other fractures, although non-operative treatment should usually be tried first, surgery is likely to be required quite often, for example, Bennett's fracture subluxations. As surgery typically costs more both in patient's risk and health care costs, it suggests that nonoperative treatment should be the default position for the large majority of these injuries, accepting the need for clinical judgement for individual cases.

This review of the literature also highlights the dichotomies between authors recommending (at times very vigorously) a range of different treatments for the same injuries. There are many possible reasons: surgeon preference/bias; a misunderstanding of the anatomy and pathology of the injury; an overemphasis on biomechanical or cadaveric studies which may not apply in clinical practice; an overemphasis on bone union which may not affect outcome; an overemphasis on anatomical reduction of intra-articular fractures which may not reliably affect outcome; and possibly most of all, the variability of the injuries such that a subgroup of each type of injury does poorly with one type of treatment, often nonoperative treatment, which skews the reported/perceived outcomes of that treatment. This subset bias requires closer observation/larger series to avoid mistreatment.

I believe we should try to focus our research efforts on areas where we might make a significant difference ahead of tackling those with marginal gains. Different patterns of displaced phalangeal fractures, and PIP joint fracture subluxations or pilon fractures are two topics in hand fracture management where the optimal treatments are very unclear and where research could make a considerable difference.

This is not a diatribe against surgical treatment of these fractures or against innovation. I look forward to new, probably less invasive techniques, like intramedullary screw fixation[20-22] (see also Chapter 5) and more reliable techniques that will improve the outcomes for our patients. Until then the literature shows the outcomes of nonoperative treatment for most of these fractures is so good that there needs to be a strong argument for surgical intervention in order to justify the risks and costs of surgery. In addition, I believe this review highlights the need to identify the subgroups which do badly with nonoperative treatment (where they exist) such as through large cohort studies of nonoperative treatment or to identify new insights, for example, the role of gliding or pivoting in bony mallet injuries[58] to clarify which injuries need surgery. In addition, any future studies of these injuries that report an improvement in outcome with surgery should ideally be run as RCTs in comparison with vigilant and clearly described nonoperative treatment, as a cohort or case series of operative treatment is very unlikely to improve on the published data.

In summary, careful study of the natural history of many hand fractures shows that the outcome of nonoperative treatment is so good that surgery is rarely required, for example, for spiral/long oblique metacarpal fractures, metacarpal neck fractures, and bony collateral ligament avulsions of the thumb and finger MP joints. In others, there is a clear role for nonoperative treatment such as for Bennett's fracture subluxations and most bony mallet injures. There are clearly other injuries which typically (but not necessarily always) require surgical stabilization. One of our aims as clinicians should be to define the subgroups better in order to advise more reliably where surgery is likely to be beneficial and where it is not. Future novel techniques may completely change how we treat these injuries.

References

[1] Diwaker HN, Stothard J. The role of internal fixation in closed fractures of the proximal phalanges and metacarpals in adults. J Hand Surg [Br]. 1986; 11(1):103–108

[2] Barton NJ. Fractures of the hand. J Bone Joint Surg Br. 1984; 66(2):159–167

[3] Al-Qattan MM. Metacarpal shaft fractures of the fingers: treatment with interosseous loop wire fixation and immediate post-operative finger mobilisation in a wrist splint. J Hand Surg [Br]. 2006; 31(4):377–382

[4] Al-Qattan MM. The use of a combination of cerclage and unicortical interosseous loop dental wires for long oblique/spiral metacarpal shaft fractures. J Hand Surg Eur Vol. 200 8; 33(6):728–731

[5] Al-Qattan MM, Al-Lazzam A. Long oblique/spiral mid-shaft metacarpal fractures of the fingers: treatment with cerclage wire fixation and immediate post-operative finger mobilisation in a wrist splint. J Hand Surg Eur Vol. 2007; 32(6):637–640

[6] Al-Qattan MM. Outcome of conservative management of spiral/long oblique fractures of the metacarpal shaft of the fingers using a palmar wrist splint and immediate mobilisation of the fingers. J Hand Surg Eur Vol. 2008; 33(6):723–727

[7] Khan A, Giddins GEB. The outcome of conservative treatment of spiral metacarpal fractures and biomechanical proof of the role of the intermetacarpal ligaments in stabilising these injuries. J Hand Surg Eur Vol. 2015; 40:59–62

[8] Low CK, Wong HC, Low YP, Wong HP. A cadaver study of the effects of dorsal angulation and shortening of the metacarpal shaft on the extension and flexion force ratios of the index and little fingers. J Hand Surg [Br]. 1995; 20(5):609–613

[9] Meunier MJ, Hentzen E, Ryan M, Shin AY, Lieber RL. Predicted effects of metacarpal shortening on interosseous muscle function. J Hand Surg Am. 2004; 29(4):689–693

[10] Strauch RJ, Rosenwasser MP, Lunt JG. Metacarpal shaft fractures: the effect of shortening on the extensor tendon mechanism. J Hand Surg Am. 1998; 23(3):519–523

[11] Wills BP, Crum JA, McCabe RP, Vanderby R, Jr, Ablove RH. The effect of metacarpal shortening on digital flexion force. J Hand Surg Eur Vol. 2013; 38(6):667–672

[12] Stern PJ. Fractures of the metacarpals and phalanges. In: Green DP, Hotchkiss RN, Pederson WC, Wolfe SW, eds. Green's Operative Hand Surgery. 5th ed. New York, NY: Elsevier, Churchill Livingstone; 2005:277–341

[13] Ali A, Hamman J, Mass DP. The biomechanical effects of angulated boxer's fractures. J Hand Surg Am. 1999; 24(4):835–844

[14] Smith RJ, Peimer CA. Injuries to the metacarpal bones and joints. Adv Surg. 1977; 11:341–374

[15] Bloem JJAM. The treatment and prognosis of uncomplicated dislocated fractures of the metacarpals and phalanges. Arch Chir Neerl. 1971; 23(1):55–65

[16] Kilbourne BC, Paul EG. The use of small bone screws in the treatment of metacarpal, metatarsal, and phalangeal fractures. J Bone Joint Surg Am. 1958; 40-A(2):375–383

[17] Diao E, Welbourn JH. Extraarticular fractures of the metacarpals. In: Berger R, Weiss A, eds. Hand Surgery. New York, NY: Lippincott Williams & Wilkins; 2004:139–151

[18] Poolman RW, Goslings JC, Lee JB, Statius Muller M, Steller EP, Struijs PA. Conservative treatment for closed fifth (small finger) metacarpal neck fractures. Cochrane Database Syst Rev. 2005(3):CD003210

[19] Orbay JL, Touhami A. The treatment of unstable metacarpal and phalangeal shaft fractures with flexible nonlocking and locking intramedullary nails. Hand Clin. 2006; 22(3):279–286

[20] Borbas P, Dreu M, Poggetti A, Calcagni M, Giesen T. Treatment of proximal phalangeal fractures with an antegrade intramedullary screw: a cadaver study. J Hand Surg Eur Vol. 2016; 41(7):683–687

[21] del Piñal F, Moraleda E, Rúas JS, de Piero GH, Cerezal L. Minimally invasive fixation of fractures of the phalanges and metacarpals with intramedullary cannulated headless compression screws. J Hand Surg Am. 2015; 40(4):692–700

[22] Giesen T, Gazzola R, Poggetti A, Giovanoli P, Calcagni M. Intramedullary headless screw fixation for fractures of the proximal and middle phalanges in the digits of the hand: a review of 31 consecutive fractures. J Hand Surg Eur Vol. 2016; 41(7):688–694

[23] Downing ND, Davis TRC. Intramedullary fixation of unstable metacarpal fractures. Hand Clin. 2006; 22(3):269–277

[24] Faraj AA, Davis TRC. Percutaneous intramedullary fixation of metacarpal shaft fractures. J Hand Surg [Br]. 1999; 24(1):76–79

[25] Foucher G. "Bouquet" osteosynthesis in metacarpal neck fractures: a series of 66 patients. J Hand Surg Am. 1995; 20(3)(p)(t 2):S86–S90

[26] Margić K. External fixation of closed metacarpal and phalangeal fractures of digits. A prospective study of one hundred consecutive patients. J Hand Surg [Br]. 2006; 31(1):30–40

[27] Westbrook AP, Davis TR, Armstrong D, Burke FD. The clinical significance of malunion of fractures of the neck and shaft of the little finger metacarpal. J Hand Surg Eur Vol. 2008; 33(6):732–739

[28] Strub B, Schindele S, Sonderegger J, Sproedt J, von Campe A, Gruenert JG. Intramedullary splinting or conservative treatment for displaced fractures of the little finger metacarpal neck? A prospective study. J Hand Surg Eur Vol. 2010; 35(9):725–729

[29] Bekler H, Gokce A, Beyzadeoglu T. Avulsion fractures from the base of phalanges of the fingers. Tech Hand Up Extrem Surg. 2006; 10(3):157–161

[30] Bischoff R, Buechler U, De Roche R, Jupiter J. Clinical results of tension band fixation of avulsion fractures of the hand. J Hand Surg Am. 1994; 19(6):1019–1026

[31] Teo CG, Pho RWH. Avulsion-fracture at the proximal attachment of the radial collateral ligament of the fifth metacarpophalangeal joint—a case report. J Hand Surg Am. 1982; 7(5):526–527

[32] Gross DL, Moneim M. Radial collateral ligament avulsion fracture of the metacarpophalangeal joint in the small finger. Orthopedics. 1998; 21(7):814–815

[33] Mikami Y, Takata H, Oishi Y. Kirschner wire stabilization of collateral ligament avulsion fractures of the base of the proximal phalanx. J Hand Surg Eur Vol. 2011; 36(1):78–79

[34] Schubiner JM, Mass DP. Operation for collateral ligament ruptures of the metacarpophalangeal joints of the fingers. J Bone Joint Surg Br. 1989; 71(3):388–389

[35] Shewring DJ, Thomas RH. Avulsion fractures from the base of the proximal phalanges of the fingers. J Hand Surg [Br]. 2003; 28(1):10–14

[36] Sawant N, Kulikov Y, Giddins GEB. Outcome following conservative treatment of metacarpophalangeal collateral ligament avulsion fractures of the finger. J Hand Surg Eur Vol. 2007; 32(1):102–104

[37] Sorene ED, Goodwin DR. Non-operative treatment of displaced avulsion fractures of the ulnar base of the proximal phalanx of the thumb. Scand J Plast Reconstr Surg Hand Surg. 2003; 37(4):225–227

[38] Auchincloss JM. Mallet-finger injuries: a prospective, controlled trial of internal and external splintage. Hand. 1982; 14(2):168–173

[39] Badia A, Riano F. A simple fixation method for unstable bony mallet finger. J Hand Surg Am. 2004; 29(6):1051–1055

[40] Bauze A, Bain GI. Internal suture for mallet finger fracture. J Hand Surg [Br]. 1999; 24(6):688–692

[41] Cheon SJ, Lim JM, Cha SH. Treatment of bony mallet finger using a modified pull-out wire suture technique. J Hand Surg Eur Vol. 2011; 36(3):247–249

[42] Damron TA, Engber WD. Surgical treatment of mallet finger fractures by tension band technique. Clin Orthop Relat Res. 1994(300):133–140

[43] Darder-Prats A, Fernández-García E, Fernández-Gabarda R, Darder-García A. Treatment of mallet finger fractures by the extension-block K-wire technique. J Hand Surg [Br]. 1998; 23(6):802–805

[44] Fritz D, Lutz M, Arora R, Gabl M, Wambacher M, Pechlaner S. Delayed single Kirschner wire compression technique for mallet fracture. J Hand Surg [Br]. 2005; 30(2):180–184

[45] Hiwatari R, Saito S, Shibayama M. The 'chased method' of mini screw fixation: a percutaneous surgical approach to treating mallet fractures. J Hand Surg Eur Vol. 201 4; 39(7):784–786

[46] Ishiguro T, Itoh Y, Yabe Y, Hashizume N. Extension block with Kirschner wire for fracture dislocation of the distal interphalangeal joint. Tech Hand Up Extrem Surg. 1997; 1(2): 95–102

[47] King HJ, Shin SJ, Kang ES. Complications of operative treatment for mallet fractures of the distal phalanx. J Hand Surg [Br]. 2001; 26(1):28–31

[48] Kronlage SC, Faust D. Open reduction and screw fixation of mallet fractures. J Hand Surg [Br]. 2004; 29(2):135–138

[49] Pegoli L, Toh S, Arai K, Fukuda A, Nishikawa S, Vallejo IG. The Ishiguro extension block technique for the treatment of mallet finger fracture: indications and clinical results. J Hand Surg [Br]. 2003; 28(1):15–17

[50] Rocchi L, Genitiempo M, Fanfani F. Percutaneous fixation of mallet fractures by the "umbrella handle" technique. J Hand Surg [Br]. 2006; 31(4):407–412

[51] Teoh LC, Lee JY. Mallet fractures: a novel approach to internal fixation using a hook plate. J Hand Surg Eur Vol. 2007; 32(1):24–30

[52] Stern PJ, Kastrup JJ. Complications and prognosis of treatment of mallet finger. J Hand Surg Am. 1988; 13(3):329–334

[53] Wehbé MA, Schneider LH. Mallet fractures. J Bone Joint Surg Am. 1984; 66(5):658–669

[54] Stark HH, Gainor BJ, Ashworth CR, Zemel NP, Rickard TA. Operative treatment of intra-articular fractures of the dorsal aspect of the distal phalanx of digits. J Bone Joint Surg Am. 1987; 69(6):892–896

[55] Okafor B, Mbubaegbu C, Munshi I, Williams DJ. Mallet deformity of the finger. Five-year follow-up of conservative treatment. J Bone Joint Surg Br. 1997; 79(4):544–547

[56] Handoll HH, Vaghela MV. Interventions for treating mallet finger injuries. Cochrane Database Syst Rev. 2004(3):CD004574

[57] Kim JK, Kim DJ. The risk factors associated with subluxation of the distal interphalangeal joint in mallet fracture. J Hand Surg Eur Vol. 2015; 40(1):63–67

[58] Giddins GE. Bony mallet finger injuries: assessment of stability with extension stress testing. J Hand Surg Eur Vol. 2016; 41(7):696–700

[59] Moradi A, Braun Y, Oflazoglu K, Meijs T, Ring D, Chen N. Factors associated with subluxation in mallet fracture. J Hand Surg Eur Vol. 2017; 42(2):176–181

[60] Giele H, Martin J. The two-level ulnar collateral ligament injury of the metacarpophalangeal joint of the thumb. J Hand Surg [Br]. 2003; 28(1):92–93

[61] Dinowitz M, Trumble T, Hanel D, Vedder NB, Gilbert M. Failure of cast immobilization for thumb ulnar collateral ligament avulsion fractures. J Hand Surg Am. 1997; 22(6):1057–1063

[62] Kuz JE, Husban, d JB, Tokar N, McPherson SA. Outcome of avulsion fractures of the ulnar base of the proximal phalanx of the thumb treated nonsurgically. J Hand Surg Am. 1999; 24(2):275–282

[63] Kozin SH, Bishop AT. Tension wire fixation of avulsion fractures at the thumb metacarpophalangeal joint. J Hand Surg Am. 1994; 19(6):1027–1031

[64] Edelstein DM, Kardashian G, Lee SK. Radial collateral ligament injuries of the thumb. J Hand Surg Am. 2008; 33(5):760–770

[65] Katz V, Loy S, Alnot JY. Sprains of the radial collateral ligament of the metacarpophalangeal joint of the thumb. A series of 14 cases. Ann Chir Main Memb Super. 1998; 17(1):7–24

[66] Melone CP, Jr, Beldner S, Basuk RS. Thumb collateral ligament injuries. An anatomic basis for treatment. Hand Clin. 2000; 16(3):345–357

[67] Smith RJ. Post-traumatic instability of the metacarpophalangeal joint of the thumb. J Bone Joint Surg Am. 1977; 59(1):14–21

[68] Camp RA, Weatherwax RJ, Miller EB. Chronic posttraumatic radial instability of the thumb metacarpophalangeal joint. J Hand Surg Am. 1980; 5(3):221–225

[69] Doty JF, Rudd JN, Jemison M. Radial collateral ligament injury of the thumb with a Stener-like lesion. Orthopedics. 2010; 33(12):925

[70] Köttstorfer J, Hofbauer M, Krusche-Mandl I, Kaiser G, Erhart J, Platzer P. Avulsion fracture and complete rupture of the thumb radial collateral ligament. Arch Orthop Trauma Surg. 2013; 133(4):583–588

[71] Edwards GA, Giddins GE. Management of Bennett's fractures: a review of treatment outcomes. J Hand Surg Eur Vol. 2017; 42(2):201–203

[72] Livesley PJ. The conservative management of Bennett's fracture-dislocation: a 26-year follow-up. J Hand Surg [Br]. 1990; 15(3):291–294

[73] Leclère FM, Jenzer A, Hüsler R, et al. 7-year follow-up after open reduction and internal screw fixation in Bennett fractures. Arch Orthop Trauma Surg. 2012; 132(7):1045–1051

[74] Cannon SR, Dowd GS, Williams DH, Scott JM. A long-term study following Bennett's fracture. J Hand Surg [Br]. 1986; 11(3):426–431

[75] Griffiths JC. Fractures at the base of the first metacarpal bone. J Bone Joint Surg Br. 1964; 46:712–719

[76] Kjaer-Petersen K, Langhoff O, Andersen K. Bennett's fracture. J Hand Surg [Br]. 1990; 15(1):58–61

[77] Oosterbos CJ, de Boer HH. Nonoperative treatment of Bennett's fracture: a 13-year follow-up. J Orthop Trauma. 1995; 9(1):23–27

4 K-wire Fixation, Intraosseous Wiring, Tension Band Wiring

Lindsay Muir, Anuj Mishra, Zafar Naqui

Abstract

We have at our disposal ever more sophisticated plate and screw systems for use in the treatment of hand fractures. While the most modern of these are excellent, there are still circumstances where the use of more traditional methods may offer an advantage. It is important for the hand surgeon to have a mastery of all methods, in order to be able to tailor the implant to the situation. Whereas plates and screws can achieve rigid fixation, Kirschner's wires (K-wires) and cerclage techniques may cause less soft tissue injury and stripping and should not be forgotten about in an understandable urge to achieve impressive postoperative X-rays.

This chapter considers the role of intraosseous wiring and K-wires in the management of hand fractures. It will examine techniques and applications in intraosseous wiring. It will review the history and theory of K-wiring and various applications for the technique. It will also outline some of the potential complications.

Keywords: hand, fracture, K-wire, cerclage wire, intraosseous wire

4.1 Intraosseous and Cerclage Wiring

Intraosseous wire can be used alone or as an adjunct to K-wire fixation. The advantages include that it requires minimal exposure, is less prominent than screws and plates, and decreases the risk of adhesions to overlying tendons. The technique is most frequently used for transverse phalangeal and metacarpal fractures and in digital replantation.

Different intraosseous wire configurations have been proposed. Lister's loop was initially described in 1978 where a single interosseous wire is used with a K-wire.[1] Double interosseous wire has been used in parallel and perpendicular configurations (90–90 wiring) for transverse metacarpal/phalangeal fractures, replantations, and arthrodesis (▶Fig. 4.1). More recently, a "theta" (θ) configuration has been described which is similar to Lister's loop (▶Fig. 4.1).[2]

4.1.1 Metacarpal and Phalangeal Fractures

Cerclage (circumferential) wiring with 24-gauge stainless steel wire can be successfully used for oblique and spiral metacarpal shaft fractures. The technique was originally described to include scoring of the cortical bone with a side-cutting burr so that wire migration would not occur (Lister 1978). In a series of 100 cases, Lister achieved a 100% union rate in the case of transverse fractures. Overall, 83.2% of the maximum attainable total active range of motion (TAM) was achieved in the 100 cases.

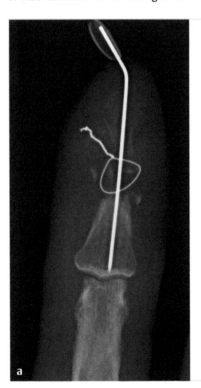
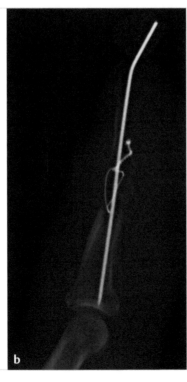

Fig. 4.1 (a, b) "Theta loop" wiring, which is similar to Lister's wire technique. In this case, for a distal interphalangeal arthrodesis following a chain saw injury. In this case, the soft bone meant that the ideal placement of the wire 3- to 4-mm away from the bone ends was not achievable.

Gingrass et al[3] achieved six excellent or good results in seven metacarpal fractures treated by double 26-gauge interosseous wires placed in a dorsal–volar direction. A single Kirschner pin was added in five of seven cases to augment stability. These authors suggest that intraosseous wiring without supplemental K-wire fixation is generally unsuitable for metacarpal shaft fractures because wire loosening and subsequent loss of reduction are real possibilities.

Gropper et al[4] used cerclage wires for the management of metacarpal shaft oblique and spiral fractures. All 21 metacarpal fractures were followed up until the patient was ready to return to work, which occurred an average of 7 weeks after surgery. Seventeen patients had no restriction of range of motion (ROM), with normal anatomical restoration of the metacarpal. Three patients lost 15 degrees of total active finger motion, and one had an extension lag of 10 degrees at the metacarpophalangeal (MCP) joint.

Al-Qattan[5] reported treatment of 36 metacarpal shaft fractures with intraosseous loop wire fixation alone. In contrast to Gingrass, he concluded that intraosseous wiring without K-wire fixation is rigid enough for immediate postoperative finger mobilization. Of 36 patients, 34 regained full ROM. Al-Qattan suggested, however, the use of supplementary K-wires if the fracture is comminuted.

In a series of 19 cases of midshaft oblique or spiral metacarpal fractures showed that cerclage wire fixation can be sufficient without scoring of bone or finger immobilization.[6]

Immediate postoperative mobilization is key to regaining the full ROM in all hand fracture patients. A review of fixation techniques of metacarpal shaft fractures found that regardless of the method of internal fixation, the majority of the patients regain a full ROM, provided a protocol of immediate postoperative mobilization is used.[5]

In long oblique or spiral fractures, lag screws have traditionally been used. Al-Qattan and Al-Zahrani[7] have described the use of intraosseous and/or cerclage dental wires for primary use or as a salvage because of the problems encountered with lag screws. The use of dental loop wires has not gained popularity because it is not believed to be rigid, based on several in vitro biomechanical studies which showed the superior stability of lag screws for long oblique and spiral metacarpal fractures.[5,8–11] The use of the combination of intraosseous and cerclage dental loop wires was described by Al-Qattan.[11] He highlighted the different roles for each technique. The intraosseous wire, although unicortical, prevents axial migration (shortening) at the fracture site, which is known to occur in long oblique/spiral metacarpal shaft fractures. It also aligns the fragments exactly and thus avoids any rotational problems, and prevents the migration of the cerclage wires, which compress the fracture site.

Al-Qattan and Al-Zahrani[7] performed a prospective study of 15 cases of long oblique or spiral fractures of proximal phalanx which were treated with cerclage wires. All fractures united. Full movement (> 260 degrees) was achieved in 12 patients. Fixed flexion deformity of 5 to 15 degrees at the proximal interphalangeal joint (PIPJ) occurred in three cases. One prominent wire was removed. No infection, complex regional pain syndrome (CRPS), loss

of fracture position, wire migration, or extrusion occurred. An average return to work of 8 weeks (7–11) was achieved.

Al-Qattan[11] showed better results with open reduction and interosseous wires when compared with closed reduction and K-wire in 78 industrial injuries with displaced unstable transverse fractures of the proximal phalanges. Forty fractures were treated with closed reduction and K-wiring that crossed the MCP joint, 38 with open reduction and interosseous loop wire fixation, 10 patients in each group were compound.

All fractures were united. Final range of movement (total active movement, TAM) was graded as excellent (> 240 degrees), good (220–239 degrees), fair (180–219 degrees), poor (< 180 degrees). For intraosseous wires, the results were excellent in 39%, good in 42%, fair in 8%, and poor in 11%. For K-wires, the results were excellent in 13%, good in 50%, fair in 25%, and poor in 13%. Thus, movement was better for intraosseous wires (19% fair and poor against 38% for K-wires). Return to work was 15 (12–30) weeks for K-wires, 14 (11–26) for interosseous wires. Complications for K-wires were fracture redisplacement in 2 cases, CRPS in 1, rotational malalignment in 1, infection in 2, and wire migration in 5, versus 3, 0, 0, 0, and 1, respectively, for intraosseous wires.

Thomas et al[2] treated 10 patients with open transverse fractures of the proximal phalanx, with a Lister loop and oblique K-wire (they named this "theta fixation") (▶Fig. 4.1). All fractures were united. Patient outcomes were assessed with the Belsky score, with 90% excellent, and 10% good results. Radiological union was achieved in 6.1 weeks. All patients returned to their preaccident employment at a mean of 11.3 weeks.

4.1.2 Fracture Dislocation around Joints

Comminuted fractures around joints are problematic. Direct fracture fixation with multiple K-wires or cerclage wires can be effective in stabilizing tenuous reductions of these fractures. Weiss[12] used cerclage wiring for PIPJ fracture dislocations. Twelve patients were treated by the volar cerclage wiring technique (▶Fig. 4.2).

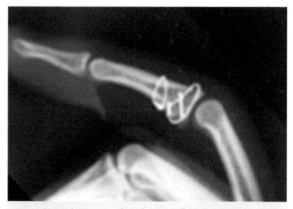

Fig. 4.2 Cerclage wiring for a fracture of the base of the middle phalanx.

At an average follow-up examination of 2.1 years, 11 of 12 patients were noted to have no radiological degenerative joint changes, with only 1 patient having evidence of early volar articular surface beaking. Average final active arc of motion at the PIPJ was 89 degrees (range 72–109 degrees). The average extension loss at the PIPJ was 8 degrees (range 0–16 degrees). There were no complications involving implant failure, irritation, or infection. The advantage of this technique was to avoid fracture fragment stripping, stable restoration of the articular surface, and palmar buttress of the middle phalanx at the PIPJ. Aladin and Davis[13] compared this technique with other open reduction and internal fixation techniques and did not show good results. Patients treated by cerclage wire fixation reported more cold intolerance and had a significantly larger fixed flexion deformity (median 30 degrees, range 18–38 degrees) and a smaller arc of motion (median 48 degrees, range 45–60 degrees) at the PIPJ, despite having the best radiological outcomes.

4.1.3 Surgical Technique

Intraosseous wires (25- or 26-gauge/0.35–0.45 mm) are useful for the fixation of unstable transverse phalangeal/metacarpal shaft fractures. The holes for the wire should ideally be drilled at least 3 to 4 mm from the fracture edge so that the wire does not cut out when it is being tightened. Kinking of the wire should be avoided because tightening becomes impossible. Additional fixation with an oblique K-wire may provide additional stability, particularly in the phalangeal diaphysis, where the bending moment is greatest (Lister's loop) (▶Fig. 4.3).[1]

4.2 K-wire Fixation

4.2.1 History

K-wire fixation has long been a principle method of fracture stabilization. Initially described by Kirschner for the application of traction in 1909, it was first used for fracture fixation by Otto Loewe in 1932. Bunnell first described the use of K-wires for transfixation of joints in the hand in the 1940s.[14] The small size of the bones of the hand with their small soft tissue envelopes coupled with the need for early mobilization of the fingers have ensured that K-wire fixation for hand fractures remain a central part of the surgeon's armamentarium.

4.2.2 Wire Design

K-wires are thin, smooth, and made of stainless steel or nitinol (nickel titanium). Their diameter is typically between 0.9 and 1.5 mm.[15] Larger diameter implants are referred to as "pins" and are too big for the hand and wrist. The end of the wire can be either diamond (two faced) or a trocar tip which has three faces (▶Fig. 4.4).

The trocar tip has been found to have the highest pullout force immediately after drilling, requiring the most torque to penetrate the bone during insertion; it does, however, generate the most heat.[16,17] Therefore, a trocar tip inserted at low speed is recommended for the strongest fixation in bone. Screw tipped or threaded wires have not been shown to have superior grip power but are less strong and have largely therefore been abandoned. Wires can be single or double ended.

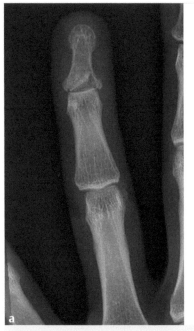
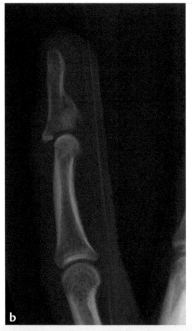
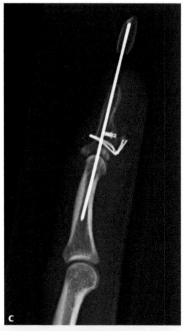

Fig. 4.3 (a–c) Leddy and Packer type Vb flexor digitorum profundus avulsion fixed with cerclage wire and longitudinal K- wire.

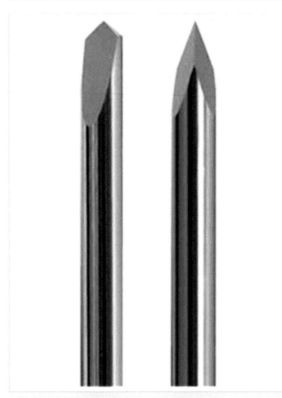

Fig. 4.4 Diamond (*left*) and trocar (*right*) K-wire tips.

Double-ended wires can be passed through back and forth, but care needs to be taken to avoid injury to the surgeon.

4.2.3 Indications

K-wires may be used effectively for many varied indications, including extra- and intra-articular fractures, joint dislocation, closed and open fractures, definitive or temporary intraoperative fixation, as well as being uses for guiding other implants. While wires can be used to pull fragments together, they can also be used to maintain a joint space between two bones. The management of specific injuries are dealt with later in this chapter. The advantages of K-wires over other techniques include their low cost, ready availability, versatility in many different fracture configurations, the requirement for only minimal dissection, and percutaneous insertion. Compared to other fracture implants, there is little implant load, which is an important consideration for the bones of the carpus and hand. It is often said that K-wires are also easy to insert and while this is true from a purely conceptual perspective, the efficient use of this technique to hold a fracture, while avoiding osteonecrosis and soft tissue injury requires skill and experience.

4.2.4 Technique: General Principles of K-wire Fixation at the MHC

We prefer to perform the procedure under local or regional anesthesia. Patients often watch the image intensifier; this helps them understand what has been done and the postoperative rehabilitation can be clearly reinforced to the patient. The role of intravenous antibiotics has not been defined.[18] A tourniquet is applied but is seldom inflated; it is preferable to allow some bleeding to help mitigate the heat generated from the wire insertion.

Most metacarpal and phalangeal fractures are amenable to smooth K-wires of between 1 and 1.3 mm in diameter, the smaller sizes being used more distally. Wires smaller than 1 mm have significantly less stiffness. For the carpus, we prefer using 1.25-mm wires.

Fractures should initially be reduced, if possible, closed, if not, then open with care taken to address any rotational deformity of the fingers, which is usually poorly tolerated. Intra-articular fractures may require open reduction, as any articular step of more than 1 mm should be avoided.

K-wires should be placed with as few passes as possible to minimize soft tissue trauma and osteonecrosis. It is helpful to take an X-ray with the fluoroscan while placing the wire over the hand in the position you will aim to drive the wire. The entry point and direction of the wire can then be marked on the skin. Plan in advance where you will place the other wire(s) and allow for this before inserting your first wire (▶ Fig. 4.5).

Ideally, the wire should be inserted perpendicular to the fracture site. Planning these steps cannot be overemphasized in reducing the number of unnecessary passages of the wire. This is especially of importance in the tubular metacarpal and phalangeal bones, which have a narrow diameter, and where repeated passage

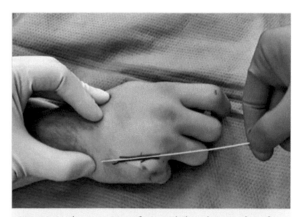

Fig. 4.5 Mark out position of wire to help reduce number of passes.

of wires can lead to osteonecrosis, loss of cortex, and weakening of the bone.

A stab incision is made where the wire will be inserted followed by blunt dissection down to the bone to protect neurovascular structures. The wire should be advanced slowly and the position checked regularly using the intensifier, this will again reduce inadvertent tissue damage and reduce the overall radiation dosage. We gently apply saline to cool the wire, taking care to avoid inadvertent splash back into the eye. A recent study has found that driving the wire using an oscillation setting as opposed to forward setting reduces the temperature also.[19] Hammering K-wires has been shown to give the strongest fixation with the minimum of thermal damage, however, it then requires great force to remove the wire should the position need changing.[20]

It may not be possible to maintain the fracture reduction and drive the K-wire across the fracture simultaneously. It is better to wire one fragment, then hold the fracture reduced, and then cross the fracture. Joysticking one fragment of the bone to the other is a very useful technique.

Maintaining reduction while wiring without the surgeon's hands being irradiated is important. Distraction of the finger by the use of a Chinese finger trap (►Fig. 4.6) or by applying a sponge holder over the fingertip wrapped with cotton gauze (►Fig. 4.7) is helpful in our experience.

Attention is required to avoid inadvertent flex on the wire while inserting. Keeping the drill and wire in line with the direction of advancement is important. An overlong length of wire between the hand and the drill will introduce whip and a tendency to bend the wire. As always, theater setup is important to reduce fatigue. It is more difficult to insert a wire back toward yourself starting from the opposite side of the table. It is therefore important to plan the direction of your wire using the preoperative X-ray before starting the procedure, so you can sit on the optimal side of the hand table and have the image intensifier and screen in the correct position.

If the direction of the wire is not perfect, do not try and adjust it by angling on the wire. It is best to back the wire out to the cortex and then reposition the wire. This prevents repeated passes of the wire through the previous track that has been created. Remember also that wires become blunt; it may be preferable to discard a wire and use a fresh one if the bone is hard.

Once the K-wire is engaged with the far cortex, care should be taken not to protrude the tip beyond the cortex as this will help maintain position and prevent migration of the wire. Occasionally, it is better for the wire to run across the bone and sit out through the skin on the opposite side of insertion, so that the wire is in a more

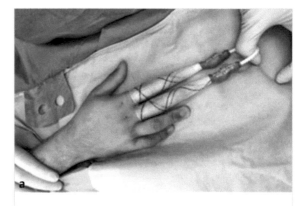

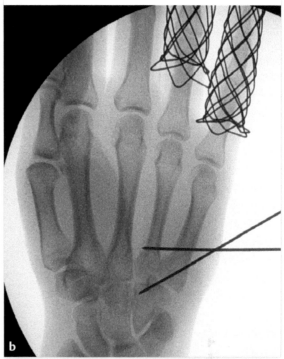

Fig. 4.6 (a) Chinese finger traps to apply traction and protect fingers from irradiation. By coning in the image intensifier field, the surgeon's fingers can be kept out of the beam. (b) Similar with metal finger traps.

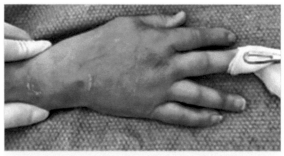

Fig. 4.7 Sponge holder and gauze for more distal fractures.

convenient place. Once the wires have been inserted, fracture reduction and finger alignment can be assessed. We use the tenodesis technique to assess finger rotation both in extension and flexion.

Wires need to be bent (retroflexed) and cut allowing for adequate space between the wire end and the skin so as not to cause skin maceration or pressure, which may facilitate pin site infection. There are various techniques of applying pin protectors or beads to keep the cut end of the wire safe.[21]

Following this, a plaster slab is applied taking care to cover the wires but leaving free as many joints as possible. The plaster is changed to a splint after 3 days. We usually remove the wires at 4 weeks to minimize the chance of infection. If a patient develops a pin track infection, the site needs to be cleaned daily and oral antibiotics commenced. If wires need to be in place for longer than 4 weeks, such as in the carpus, then they are buried. All patients are reviewed in our dressing clinic within the week and directed physiotherapy started to obviate any joint stiffness.

4.2.5 Published Studies on Use of K-wires in Carpus and Hand

Carpal Fractures

Improvements in small headless compression screw design have seen the K-wire being largely replaced for isolated fractures of the carpal bones, particularly in the scaphoid. Advantages of screw fixation include the compression achieved at the fracture site,

no potentially exposed metalwork and early mobilization resulting in less stiffness. Multiple percutaneous wires can be used as an alternative to screw fixation (which is a relatively large implant load) for scaphoid nonunion (▶ Fig. 4.8).

However, K-wires still have a place in the management of fracture/ligament dislocations of the carpus, being particularly useful in perilunate injury pattern.[22] Typically, wires can be introduced from scaphoid into lunate and scaphoid into capitate to stabilize the carpus in this complex injury. We use 1.25-mm wires, taking care to dissect on to the bone before proceeding to wire (▶ Fig. 4.9). Stiffness is a recognized sequalae of this injury and K-wire immobilization does not help obviate this.

Bennett's Fracture

For fractures at the base of the first metacarpal involving less than 20% of the articular process, closed reduction and percutaneous pinning have been found to give good long-term outcomes equal to those of open reduction and internal fixation.[23] However, this is predicated on achieving an articular step-off of less than 1 mm. Reduction can be achieved by applying traction on the thumb in pronation and adduction. The first wire can be passed from metacarpal into the trapezium and the second wire from first metacarpal into the second.[24] If a good reduction of the articular surface is not possible, then open reduction should be performed. Where a fragment is too small to accept a screw, K-wires can still be used to reduce and hold the fracture (▶ Fig. 4.10).

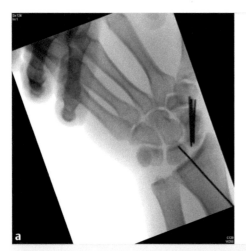
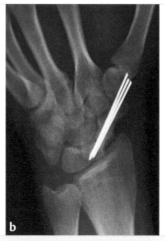
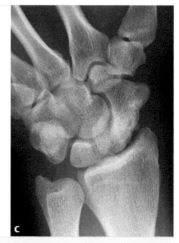

Fig. 4.8 (a–c) K-wires for stabilization after grafting for scaphoid nonunion. (These images are provided courtesy of Dr. Clara Wong.)

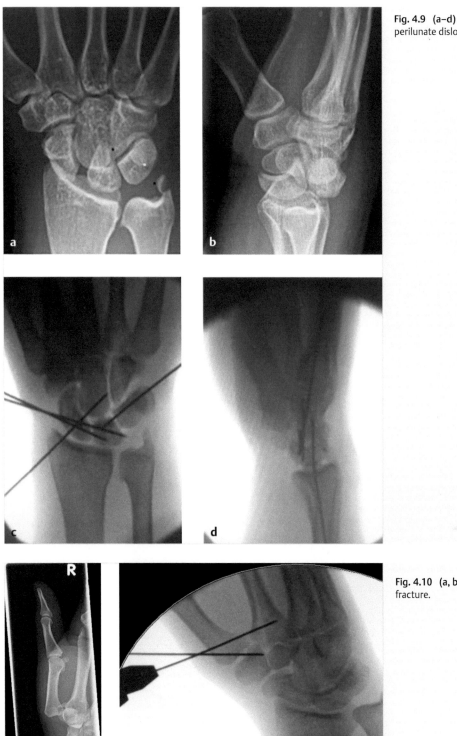

Fig. 4.9 (a–d) Use of K-wires in perilunate dislocation of the wrist.

Fig. 4.10 (a, b) K-wiring for Bennett's fracture.

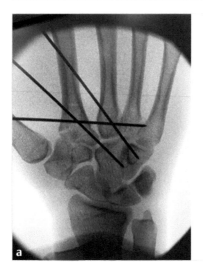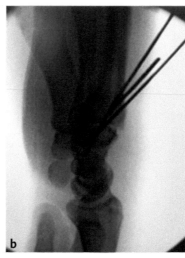

Fig. 4.11 (a, b) K-wire fixation of multiple metacarpal base fractures.

Metacarpal Shaft Fractures

K-wires can be used in nearly all shaft fractures, whether the pattern is transverse, oblique, spiral, or comminuted. Wires can be placed transversely, thereby using neighboring metacarpals to splint the fracture,[25] two distal wires and one proximal wire is the usual combination. Care must be taken not to distract the fracture. Wires are particularly useful for base of metacarpal and carpometacarpal joint dislocation (▶ Fig. 4.11).

A crossed K-wire combination is also popular; it can be technically demanding to have the wires cross at the fracture site and vigilance is required to keep extensor tendons and the MCP joint free from impalement.

Intramedullary, K-wire fixation, using multiple prebent wires (0.8 or 0.9 mm) may provide internal three-point fixation, thereby controlling rotation. Wires are introduced antegrade from the base of the metacarpal, via a small hole fashioned using an awl.[26] An advantage of this technique is that the wires may be left in the bone, obviating the need for a second procedure.

Metacarpal Neck Fractures

A nonrandomized comparison between percutaneous transverse K-wire and intramedullary K-wire for fractures of the neck of the little finger metacarpal showed no difference in outcomes.[27] It was noted that the potential complication of the transverse configuration of tethering of the sagittal bands of the extensor mechanism

was mitigated by maintaining distance between the metacarpals when drilling. For the intramedullary technique wire migration and metacarpal head perforation were best avoided by using the Foucher bouquet configuration allowing a three-point fixation within the metacarpal (▶ Fig. 4.12).[28]

Phalangeal Fractures

Long oblique fractures of the phalanges have been managed well with closed reduction and percutaneous midlateral K-wires perpendicular to the fracture. Green and Anderson[2,9] achieved full ROM in 18 of 22 patients in their series (▶ Fig. 4.13).[30]

Proximal Interphalangeal Joint Fracture Dislocation

de Haseth et al[31] described the use of K-wire pinning for these complex injuries. They believed this to be an effective, yet minimally invasive, and simple technique. K-wires were removed at 4 weeks (▶ Fig. 4.14).

Mallet Fracture

K-wires can also be used to hold fractures by way of buttressing the fragments. This technique is particularly useful for extension blocking of mallet finger fractures (▶ Fig. 4.15).[32,33]

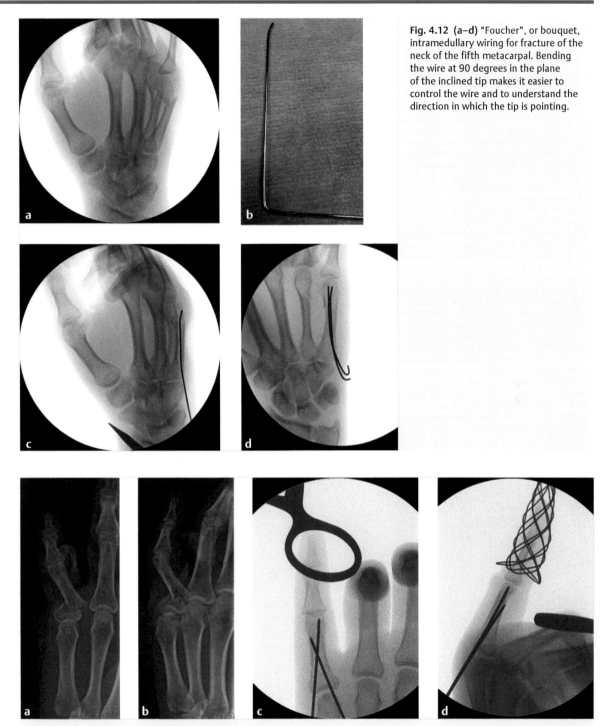

Fig. 4.12 (a–d) "Foucher", or bouquet, intramedullary wiring for fracture of the neck of the fifth metacarpal. Bending the wire at 90 degrees in the plane of the inclined tip makes it easier to control the wire and to understand the direction in which the tip is pointing.

Fig. 4.13 (a–d) Percutaneous K-wiring of a fracture of the proximal phalanx.

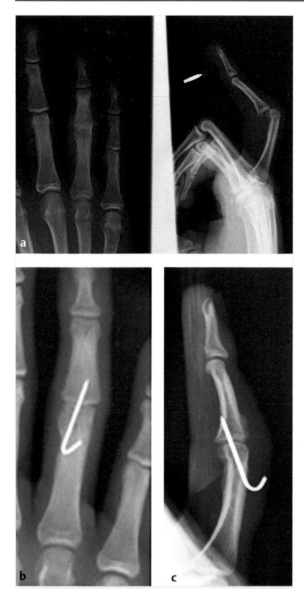

Fig. 4.14 (a–c) Simple use of K-wire to hold reduced volar PIPJ dislocation for a period of no more than 3 weeks. Full range of motion was achieved at 6 weeks.

4.2.6 Complications

As with all surgical treatments, K-wire fixation has the potential for complications. These include wire breakage, osteonecrosis, and wire track infection (▶Fig. 4.16), loss of fixation (▶Fig. 4.17), migration, fracture nonunion, fracture malunion, and nerve injury.

K-wire placement can tether the extensor apparatus and therefore also limit joint flexion.[34] Care needs to be taken to keep wires remote from the extensor tendons. Sparing of the finger joints is also important when wiring metacarpal and phalangeal fractures. In Al-Qattan's series of 35 patients with unstable transverse proximal phalangeal fractures, joint movement was significantly improved when not wiring the joint as compared to his previous study.[35]

K-wires create a potential pathway for bacterial infection through the skin and into the bone. An incidence of 7% was established in a retrospective review of 1,213 patients.[36] Although in their study Stahl and Schwartz[37] did not find a difference in infection rate between buried and exposed wires, it is generally accepted that leaving wires exposed for more than 4 weeks carries risk of infection and so if a longer duration is required, then wires should be buried. The use of K-wires in digital fractures that are comminuted and unstable whereby additional splint immobilization is offered may result in joint stiffness and tendon adhesions.[38]

4.2.7 Summary

The management of hand fractures is complex and requires skill and thought to achieve optimum results. Having a mastery of multiple treatment techniques will help the surgeon match the operation to the fracture and the patient. We consider that intraosseous wiring and K-wiring, while long established, retain a valuable place alongside plate and screw fixation. However, their use should command the same skill, concentration, and attention to detail as any other form of treatment in order to avoid complications.

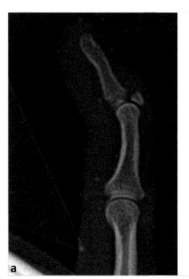
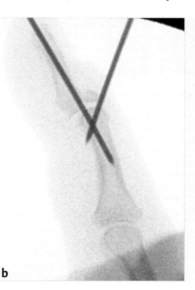

Fig. 4.15 (a, b) Extension block wiring for mallet fracture.

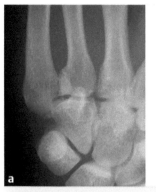
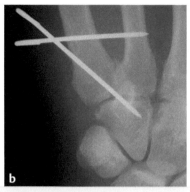
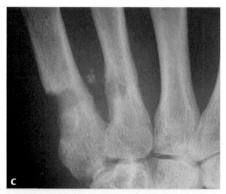

Fig. 4.16 (a–c) Complications: Osteomyelitis following K-wire fixation of a fracture of the proximal end of the fifth metacarpal (reverse Bennet's fracture).

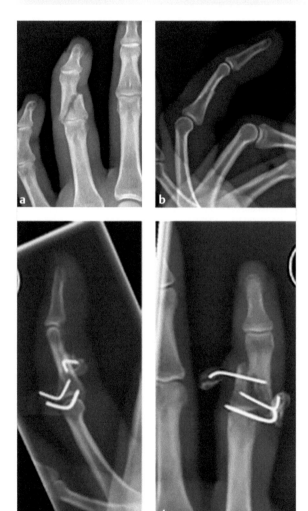

References

[1] Lister G. Intraosseous wiring of the digital skeleton. J Hand Surg Am. 1978; 3(5):427–435

[2] Thomas BP, Sreekanth R, Pallapati SC. Open proximal phalangeal shaft fractures of the hand treated by theta fixation. Indian J Orthop. 2015; 49(3):312–316

[3] Gingrass RP, Fehring B, Matloub H. Intraosseous wiring of complex hand fractures. Plast Reconstr Surg. 1980; 66(3):383–394

[4] Gropper PT, Bowen V. Cerclage wiring of metacarpal fractures. Clin Orthop Relat Res. 1984(188):203–207

[5] Al-Qattan MM. Metacarpal shaft fractures of the fingers: treatment with interosseous loop wire fixation and immediate postoperative finger mobilisation in a wrist splint. J Hand Surg [Br]. 2006; 31(4):377–382

[6] Al-Qattan MM, Al-Lazzam A. Long oblique/spiral mid-shaft metacarpal fractures of the fingers: treatment with cerclage wire fixation and immediate postoperative finger mobilisation in a wrist splint. J Hand Surg Eur Vol. 2007; 32(6):637–640

[7] Al-Qattan MM, Al-Zahrani K. Open reduction and cerclage wire fixation for long oblique/spiral fractures of the proximal phalanx of the fingers. J Hand Surg Eur Vol. 2008; 33(2):170–173

[8] Firoozbakhsh KK, Moneim MS, Howey T, Castaneda E, Pirela-Cruz MA. Comparative fatigue strengths and stabilities of metacarpal internal fixation techniques. J Hand Surg Am. 1993; 18(6):1059–1068

[9] Matloub HS, Jensen PL, Sanger JR, Grunert BK, Yousif NJ. Spiral fracture fixation techniques. A biomechanical study. J Hand Surg [Br]. 1993; 18(4):515–519

[10] Prevel CD, Morgan R, Molnar J, Eppley BL, Moore K. Biomechanical testing of titanium self-tapping versus pretapped lag screw fixation of spiral metacarpal fractures. Ann Plast Surg. 1996; 37(1):34–40

[11] Al-Qattan MM. Closed reduction and percutaneous K-wires versus open reduction and interosseous loop wires for displaced unstable transverse fractures of the shaft of the proximal phalanx of the fingers in industrial workers. J Hand Surg Eur Vol. 2008; 33(5):552–556

[12] Weiss AP. Cerclage fixation for fracture dislocation of the proximal interphalangeal joint. Clin Orthop Relat Res. 1996(327):21–28

[13] Aladin A, Davis TR. Dorsal fracture-dislocation of the proximal interphalangeal joint: a comparative study of percutaneous Kirschner wire fixation versus open reduction and internal fixation. J Hand Surg [Br]. 2005; 30(2):120–128

Fig. 4.17 (a–d) Complications: K-wires are not infallible and need to be inserted with care and thought. This fracture in a young patient referred from another center fell apart within 2 weeks of surgery.

[14] Huber W. Historical remarks on Martin Kirschner and the development of the Kirschner (K)-wire. Indian J Plast Surg. 2008; 41(1):89–92

[15] Harasen G. Orthopedic hardware and equipment for the beginner: part 1: pins and wires. Can Vet J. 2011; 52(9):1025–1026

[16] Namba RS, Kabo JM, Meals RA. Biomechanical effects of point configuration in Kirschner-wire fixation. Clin Orthop Relat Res. 1987(214):19–22

[17] Piska M, Yang L, Reed M, Saleh M. Drilling efficiency and temperature elevation of Kirschner-wire point. J Bone Joint Surg Br. 2002; 84(1):137–140

[18] Gulati A, Dixit A, Williamson DM. The role of prophylactic antibiotics for percutaneous procedures in orthopaedic surgery surg science. 2011; 2:248–352

[19] Anderson SR, Inceoglu S, Wongworawat MD. Temperature rise in Kirschner wires inserted using two drilling methods: forward and oscillation. Hand (NY). 2017:1558944717708052

[20] Franssen BBGM, Schuurman AH, Mink Van Der Molen AB, Kon M. Hammering versus drilling of sharp and obtuse trocar-point k-wires. J Hand Surg Eur Vol. 2009; 34(2):215–218

[21] Vishwanath G. Managing the cut end of a K wire. Indian J Plast Surg. 2010; 43(1):117–118

[22] Herzberg G, Forissier D. Acute dorsal trans-scaphoid perilunate fracture-dislocations: medium-term results. J Hand Surg [Br]. 2002; 27(6):498–502

[23] Lutz M, Sailer R, Zimmermann R, Gabl M, Ulmer H, Pechlaner S. Closed reduction transarticular Kirschner wire fixation versus open reduction internal fixation in the treatment of Bennett's fracture dislocation. J Hand Surg [Br]. 2003; 28(2):142–147

[24] van Niekerk JL, Ouwens R. Fractures of the base of the first metacarpal bone: results of surgical treatment. Injury. 1989; 20(6):359–362

[25] Galanakis I, Aligizakis A, Katonis P, Papadokostakis G, Stergiopoulos K, Hadjipavlou A. Treatment of closed unstable metacarpal fractures using percutaneous transverse fixation with Kirschner wires. J Trauma. 2003; 55(3):509–513

[26] Faraj AA, Davis TR. Percutaneous intramedullary fixation of metacarpal shaft fractures. J Hand Surg [Br]. 1999; 24(1):76–79

[27] Wong TC, Ip FK, Yeung SH. Comparison between percutaneous transverse fixation and intramedullary K-wires in treating closed fractures of the metacarpal neck of the little finger. J Hand Surg [Br]. 2006; 31(1):61–65

[28] Foucher G. "Bouquet" osteosynthesis in metacarpal neck fractures: a series of 66 patients. J Hand Surg Am. 1995; 20(3 pt 2):S86–S90

[29] Green DP, Anderson JR. Closed reduction and percutaneous pin fixation of fractured phalanges. J Bone Joint Surg Am. 1973; 55(8):1651–1654

[30] Greene TL, Noellert RC, Belsole RJ, Simpson LA. Composite wiring of metacarpal and phalangeal fractures. J Hand Surg Am. 1989; 14(4):665–669

[31] de Haseth KB, Neuhaus V, Mudgal CS. Dorsal fracture-dislocations of the proximal interphalangeal joint: evaluation of closed reduction and percutaneous Kirschner wire pinning. Hand (NY). 2015; 10(1):88–93

[32] Darder-Prats A, Fernández-García E, Fernández-Gabarda R, Darder-García A. Treatment of mallet finger fractures by the extension-block K-wire technique. J Hand Surg [Br]. 1998; 23(6):802–805

[33] Chung DW, Lee JH. Anatomic reduction of mallet fractures using extension block and additional intrafocal pinning techniques. Clin Orthop Surg. 2012; 4(1):72–76

[34] Sela Y, Peterson C, Baratz ME. Tethering the extensor apparatus limits PIP flexion following K-wire placement for pinning extra-articular fractures at the base of the proximal phalanx. Hand (NY). 2016; 11(4):433–437

[35] Al-Qattan MM. Displaced unstable transverse fractures of the shaft of the proximal phalanx of the fingers in industrial workers: reduction and K-wire fixation leaving the metacarpophalangeal and proximal interphalangeal joints free. J Hand Surg Eur Vol. 2011; 36(7):577–583

[36] van Leeuwen WF, van Hoorn BT, Chen N, Ring D. Kirschner wire pin site infection in hand and wrist fractures: incidence rate and risk factors. J Hand Surg Eur Vol. 2016; 41(9):990–994

[37] Stahl S, Schwartz O. Complications of K-wire fixation of fractures and dislocations in the hand and wrist. Arch Orthop Trauma Surg. 2001; 121(9):527–530

[38] Pun WK, Chow SP, So YC, et al. A prospective study on 284 digital fractures of the hand. J Hand Surg Am. 1989; 14(3):474–481

5 Intramedullary Screw Fixation of the Metacarpals and Phalanges of the Hand

Maurizio Calcagni, Lisa Reissner, Christoph Erling, Thomas Giesen

Abstract

The development of headless compression screws in the 1980s opened new possibilities for the internal fixation of carpal bones, rapidly becoming the standard. In fingers and metacarpals, their use was limited for a long time to the arthrodesis of the distal interphalangeal (DIP) joint or for the treatment of phalanges nonunion. The first reports were published about the fixation of transverse fresh fractures treated with intramedullary headless screws only after 2010. The technique is therefore relatively recent and not refined enough to give absolute indications. Ideally, the fracture should be transversal and with minimal comminution, although in some cases the intramedullary screw can also be used as strut to restore axis and length of the bone. The procedure is based on a few steps that must be adapted to the different anatomical sites: closed reduction of the fracture, insertion of an axial guidewire, and fixation with a compression headless screw, with or without predrilling. In the published case series, the results are very good in terms of bone healing and range of motion. The area of damaged articular surface was calculated by several papers with different methods, with results varying between 4 and 20% depending on the involved joint and the size of the screw.

Intramedullary screw fixation of metacarpal and phalangeal fractures is a relatively new technique with good reproducible results and low complication rate.

Keywords: intramedullary screw, osteosynthesis, hand fractures, headless screws

5.1 Introduction

The treatment of hand fractures has been debated for a very long time, often with diverging opinions among surgeons about conservative treatment versus surgical fixation for the same pattern of hand fracture. The use of casts or splints might reduce hardware associated complications, but sometimes it does not allow for true early rehabilitation and can cause stiffness and therefore prolonged sick leave. In hand fractures, the use of osteosynthesis material applied on the outer surface of the bone or protruding through the skin is associated with a high rate of complications.[1,2] Some of the described complications are those related to surgery such as infection, iatrogenic nerve lesions or malposition, but most complications are related to the fixation material itself: allergic reactions, pin tract infections, tendon adhesions, joint stiffness, and hardware intolerance are the most common.

The hand is very sensitive to the volume of the inserted hardware as the hand bones are in the vicinity of gliding structures; tendons, ligaments, intrinsic muscles, and nerves that during healing time can become tethered with surgical scars and/or plates and screws. The evolution of materials and manufacturing techniques contributed greatly to the reduction of those problems; modern plates are made of titanium with higher tissue compatibility, have a lower profile, and screws no longer have any sharp edges, reducing volume-associated complications. Nevertheless, hardware placed on the outer surface of the bones of the hand often needs to be removed and the aforementioned structures released from the scar, leading the patient to a second operation with the potential of new complications.

In the 1930s, the use of the intramedullary nail was popularized in Germany for the lower extremities with a high rate of success, starting the development of this kind of osteosynthesis. Kirschner wires (K-wires), percutaneous and not, were widely used intramedullary for finger and metacarpal fractures, but still had some complications and limitations.

Looking for a better intramedullary fixation, in 1977, Foucher[3] presented the bilboquet technique which is probably the first example of a stable intramedullary fixation in the phalanx of the hand. For the bilboquet technique, special intramedullary pins were used, and sometimes they were also cemented. Later the wires were modified in different fashions: with or without a thread or with a small hole for locking, in the case of phalangeal fractures. Unfortunately, this new material was difficult to use and never had much success.

Later, the headless compression screw was introduced for the treatment of scaphoid fractures,[4] adding the feature of compression to the intramedullary position of the hardware. Despite their rapid success for the carpal bones, this concept was only recently also extended to the treatment of metacarpals and phalanges.

The first use of headless compression screws in the fingers was limited to the arthrodesis of the DIP joint[5] or for the treatment of phalanges nonunion.[6] The limitation of the use of the first generation of headless screws was the need for an external jig for drilling and compression.

In the next generations, headless screws were cannulated for a guidewire, for much easier insertion. As a last evolution, the screws were manufactured by different brands as self-drilling and self-tapping, reducing the need for drilling before insertion of the screw and further simplifying the surgical procedure and reducing the needed exposure.

In 2010, the first case report of a transverse fresh fracture treated with an intramedullary cannulated headless screw was published.[6] Ruchelsman et al[7] presented the first clinical case series after a theoretical work on the volume needed by the screw head and on the area of damaged cartilage surface.[8] This paper was followed by few others[9-11] presenting more cases, although with short follow-up.

5.2 Indications

The technique is relatively recent and not refined enough to give absolute indications. Ideally, the fracture should be transversal and with minimal comminution, even though in some cases the intramedullary screw can also be used as a strut to restore axis and length of the bone. In comminuted metacarpal fractures, the use of two converging screws in order to lock the compression has been proposed.[9]

There is no data about the maximal acceptable angle of the fracture line that is amenable to this type of osteosynthesis, but we do not recommend fixing true oblique or spiral fractures. As a rule of thumb, we switch to lag screw fixation when at least two can be safely placed.

Both bone fragments must be big enough to accommodate the threaded heads without impinging the fracture line and preventing compression.

5.3 Surgical Technique

The procedure is based on a few steps that are common among the different anatomical sites.

Before surgery, it is mandatory to measure the width of the medullary canal in the two planes to choose the appropriate screw size. The canal is not symmetrical and the lateral view is the one to consider for accurate measurements. Normally, the distal head of the screw will lie at the isthmus, the narrowest point of the medullary canal, and this value is the one to consider. The choice is usually between 2.2 and 3 mm, but it might be different according to the brand of screw being used by the surgeon. For distal phalanx fractures, some brands do not provide a screw small enough.

For metacarpals, they might sometimes have a diameter of 4 mm or more, and a larger screw might be necessary. Nevertheless in such cases of large intramedullary canal, a smaller screw will work as an elastic fixation (▶Fig. 5.1).

The fracture is reduced under the fluoroscope and the skin is incised by 2 to 4 mm depending on the size of the planned screw, in a site that will allow for central placing in the medullary canal of the guidewire. The site of introduction varies between different bones as described below. The wire is then drilled across the fracture line. After controlling the proper position of the wire in both planes, the screw is advanced (in most cases without predrilling if the screw allows it) for optimal compression. The head must be accurately countersunk in the subchondral bone to avoid secondary joint damage.

The length of the screw is calculated on the X-rays before surgery in order to spare time during the procedure. Compression is achieved by advancing the screw, therefore, when treating short bones or fractures near to a joint, a few millimeters should be detracted from the length in order to avoid protrusion of the screw into the joint space.

There are no data about the superiority of one brand over the others, as long as the screws have particular

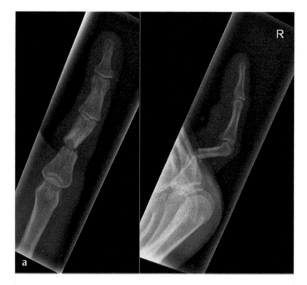

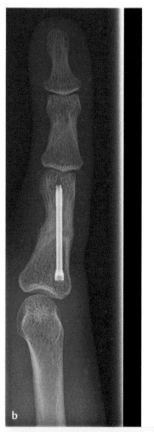
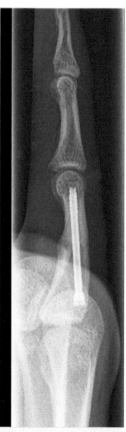

Fig. 5.1 (a, b) Displaced shaft fracture of the proximal phalanx treated with an anterograde intramedullary screw with the intra-articular technique.

characteristics. In our experience, the screw must be cannulated to allow percutaneous fixation and the different pitch of the threads should be enough to achieve good compression without the need for external devices like compression-jigs or broad-head screwdrivers. The diameter of the screwdriver itself is also very important, because it must be of the same size or even smaller than the screw itself to avoid greater damage to the bone and cartilage at the insertion site.

Each bone requires an adaptation of this basic technique, especially the placement of the skin incision, to achieve optimal results.

5.3.1 Distal Phalanx

The skin incision is placed at the hyponychium and the bone tuft exposed. The wire is placed in a central position and the screw advanced. It is very important to manually compress the fracture before crossing it with the screw since there is very little space for advancing the screw to achieve compression. The screw must be long enough but not too long in order to avoid perforation of the DIP joint.[12] The distal phalanx is very small and only the 2.2 mm or smaller screws fit in the bone.[13,14]

5.3.2 Middle Phalanx

There are two approaches: through the DIP joint in a retrograde manner and through the proximal interphalangeal

(PIP) joint in an anterograde fashion. We prefer the retrograde approach in case of open fractures where the DIP joint is already exposed, or distal fractures of the P2, head and neck for example.

In these cases, the DIP joint is flexed and the fracture reduced. A 2-mm skin incision is made at the DIP joint and through the extensor tendon. Under fluoroscopic control, a guidewire is advanced through the head of the middle phalanx across the fracture into the proximal fragment. The wire should be as central as possible to prevent secondary dislocation during positioning of the screw. This can be difficult in stiff joints when flexion of the DIP is limited. The length of the screw is then determined on the X-ray or directly with the dedicated instrument. The screw must be long enough, but not too long in order to avoid perforation of the PIP joint. The screw is finally advanced until a good compression is achieved and the second thread is in a subchondral position.

In shaft fractures, we insert the screw through the PIP joint. The PIP joint is flexed as much as possible and the wire is inserted from the dorsal aspect of the distal proximal phalanx (▶Fig. 5.2).

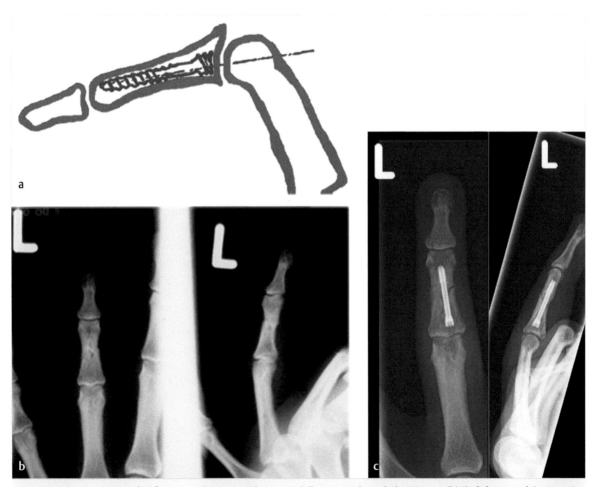

Fig. 5.2 (a) Management of P2 fracture with anterograde intramedullary screw through the PIP joint. **(b)** Shaft fracture of the P2 with a rotational deformity, treated with an anterograde screw **(c)**.

Then the screw is advanced along the wire without predrilling and the fracture fixed.

5.3.3 Proximal Phalanx

For this bone, there are two possible approaches.

Intra-articular Approach

At the dorsal side of the metacarpophalangeal (MP) joint, a 2- to 3-mm incision is made through the skin and the extensor hood. Under fluoroscopic control, a guidewire of appropriate size is then centrally inserted from dorsal into the base of the proximal phalanx along the longitudinal axis through the MP joint held in about 60 degrees of flexion. To facilitate the intra-articular insertion of the wire, the base of the proximal phalanx can be gently pushed dorsal manually. Afterward, a cannulated headless compression screw of appropriate length is inserted with a cannulated screwdriver without predrilling, until the screw head is fully underneath the cartilage level. In some cases, when the fracture is slightly oblique, the insertion point can be eccentric making the positioning of the wire less difficult (▶ Fig. 5.3).

Transmetacarpal Approach

A small skin incision is placed slightly proximal to the metacarpal head.[10,11] The extensor hood is also incised, and under fluoroscopic control, a guidewire adapted to the selected screw is centrally inserted from dorsal in an anterograde direction, through the metacarpal head. The MP joint is held in flexion and the fracture is reduced and aligned with the wire. This is placed in the proximal phalanx across the fracture line. The screw is then advanced through the metacarpal head until the trailing end is fully underneath the cartilage of the phalanx base. In this case, the size of the screwdriver is crucial to avoid damage to the MP joint and it must be the same size of the screw or smaller. Manipulation should be very careful until complete removal of the wire to avoid bending or breakage.

5.3.4 Distal Approach from the PIP Joint

As described by del Piñal et al,[9] a retrograde technique is possibly easy to perform and in our practice the best solution for fracture to the distal third of the proximal phalanx.

5.3.5 Metacarpals

Stab incision distal to the MP joint through the extensor hood. The fracture is reduced under fluoroscopic control and a guidewire of the proper size is drilled. The screw is then advanced across the fracture line. The length of the screw should have good purchase at the isthmus

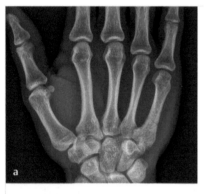
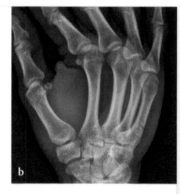
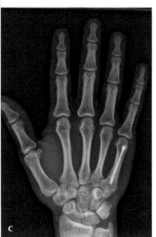
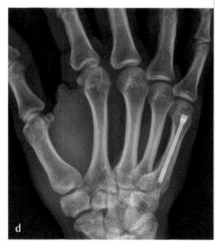

Fig. 5.3 (a, b) Refracture of a fifth metacarpal shortly after plate removal. Fixation with retrograde intramedullary screw (c, d). The patient was immediately mobilized after surgery.

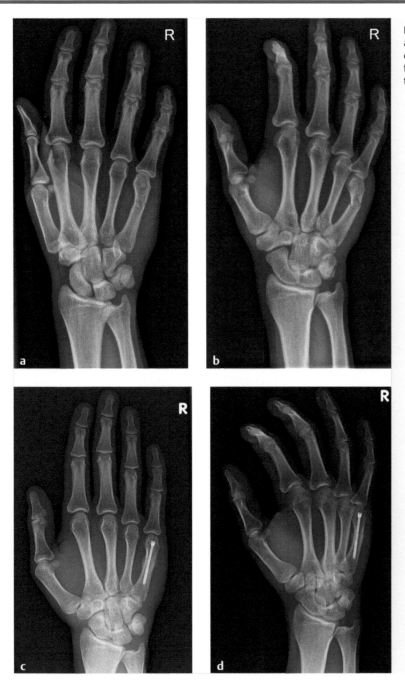

Fig. 5.4 (a–d) Intramedullary fixation of a large metacarpal with screw. Note the evident callus due to the merely elastic fixation with no compression provided by the screw.

of the bone to ensure optimal compression (▶ Fig. 5.4). In the case of comminution, compression should be avoided and the screw will just secure the axis of the bone, functioning as a strut. del Piñal et al[9] also proposed the use of a second converging screw creating a "Y-shaped" fixation that cannot collapse with shortening of the segment.

5.3.6 Postoperative Treatment

For finger fractures, an active motion protocol is initiated with buddy taping to the adjacent healthy finger. At night, a rest splint in extension is applied to prevent PIP contracture. Distal phalanx fractures are protected for 4 weeks to avoid striking the finger during activity, but active exercises are started immediately.

In metacarpal fractures, a brace (with wrist and MP joints free) and buddy taping to the adjacent finger are applied. Mobilization is started immediately. After 4 to 6 weeks, unprotected load is allowed depending on clinical and X-ray judgment.

Additional care is necessary when the compression achieved intraoperatively is insufficient. In these cases, mobilization can be delayed and tenodesis exercises initiated immediately.

5.4 Results

In the published case series,[7,9–11] the results are very good in terms of bone healing and range of motion. More than 90% of the patients healed uneventfully. In some cases, with a large intramedullary canal diameter a hypertrophic callus was observed, but no nonunion was reported.

The percentage of damaged articular surface was calculated with different approaches and in different locations, making a comparison impossible. A computed tomography (CT) scan simulation study[8] of the metacarpal head showed that the area of cartilage surface damaged by the screw head ranged from 4 to 12%, depending on the diameter of the screw. del Piñal[9] analyzed the head of the proximal phalanx and reports about 13 to 22% of damaged area. Borbas et al[15] performed a cadaver study on the damaged articular surface of the base of the proximal phalanx and reported values of 4.5% with the 2.2-mm screws and 8.3% with the 3-mm screws. All these measurements demonstrate very limited chondral damage. Moreover, the position of the screw is central in the phalanx heads, between the condyles, where the load is reduced.[16] At the metacarpal head, the insertion of the screw is in a dorsal eccentric position in the axis of the medullary canal where the load is minimal.[8]

5.5 Complications

The complications reported were minimal and mainly related to concomitant soft tissue involvement. Giesen et al[10] report an average extension-lag of 2 degrees at the MP joint and of 8 degrees at the PIP joint (depending on the treated segment). No other complications were reported.

Removal of the screw was needed in an extremely low percentage of cases (1.5–3%) where an intra-articular protrusion was observed. Shortening of the bone was also produced in the case of major comminution. Intraoperative complications that led to a different fixation are also reported (breakage of the screw or lack of compression).

All published series have a limited follow-up, thus leaving unanswered the question about osteoarthritis at the insertion site, particularly if a transmetacarpal approach is chosen. There is only one article about a very similar condition[17] where the scaphoid is fixed through the trapezium. In this study, only two (5.4%) cases of symptomatic scaphotrapeziotrapezoidal (STT) joint osteoarthritis were observed.

5.6 Conclusions

The intramedullary screw fixation of metacarpal and phalangeal fractures is a new technique with good, reproducible results and low complication rate. In our unit, it is the standard for finger and metacarpal fractures with small comminution. The ideal indications are transverse or short oblique fractures with minimal comminution. As a rule, when the fracture is oblique enough for lag screw fixation, then this is the technique of choice. A learning curve is necessary to select proper indications and to avoid some problems that can jeopardize the functional result. Particularly important is the choice of screw diameter to accommodate the medullary canal and achieve adequate compression.

Complication rate is low, but only longer follow-up studies and comparison with other fixation techniques will allow for a better definition of indications and limitations.

References

[1] Fusetti C, Meyer H, Borisch N, Stern R, Santa DD, Papaloïzos M. Complications of plate fixation in metacarpal fractures. J Trauma. 2002; 52(3):535–539

[2] Page SM, Stern PJ. Complications and range of motion following plate fixation of metacarpal and phalangeal fractures. J Hand Surg Am. 1998; 23(5):827–832

[3] Foucher G, Merle M, Michon J. [Internal fixation in the stabilisation of fractures of the metacarpus and phalanges (author's transl)] Ann Chir. 1977; 31(12):1065–1069

[4] Herbert TJ, Fisher WE. Management of the fractured scaphoid using a new bone screw. J Bone Joint Surg Br. 1984; 66(1):114–123

[5] Faithfull DK, Herbert TJ. Small joint fusions of the hand using the Herbert bone screw. J Hand Surg [Br]. 1984; 9(2):167–168

[6] Boulton CL, Salzler M, Mudgal CS. Intramedullary cannulated headless screw fixation of a comminuted subcapital metacarpal fracture: case report. J Hand Surg Am. 2010; 35(8):1260–1263

[7] Ruchelsman DE, Puri S, Feinberg-Zadek N, Leibman MI, Belsky MR. Clinical outcomes of limited-open retrograde intramedullary headless screw fixation of metacarpal fractures. J Hand Surg Am. 2014; 39(12):2390–2395

[8] ten Berg PW, Mudgal CS, Leibman MI, Belsky MR, Ruchelsman DE. Quantitative 3-dimensional CT analyses of intramedullary headless screw fixation for metacarpal neck fractures. J Hand Surg Am. 2013; 38(2):322–330.e2

[9] del Piñal F, Moraleda E, Rúas JS, de Piero GH, Cerezal L. Minimally invasive fixation of fractures of the phalanges and metacarpals with intramedullary cannulated headless compression screws. J Hand Surg Am. 2015; 40(4):692–700

[10] Giesen T, Gazzola R, Poggetti A, Giovanoli P, Calcagni M. Intramedullary headless screw fixation for fractures of the proximal and middle phalanges in the digits of the hand: a review of 31 consecutive fractures. J Hand Surg Eur Vol. 2016; 41(7):688–694

[11] Itadera E, Yamazaki T. Trans-metacarpal Screw Fixation for Extra-articular Proximal Phalangeal Base Fractures. J Hand Surg Asian Pac Vol. 2017; 22(1):35–38

[12] Henry M. Variable pitch headless compression screw treatment of distal phalangeal nonunions. Tech Hand Up Extrem Surg. 2010; 14(4):230–233

[13] Mintalucci D, Lutsky KF, Matzon JL, Rivlin M, Niver G, Beredjiklian PK. Distal interphalangeal joint bony dimensions related to headless compression screw sizes. J Hand Surg Am. 2014; 39(6):1068–74.e1

[14] Wang WL, Darke M, Goitz RJ, Andrews CL, Fowler JR. A comparison of plain radiographs and computed tomography for determining canal diameter of the distal phalanx. J Hand Surg Am. 2015; 40(7):1404–1409.e1

[15] Borbas P, Dreu M, Poggetti A, Calcagni M, Giesen T. Treatment of proximal phalangeal fractures with an antegrade intramedullary screw: a cadaver study. J Hand Surg Eur Vol. 2016; 41(7):683–687

[16] Weiss AP. Intramedullary Herbert screws for treatment of phalangeal nonunion. Tech Hand Up Extrem Surg. 1997; 1(1):41–47

[17] Geurts G, van Riet R, Meermans G, Verstreken F. Incidence of scaphotrapezial arthritis following volar percutaneous fixation of nondisplaced scaphoid waist fractures using a transtrapezial approach. J Hand Surg Am. 2011; 36(11):1753–1758

6 Plate and Screw Fixation of Hand and Carpal Fractures

Philippe Cuénod

Abstract

Plates and screws allow fixation of carpal and hand fractures in a rigid fashion to allow early mobilization. Described in the early 20th century, the technique has developed to allow nowadays to treat all kinds of fractures with good results. It, however, requires a precise technique, is more demanding than other methods, and yields risks of complications. It is essential to bear in mind that this option is only one of the possibilities to treat fractures, mostly when they cannot be treated conservatively or by less invasive techniques. The general principles of screw and plate fixation are exposed. The main indications and techniques are discussed, with the help of clinical cases.

Keywords: hand fracture, carpal fracture, plate and screw fixation, osteosynthesis, internal fixation

6.1 Introduction and Historical Perspective

Open reduction with plate and screws fixation has become a standard technique in the management of hand and carpal fractures. It requires a good knowledge of bone healing biology, implants, indications and surgical technique, as well as potential complications. This chapter exposes the general principles of osteosynthesis, as coined by Lambotte in 1907[1] and their clinical applications.

The natural healing of a fractured bone occurs through the formation of a callus secondary to interfragmentary movements, the so-called indirect bone healing. Lucas-Championnière in 1895 advised movements rather than immobilization for fracture healing and functional recovery.[2]

When the fracture is absolutely stable, for example, by screw and plate fixation, the consolidation of the bone takes place without any external callus formation but, instead, by direct osteonal remodelling.[3,4]

Hansmann in Germany is credited of the first fracture treatment with a plate in 1886. After he had advocated conservative treatment, Perkins from England in 1940 also started to fix the fractures to allow early mobilization.[2] In 1949, Robert Danis from Belgium, exposed his theory of osteosynthesis: the fracture should be rigidly stabilized to allow early motion and rehabilitation.[5] He called the healing of the bone without external callus formation, "soudure autogène" (autogenous welding).[5]

Further development of internal fixation was subsequently based on experimental and clinical studies conducted by the AO foundation (Arbeitsgemeinschaft für Osteosynthesefragen), created in 1958 by Swiss surgeons Maurice Müller, Martin Allgöwer, Robert Schneider, and Hans Willenegger.[2]

6.2 Implants and Technical Principles

6.2.1 The Plates and Their Applications

Compression at the fracture site increases the rigidity of fixation and allows direct bone healing. The dynamic compression plate (DCP) has eccentric holes with a sloping surface on the side away from the fracture. When the screw is tightened, its head moves down the slope and shifts the plate in relation to bone resulting in compression at the fracture site.[2] The plates currently available for metacarpal and phalangeal fixation have oval holes without any sloping inner surface. The compression is achieved by first drilling a hole close to the fracture line and inserting a screw engaging the far cortex but without tightening it. The plate is then pulled toward the other fragment. The first screw then occupies an eccentric load position. The second screw is then inserted as a load screw at the distalmost edge of the hole in relation to the fracture. The screws are then tightened alternately to produce the interfragmentary axial compression (▸Fig. 6.1).

To decrease the pressure on the bone surface that causes necrosis, the plates are carved on their undersurface to decrease the areas of pressure on the underlying bone without decreasing the amount of metal at any transverse section of the plate. These plates are referred as limited-contact dynamic compression plate (LC-DCP).[2]

In single-plane fracture, any strain or movement will concentrate on that plane with a risk of failure. Therefore, if it is only supported with a plate in axial compression, a gap may open at the opposite cortex due to the elasticity of the plate. This pitfall may be prevented by inserting a lag screw through the fracture plane or by prestressing the plate with an overbending, the natural tendency of the plate to return to its original shape resisting the opening of the other cortex.[2]

When the fracture is multiplanar, one must not try to achieve absolute rigid fixation that might jeopardize the blood supply. The rule is never to sacrifice the biology of the fracture site to achieve a reduction and fixation.[6] The multiple fragments are aligned and the minor residual instability between them will result in motion of relatively low amplitude, evenly distributed between fracture planes. A biological osteosynthesis is done with a plate bridging the fracture, restoring the length, the axis, the rotation, respecting the biology.[2,6] Bony fragments without bony attachment, too small or missing, can be replaced in hand fracture by bone graft and plate bridging.[6,7]

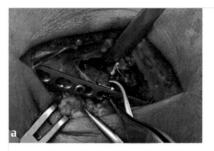
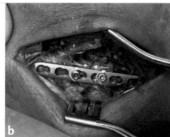
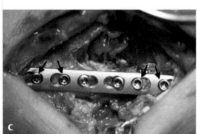

Fig. 6.1 Principle of compression plate for metacarpal and phalangeal fractures. (a) The first screw is inserted in the hole close to the fracture line, engaging the far cortex, without tightening it. The plate is pulled toward the other fragment, to bring the first screw to an eccentric load position. (b) The second screw is inserted at the distalmost edge of the hole in relation to the fracture and the screws are tightened alternatively, producing the interfragmentary axial compression. (c) The remaining screws are inserted in neutral position, or, in the locking technique in the threaded holes (*black arrows*).

The traditional technique of plate fixation to the bone surface by screws engaging both cortices create frictional forces between the plate and the bone that neutralize the destabilizing forces.[2] They are indicated when compression at the fracture site is required, in multiple ipsilateral metacarpal fractures, for nonunions that require absolute stability, in marked comminution, and for periarticular fractures.[8,9] A screw purchase decreased by poor bone quality (osteoporosis, high comminution, bone loss, metaphyseal or pathological bone) yields a risk of screw anchorage loosening and implant failure.[2,10,11] Attempts at increasing the plate-bone friction may jeopardize the fracture site and periosteal biology.[10] New concepts have therefore been developed where the screws, locked in threaded holes in the plate, create a frame with angular stability that acts as an internal–external fixator.[2,10] The plate is then no longer compressed against the bone, but "hovers" over it with a slight space between the plate and the bone that preserve periosteal blood supply.[2,4,10] The stability achieved in a locked plate system do not rely on the fixation strength of a single screw but on the sum of the strength of all screw-bone interfaces.[8,10] This locking compression plate (LCP) seems to provide more stable fixation than conventional nonlocking plates as it has been shown in multiple laboratory and clinical studies, although data are sometimes confusing.[10,11] Its use is, however, recommended for indirect fracture reduction, periarticular metacarpal and phalangeal fractures, in particular with comminution, for diaphyseal fractures with bone loss or poor quality bone, for nonunion or corrective osteotomy fixation, in severe fracture to prevent fragment devitalization, for plating where anatomical constraints prevent insertion on the tension side of the bone and for small joints fusion.[8–10] Experimentally, metacarpal fracture dorsal plate fixation with four bicortical locking screws has equivalent biomechanical properties as a plate with six bicortical nonlocking screws, thus decreasing the dissection and allowing stable plate fixation in very proximal and distal fractures.[12] It has been assumed that unicortical plate fixation could be strong enough with the advantage of decreasing the risks of damage to the volar structure such as flexor tendons, compared to the traditional bicortical fixation.[13,14] Other biomechanical studies have shown, however, that bicortical was superior in metacarpals and phalanges.[15,16] The modern locking plates can be used either with locking or conventional screws with the compression effect, owing to the double circular holes, one with a thread, the other eccentric and smooth (▶ Fig. 6.2).

In addition to straight plates, a wide range of shapes are proposed to adapt to the various patterns of fractures that can be encountered. The plates can be T- or Y-shape, with a double row or a perpendicular blade for bone anchoring.

6.2.2 Screws

The screws that are used for metacarpal and phalangeal fixation are of self-tapping cortical type. They are used either to anchor the plate or for direct bone fixation. A screw can be defined as a device composed of a central core surrounded by an helicoidal thread, that converts rotational force into linear motion causing the screw to move along the longitudinal axis of its shaft.[17] The effective thread depth of the helix purchases in the bone to promote this motion. The pitch is the height travelled by the screw with each 360-degree turn of the helix. Therefore, the shorter the distance, the finer the pitch, the longer the distance, the coarser the pitch. With a finer pitch, more turns engage in the cortex (▶ Fig. 6.3a).

When a screw is fully inserted, its head contacts the bone and resists further longitudinal motion. Therefore, more drive will create a tensile force in the core, balanced by an equal compression force at the screw head/bone interface. Countersink of the cortex beneath the screw head will increase the area of compression, decreasing the local pressure, thus the risk of bone failure. If the screw is inserted across a fracture plane with purchase in both cortices, the compression does not pass across the fracture plane, unless the reduced bone fragments are held under compression by a reduction clamp, before inserting the screw, as shown by Roth et al.[18] The technique of lag screw is, however, commonly used in order to allow compression forces to pass across the fracture plane. Owing to the small size of metacarpal and phalangeal bones, the technique of lag screw insertion may slightly differ in hand than in larger bones. After fracture reduction, the pilot hole, at a diameter slightly bigger than the core, is drilled in both cortices. To drill first, both cortices prevent the risk of axial deviation, but require a good inspection of the fragments

prior to reduction to aim correctly when the fracture is reduced. A gliding hole is then drilled in the proximal cortex at a diameter greater than the outer diameter of the screw. The hole in the near cortex is countersunk and the screw inserted with its tip protruding slightly beyond the outer cortex, in order to have a maximum of purchase in the bone. In this manner, the screw glides through the inner cortex and purchases in the outer cortex. When its head abuts against the proximal cortex, it creates a compressive force through the fracture line (▶ Fig. 6.4).

A lag screw inserted perpendicularly to the long axis of the bone will give a maximum resistance to shearing forces generated by axial loading. If the screw is inserted perpendicularly to the fracture plane, it produces a maximal interfragmentary compression. Therefore, to meet both types of stability, different options can be used: either insert two screws, one perpendicular to the bone long axis and one perpendicular to the fracture plane. Another option is to insert one or more lag screws perpendicular to the fracture plane, yielding interfragmentary compression, and neutralize the shear forces by a so-called neutralizing or protection plate.[2,6,19]

Two more important points must be observed in screw insertion: First, the holes in both fragments must be coaxial, otherwise the reduction will be lost. Secondly, the interfragmentary screw should pass perpendicularly to the fracture plane and the holes should seat in the center of each fragment, which is sometimes difficult to achieve in the small bones of the hand.

Another way to achieve fragment compression is the headless compression screw designed by Timothy Herbert to achieve compression by use of a differential thread pitch between its proximal and distal ends, the proximal one being narrower than the distal. Therefore, by inserting the screw, the distal thread progresses quicker than the proximal, compressing the fragments as would a lag screw do[20–22] (▶ Fig. 6.3b). Further development with a central cannulation simplify the insertion over a guiding K-wire and another design with a conical shape with a progressively shorter thread has also been proposed (▶ Fig. 6.3c).

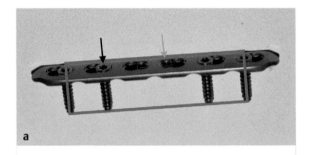

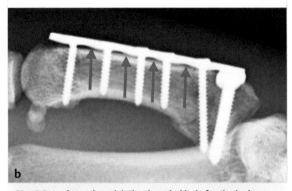

Fig. 6.2 Locking plate. (a) The threaded hole for the locking screw (*blue arrow*). The screw locked in place (*black arrow*). The plate and the screws act as a functional frame that increases the stability (*red frame*). (b) The plate lies on the bone with a slight interval to preserve the periosteal blood supply (*red arrows*).

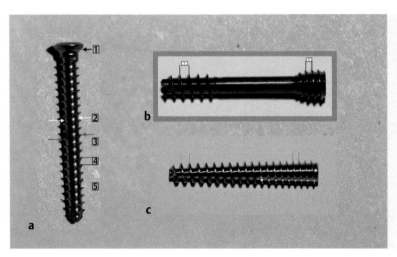

Fig. 6.3 Various types of screws for carpal, metacarpal, and phalangeal fractures. (a) Cortical screw. 1. Head; 2. Core diameter; 3. Outside diameter or thread; 4. Pitch: distance the screw advances for each 360-degree turn; 5. Effective thread depth. (b) Headless compression screw with double thread with different pitch. The distal thread with a coarse pitch progresses more quickly than the proximal, finer, pitch, creating interfragmentary compression. (c) The same principle of compression with the conical screw with progressively finer pitch from distal to proximal.

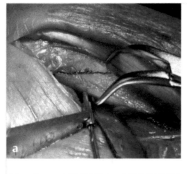
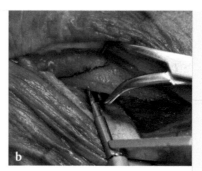
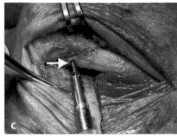

Fig. 6.4 Principles of lag screw insertion. **(a)** After fracture reduction, the pilot hole, slightly larger than the core diameter, is drilled perpendicular to the fracture plane. **(b)** After screw length measurement with a depth gauge, the gliding hole is drilled in proximal cortex at a diameter greater than the screw's outer diameter. **(c)** The screw is inserted after countersinking of proximal cortex (*yellow arrow* showing the bevel of the hole).

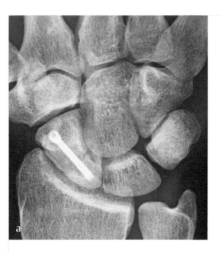
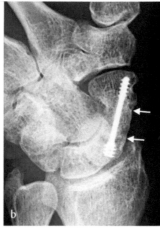
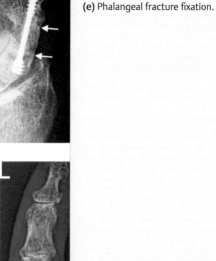
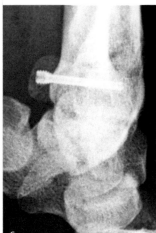
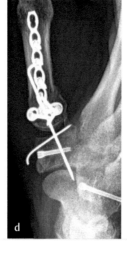
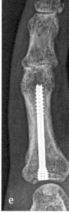

Fig. 6.5 Examples of headless screw use. **(a)** Retrograde scaphoid fixation (waist fracture). **(b)** Bone graft (*white arrows*) and anterograde scaphoid fixation for nonunion. **(c)** Uncinate process of the hamate fixation. **(d)** Trapezium fracture. **(e)** Phalangeal fracture fixation.

Although designed initially for the scaphoid fracture and nonunion, increasing the fusion rate and allowing early mobilization, it can also be used for fracture of other carpal bones as capitate or uncinated process of the hamate, as well as hand fractures as more recently described[23-26] (▶Fig. 6.5).

6.3 General Considerations and Indications

This part is based on the literature, but also and foremost on the author's clinical experience through years of good results and disappointing failures. Evidence-based guidelines would be in theory beneficial, but are lacking (see also Chapter 2).[27] Moreover, even if the strategy is evidence based, the outcome is not surely good, depending on the technique, the patient's healing biology, the quality of the rehabilitation, and patient's ability to cooperate. Indications to use plate and screw fixation are summarized in ▶Table 6.1.

This chapter focuses mostly on fracture treatment with plate and screws. The technique of osteosynthesis, however, is also used in nonunion, malunion, or bone

reconstruction following excision for tumor or other pathological bony conditions. As the general principles of fixation follow the same rules as in fracture treatment, these other indications are not developed here, as they are exposed in other,[1] more specific, chapters.

General indications for metacarpal or phalangeal fractures' operative treatment are unstable or unreducible fractures, displaced or unstable comminuted, multiple fractures, fractures associated with polytrauma or open fractures, fractures with bone loss.[6,28-31]

In carpal trauma, the main indication for screw fixation is the scaphoid fracture. Although a conservative treatment with cast is possible, multiple series has shown that long immobilization is no longer necessary and that percutaneous fixation of scaphoid may be the routine treatment to decrease the out of work time and increase the union rate.[32] Uncinate process of hamate fracture, although less common, or less frequently diagnosed, is also a good indication for percutaneous screw fixation, as are other carpal bone, capitate, trapezium, as well as combined carpal fractures.

Arthritis of the carpus secondary to scaphoid nonunion advanced collapse (SNAC wrist) may require either partial of complete fusion. Although fixation may be achieved by K-wires or specially designed plates, headless compression screws are also an option for intracarpal fusions. If the degenerative changes are too extensive, a total wrist fusion may be required, when prosthetic arthroplasty is contraindicated. A specially designed plate either dorsally bent or straight is generally used.

When considering an operative fixation, some rules have to be followed: do not treat X-rays, but a patient according to his or her needs; choose plate and screws fixation because it is indicated not because it is a nice operation to perform. The technique must be tailored to the patient and not the patient to a preoperatively planned operation. This must be kept in mind when deciding to go to the operation theater. A less invasive method of fixation may create less soft tissue damage than a formal open approach. It is nowadays sometimes possible to use mini-invasive technique to fix a fracture with percutaneous screw, be cannulated or not. Once again, conservative treatment must always be considered if possible.

In situation where plate and screws' fixation is indicated, it must be used only when a complete ancillary set is available, the operating theater conditions good, and the surgeon is well trained in this technique. Failure to observe these prerequisites could do more damage to the patient's hand than a conservative treatment.

The principles of hand fracture operative management, anatomical reposition of the fracture, stable fixation preserving soft tissues, and institution of early motion have to be followed.[27]

As the size of the screws varies greatly between the manufacturers, it is not specified in the text. The screw of diameters between 1 and 2.5 mm are currently available. The screw diameter depends on the size of the fracture fragments, as well as the size of the plate, if any.

Table 6.1 Indications to internal fixation with plate and/or screw

Phalanges and metacarpals		
	Fractures	Unstable Displaced Comminuted Unreducible Open Multiple With bone loss Associated with polytrauma
	Nonunion	With cortical bone graft Without bone graft
	Bone reconstruction	With cortical bone graft Without bone graft
	Posttraumatic arthritis	Fusion with or without bone graft
Carpus		
	Fractures	Scaphoid, except distal pole Uncinate process of hamate Capitate Fracture(s) in carpal dislocation Trapezium Dorsal avulsion of triquetrum with large fragment
	Nonunion	Fixation without bone graft Reconstruction with bone graft • Conventional iliac crest • Pedicled vascularized graft • Free vascularized graft
	Posttraumatic: SLAC/SNAC/DRF	Limited fusion Complete wrist fusion

Abbreviations: DRF, distal radius fracture; SLAC, scapholunate advanced collapse; SNAC, scaphoid nonunion advanced collapse.

6.4 Specific Indications and Procedures

This chapter is based on various textbooks and articles[6,19,33–36] that are not systematically referenced through the text.

6.4.1 Phalangeal Fractures

Distal Phalanx Fracture

The distal phalanx fractures are commonly either comminuted or transverse and better treated with K-wires. The intra-articular fracture of the phalangeal basis with a displaced dorsal fragment can, however, be fixed by two or three mini-screws after open reduction. In certain cases, when close reduction is still possible, percutaneous screw insertion may be tried. To prevent breakage of the displaced fragment, the holes are not made with a drill but with an 0.8-mm K-wire instead. A mini dorsal plate with proximal hooks may also be used.[37]

A volar avulsion fracture, as in jersey finger, as well as oblique fracture, may be indications to lag screw fixation, if the fragment is large enough.

Fractures of the Proximal and Middle Phalanges

Owing to the delicate extensor tendon mechanism running on the dorsum of the phalanges, the use of plate involves a risk of scar adhesions leading to stiffness, above all on the basal phalanx of the fifth finger. Therefore, alternative methods of fixation should be encouraged, whenever possible. The approach of the proximal and middle phalanges may be dorsal or lateral. The former requires the longitudinal split of the extensor on both phalanges, or elevating an interval between central and lateral bands on the proximal phalanx or elevation of the lateral band on the middle phalanx. It gives a better exposure of the fracture and is the preferred method of the author. The lateral approach is less damaging for the extensor apparatus, produces less adhesions, is more cosmetic, but may give a less good fracture exposure.[38] Plates, when needed, may be inserted dorsally or laterally. It depends on fracture anatomy and personal preference. Biomechanical studies seem to show that dorsally applied plates yield better stability, but results are, however, dependent on the quality of the implants that greatly differ from one

manufacturer to another.[39,40] Clinical analysis seems to confirm that there is no difference in outcome, be the plate lateral or dorsal.[41]

Transverse Fracture of the Proximal and Middle Phalanges

If an alternative method is not chosen (intramedullary pin or compression screw), the fixation is achieved by a compression plate. Approach can be lateral or dorsal. In order to prevent opening of the fracture at the opposite cortex, the plate is slightly overbent. A 5-hole plate is used leaving the central hole empty at the level of the fracture site. Care must be taken to center the plate on the long axis of the diaphysis laterally. A laterally placed plate is favored by the AO group.[17] However, dorsally placed plate is also possible following the same rules.

Short Oblique Fracture of the Proximal and Middle Phalanges

Obliquity of the fracture may be either in frontal or sagittal plane. The plate can be applied either dorsally or laterally on the phalanx, depending on the fracture plane. Fixation is achieved by a lag screw and a neutralizing plate. If the fracture is seen in the anteroposterior (AP) view, the plate is placed laterally with the lag screw inserted through the plate perpendicular to the fracture line. If the obliquity is visible in the lateral view, the plate should be applied dorsally for the same reason. The lag screw can also be inserted separately from the plate that will seat either laterally or dorsally according to the fracture plane. The use of a double row neutralization plate is a good option, but this type of facture may sometimes be treated by lag screws without plate, if the fragments are large enough (▶ Fig. 6.6).

Long Oblique Fracture of the Proximal and Middle Phalanges

This type of fracture is perfectly suitable for multiple lag screws. It is important to determine correctly the geometry of the fracture in order to place the lag screws in the middle of the fragments, otherwise the risk of displacement exists. A minimum of two screws is required for stability. A comparison of two versus three lag screws to fix this type of fracture did not show any difference in stability.[42] Screws are evenly distributed along the fracture line and their direction vary according to the need to be perpendicular to

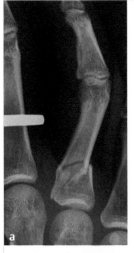
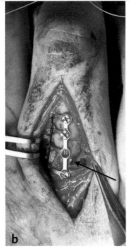
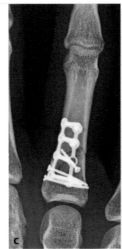

Fig. 6.6 Short oblique phalangeal base fracture: two methods of fixation. (a) Very short oblique fracture of basal phalanx. (b) Operative view: lag screw and double row neutralization plate (*arrow*). (c) Postoperative posteroanterior radiological view. (d) Short oblique fracture with longer fragments and articular extension. (e) Postoperative PA radiological view. Fixation with four lag screws.

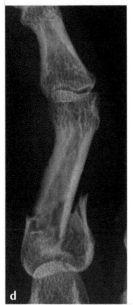
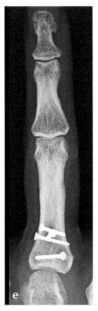

the fracture line. This technique is less invasive than plate fixation and yields good functional results.[43]

Comminuted Diaphyseal Fracture of the Proximal and Middle Phalanges

These fractures are often open and/or with soft tissue damage. Stabilization is required in order to allow early mobilization to decrease the risk of soft tissue adhesions and stiffness. The use of a bridging plate after gross alignment of fragments without too much dissection allows the fracture to heal by external callus through slight interfragmentary movements. The use of a laterally inserted condylar plate may interfere with the soft tissues and its insertion is very demanding. A straight plate either dorsally or laterally inserted with two holes on each side of the comminution is suitable to allow for fracture healing. If the comminution is too important and the viability of the fragments questionable, they can be excised and replaced by a corticocancellous graft. A T- or Y- or reconstruction plate can also be used according to the type and the anatomy of the fracture. In this occurrence, the use of locking plate is certainly indicated in order to gain stability.

Condylar Fracture of the Proximal and Middle Phalanges

Condylar fractures are very unstable and should be treated operatively. The articular surface has to be realigned and the fracture fixed either by K-wire or screws.[44] Both techniques give the same stability in laboratory.[45] The fracture may be approached dorsally or laterally with longitudinal extensor apparatus splitting. In some cases, where the fracture can be closely reduced, the screws can be percutaneously inserted. To prevent damage to the condylar fragment, a 0.8 wire can be used instead of a drill (▶ Fig. 6.7). Depending on the size of the fragment, one or more screws are used. If only one screw is used, it should be placed distally to the insertion of the collateral ligament not to interfere with joint motion.[34] Gentle handling is of utmost importance not to jeopardize the blood supply that could lead to condylar necrosis. In some difficult cases, fixation can be achieved by intra-articularly placed interfragmentary screws. In this case, the cartilage should be countersunk to a depth of 1 mm in order to completely bury the screw head under the articular surface.[46]

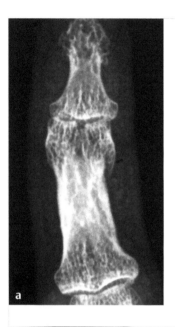
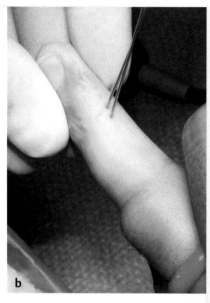
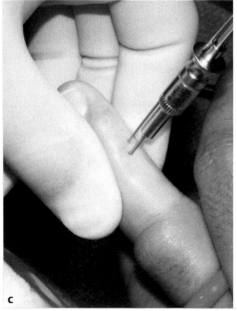
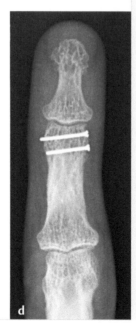

Fig. 6.7 Percutaneous fixation of condylar phalangeal fracture. **(a)** Displaced condylar fracture with articular step-off. **(b)** Percutaneous pinning for reduction by manipulation and provisional fixation. A second wire is inserted to drill the hole for the screw. **(c)** Percutaneous screw insertion. The first pin is then replaced by a screw. **(d)** Postoperative X-ray.

Other Articular Fractures of the Proximal and Middle Phalanges

Bony avulsions, if displaced, must be reduced, above all if they involve a significant amount of the articular facet. Fixation is achieved with lag screws. Articular fracture of the proximal phalanx can be exposed by a dorsal or volar approach, reduction achieved, and fragment fixed with one or two lag screws. A tip to facilitate the procedure is to insert a fine K-wire at the edge of the fragment and use it as a lever to reduce the fracture and tentatively fix it before inserting the screw.

The dorsal avulsion fracture of the middle phalanx base, if displaced, must be reduced and fixed with one or two lag screws. Reduction should be anatomical in order to prevent joint degeneration. Experience, however, has shown that this is a difficult fracture to treat, and, when the fragment is aligned with the base of the phalanx, it is better treated conservatively, if the fragment dislocation is not too important.

The volar fracture of the middle phalanx basis is often associated with multiple depressed fragments, and are difficult to treat.[47] The classical treatment is either the active mobilization with extension by an external fixator, or an open reduction and internal fixation (ORIF) through a so-called shotgun approach. Lag screws can be inserted from palmar to dorsal. In the hands of the author the active mobilization with traction does not always reduce the depressed fragments and the shotgun approach is a source of flexion contracture. An alternative is to approach the fracture by a minimally dorsal exposure, to reduce it by traction and manipulation with a dorsally inserted hook to elevate the joint surface. In addition to K-wires, a dorsally inserted lag screw can be used. This latter technique respects soft tissue and tendon gliding, allows early motion to prevent stiffness (▶ Fig. 6.8).

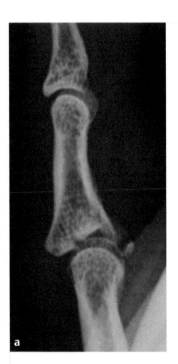
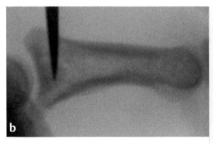
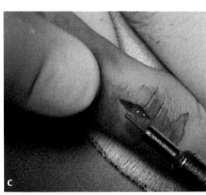
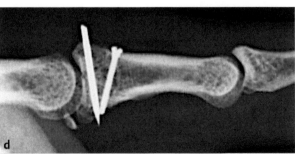

Fig. 6.8 Comminuted intra-articular fracture of middle phalanx base ("pilon fracture"). (a) Depressed and comminuted fracture of P2 base. (b) Minimally invasive approach. Longitudinal traction to align fragments and elevation of the depressed fragments with an owl. (c) Percutaneous screw insertion. (d) Postoperative lateral X-ray: screw to fix the main fragment and K-wire buttressing the subchondral bone.

6.4.2 Metacarpal Fractures

The metacarpals are approached through a dorsal incision, the fracture exposed, reduced, and tentatively fixed by a bone clamp or any other suitable methods, like K-wires, suture loop around the bone, or the assistant's fingers. In simple fractures, the reduction must be anatomical. If the fracture is comminuted, or when bone fragments are missing, an adaptation reduction should be performed, always keeping in mind the general axis, particularly rotation. As a rule, the fingers should all aim at the scaphoid tubercle while in flexion. The bone fixation will depend on the type of fracture and the available implants, but also and probably foremost on the surgeon's preferences, experience, and inspiration, as long as it follows the mechanical rules.

Transverse Metacarpal Fracture

This is the good situation for the compression plate technique: The fracture is unstable and long to heal and prone to nonunion.[48] As a lag screw cannot be used, plating must be performed with compression technique. A 4- to 5-hole plate is inserted on the dorsal aspect of the metacarpal. The plate is slightly overbent in order to compress the far cortex. The first screw is inserted near the fracture line, engaging both cortices without tightening it. The plate is moved to bring the screw to the distal border of the eccentric hole, then the second screw is inserted near the fracture line in the eccentric hole. Tightening the screws will produce axial compression. The other screws are inserted in neutral position, as shown in (▶ Fig. 6.1).

An alternative method to treat this type of metacarpal fracture is the percutaneous fixation with an intramedullary cannulated headless compression screw.[23,24] A guidewire is inserted into the diaphysis through a 1-cm incision over the maximally bent MP joint. The subchondral bone is countersunk and a 3-mm-diameter cannulated screw is inserted.

Short Oblique Metacarpal Fracture

As the fracture plane is too short to accommodate more than one screw, a neutralization plate must be used, in order to prevent implant failure. Even two screws are sometimes not enough, particularly if anatomical reduction is not achieved. The lag screw is either inserted independently of the plate, leaving empty the central hole at the level of the screw or through the plate. As a rule, the plate is inserted on the dorsal aspect of the metacarpal to better resist the mechanical constraints. Therefore, if the plane of the fracture is sagittal, the lag screw is inserted independently of the plate, since they lie in a different plane. Conversely, if the fracture plane is mainly transverse, the lag screw may be inserted through one of the plate holes. Usually, the neutralization plate should have 5 holes and perfectly adapt to the bone surface without overbending, since it is not in a compression mode. If the fracture is

at the metaphysis, the neutralization plate cannot be a 5-hole straight one, since the space is too short. In this occurrence, a reconstruction (double row) or a T-shape plate should be used instead.

Long Oblique Metacarpal Fracture

These fractures are best treated by lag screws.[17,19] The number depends on the length of the fracture. A minimum of two screws must be used, which necessitates that the length of the fracture zone be at least twice the diameter of the metacarpal bone. In case of a shorter fracture line, a single lag screw and a protection plate must be used.[17] Freeland and Jabaley propose as a tip to divide the length of the fracture according to the ratio fracture length on longest diameter of the bone at the fracture site.[19] If the fracture is twice the bone diameter, the fracture is divided into thirds and two screws can be safely inserted at equal distance. If the fracture is three times the diameter, the fracture is divided into fourths and three screws inserted. Three screws should be inserted at equal intervals and each one perpendicularly to the fracture plane, which, in spiral fractures, results in the screws following a helicoidal disposition.[19] Countersinking increases the stability.[17] According to the author's experience, if only two screws are inserted, it is safer to add a neutralization plate and the number of screws is more a matter of experience and common sense than arithmetic rules (▶ Fig. 6.9).

Comminuted Metacarpal Fracture

In this situation, the bone fragments cannot be reduced without jeopardizing their blood supply. The fracture is therefore bridged by a plate anchored in the main proximal and distal fragments without compression. The bony fragments in between are aligned as well as possible, without interfering with their blood supply. The fracture will then heal by callus formation.[17,19] If the bony destruction is too important, the fragments can be replaced by a corticocancellous graft from the distal radius, the olecranon or, if a larger graft is required, from the iliac crest, fixed with a long plate spanning the entire reconstruction.[6,7,19] This situation of spanning plate is a good indication for a locking plate that acts as an internal–external fixator.

Proximal Intra-Articular Metacarpal Fracture

The fifth metacarpal base is the most common carpometacarpal (CMC) joint fracture. It is sometimes associated with a dislocation and a fracture of the dorsal margin of the hamate. It is frequently comminuted and the cancellous bone crushed. The fragments are often too small to be fixed by plate and/or screws and K-wires are therefore preferred. However, if the fragments are

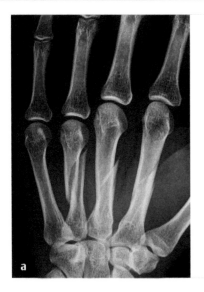
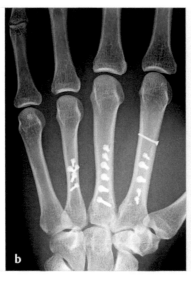

Fig. 6.9 (a) Multiple long oblique metacarpal fractures. (b) Multiple lag screw fixation.

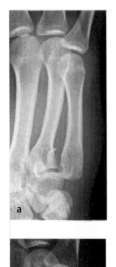
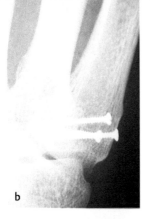
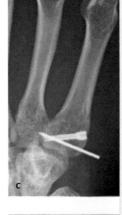

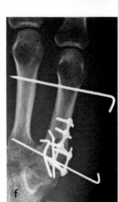

Fig. 6.10 Intra-articular fracture of the metacarpal base. (a) Metacarpal base fracture with one fragment. (b) Fixation with three lag screws. (c) Fixation with headless compression screw and antirotation K-wire. (d) Fracture of the metacarpal base with joint surface involvement. (e) Operative view: ORIF with double row plate, screws and K-wire. (f) Postoperative X-rays: inter-metacarpal suspension with K-wires to protect the stabilization.

big enough, they may be fixed, after reduction, with one or more screws, either lag cortical or headless compression screws or with a reconstruction, or an L-, T-, Y-shaped plates, according to the geometry of the fracture (▶Fig. 6.10). The volar–radial fragment, as well as all articular fragments, should be reduced first, to restore the joint surface and the plate inserted dorsally with the help of K-wires and cancellous bone graft as required. One screw is inserted first without tightening it, in order to align the plate on the diaphysis where it is anchored by the most distal screw. The second proximal screw is inserted and finally the last diaphyseal ones. As the pattern of these kind of fracture is variable, only general principles can be exposed and imagination and skills of the surgeon may sometimes replace a poorly inserted screw. It is at times possible to use a plate to bridge the fracture from the hamate to the metacarpal with some traction to align the fragments. After healing of the fracture, the plate is removed to allow rehabilitation.

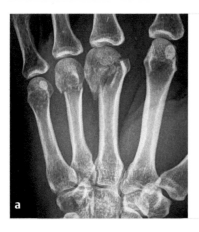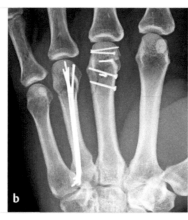

Fig. 6.11 Distal intra-articular metacarpal fracture. **(a)** Metacarpal head comminuted fracture. **(b)** Fixation with multiple lag screws. Note the subcapital fourth metacarpal fracture fixed with intramedullary K-wires.

Distal Intra-articular Metacarpal Fracture

The pattern of these fractures is more predictable. They may be simple or multifragmentary. If the fragments are too small, they are not amenable to screw fixation. If they are large enough, they can be fixed with lag screws or headless cannulated compression screws in an anterograde or retrograde fashion. In either way, it is important to bury the head in the cartilage or avoid to perforate the joint cartilage with the tip of the screw, as in the phalangeal condyles.[46] The length of the anterograde screw must be 1 mL shorter than the measured length (▶Fig. 6.11).

Subcapital Metacarpal Fracture

Although intramedullary wire fixation is the common technique to fix subcapital metacarpal fracture, intramedullary fixation with a headless cannulated compression screw has been reported with favorable outcome.[23,49] Both these techniques compared favorably to the laterally inserted condylar plate, not only in terms of stability, but because of the less invasive procedure.

First Metacarpal Fractures

Fractures of the thumb metacarpal show some typical patterns. The extra-articular fracture of the metacarpal is typically displaced in flexion, which may impair function. Open reduction and T-shape plate fixation is the usual procedure, performed through a dorsal approach. It may be done either by traction, manipulation, and provisional K-wire stabilization before inserting the plate. Alternatively, a T-shape locking plate is first fixed on the proximal fragment, before reducing the fracture using the plate as a lever. The plate must be contoured by bending the transverse limbs to adapt to the base of the metacarpal. The first two screws are inserted in the locking holes in the transverse limbs of the plate. The distal diaphyseal screw is inserted in a standard way and the remaining ones either as standard or locking screws according to the bone condition.[50] Care must be taken to properly align the plate before inserting the basal screws to be in line with the diaphysis after reposition (▶Fig. 6.12).

The intra-articular Bennett's fracture separates the volar–ulnar aspect of the base from the remaining metacarpal.[51] If the fragment is small, K-wire suspension–fixation is indicated, but if the fragment is large enough, is may be fixed by one or two headless cannulated compression screws inserted percutaneously (▶Fig. 6.13), or by open exposure using the Gedda-Moberg approach, taking care not to injure the superficial sensory nerves.

The treatment of the comminuted intra-articular Rolando fracture of the first metacarpal base (initially described as a T-shaped or Y-shaped intra-articular) is more demanding.[51,52] The main goal is to restore an articular surface to prevent arthritis. The reduction and fixation are achieved with a T-shape locking plate through a dorsal approach for T-pattern fracture in the frontal plane or a radiopalmar approach if the fracture is in the sagittal plane.[17] The articular fragments must first be reduced and tentatively fixed with K-wires before insertion of the plate.

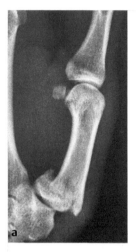
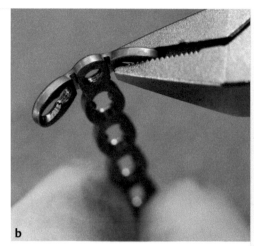

Fig. 6.12 Extra-articular metacarpal base fracture. (a) Extra-articular fracture with flexion deformity and dislocation of fragments. (b) Plate bending with pliers to accommodate the metacarpal base shape. (c) Locking plate fixed on the dorsal aspect of the metacarpal. (d) Postoperative X-rays.

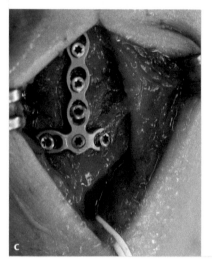
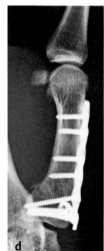

6.4.3 Carpal Fracture and Other Conditions

Percutaneous fixation of scaphoid fracture with headless compression screws has become the standard treatment in many hand centers, as the recovery is shorter and the general results are good.[21,32] As this topic, as well as scaphoid nonunion, where headless screws are widely used, are covered in Chapters 25 and 26, it will not be developed much further. Other bones are amenable to percutaneous fixation with headless compression screws, although the incidence of fracture of the other carpal bone is much lower

than the scaphoid. Fracture or nonunion of the hook of the hamate can reliably be treated by percutaneous screw fixation. The uncus is first localized by palpation and image amplifier and the guidewire inserted under fluoroscopic control. Preoperative CT scan is helpful in choosing the correct angle for pin insertion. Most commonly, it has to be inserted in a dorsoproximal direction to account for the orientation of the uncinated process. A 2.0 cannulated screw is used. Care must be taken not to deviate from the tip of the uncus while inserting the K-wire, because the ulnar neurovascular bundle lies close to the inner aspect of the hook and could be injured. This technique can be

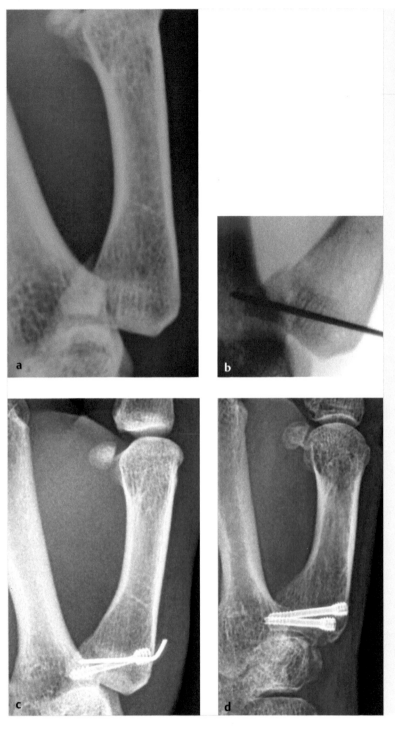

Fig. 6.13 Bennett's fracture of first metacarpal. **(a)** Bennett's fracture with large fragment. **(b)** Reduction by longitudinal traction and dorsal pressure on the metacarpal base and percutaneous pinning. **(c)** Fixation with a headless screw and an antirotation pin. **(d)** Alternative option: fixation with two headless screws.

used either for fresh fracture or nonunion. The stability of the fracture after fixation allows immediate active motion (▸Fig. 6.14). The same minimally invasive technique can also be used in multiple carpal fractures or dislocation to minimize the soft tissue damage. As an example, a combined coronal fracture dislocation of capitate and hamate has been treated with such a method with a good functional result (▸Fig. 6.15).

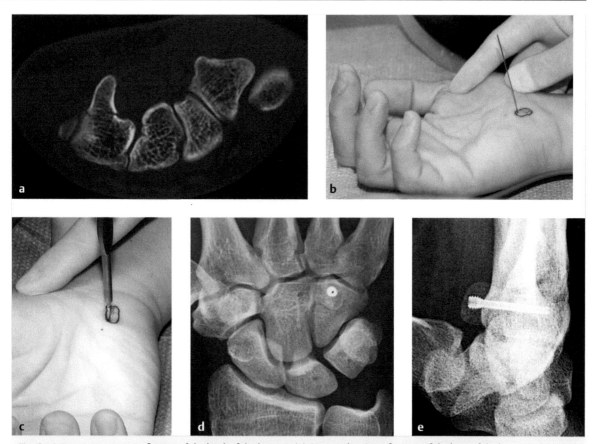

Fig. 6.14 Percutaneous screw fixation of the hook of the hamate. **(a)** CT scan showing a fracture of the base of the hamate uncinate process. **(b)** After location of the process by palpation and X-rays, a guidewire is inserted into the bone in a dorsoproximal direction. **(c)** After measurement, the adequate screw is inserted. **(d)** PA X-ray control. **(e)** Special incidence to better show the uncus and the screw position.

6.5 Complications

Complications of screw and plate fixation are not uncommon. A good technique and appropriate implants are required to get good clinical results. The fixation must be stable enough to allow early rehabilitation. Even with a proper surgical treatment, the complications as malunion, late union, or nonunion, stiffness, plate loosening or breakage, complex regional pain syndrome (CRPS) and infections may be encountered in metacarpal fractures.[52,53] Owing to the smaller implants used today and better knowledge of the technique, a complication rate, as high as 75% in some old series,[54] should no more be seen. The complication rate is higher in phalangeal fractures than in metacarpal fractures, in open lesions, associated soft tissue injury, and increasing age,[28,53,55–58] but dropped compared to previous series.[57,59–61]

As implant failure is most of the time a surgeon's technical mistake, great care must be taken to follow the general principle of plate and screw fixation to avoid complications.

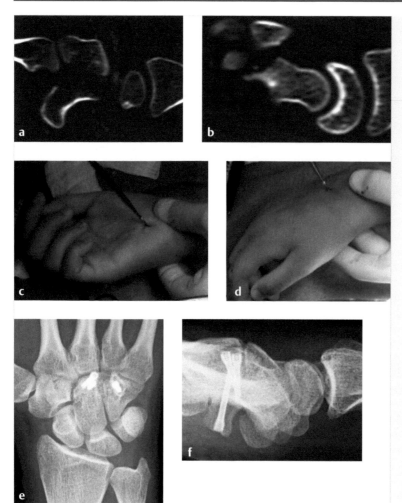

Fig. 6.15 Combined coronal fracture dislocation of hamate and capitate. **(a)** CT view of the fracture through the body of the hamate in a coronal plane. **(b)** CT view of the fracture dislocation of the capitate. **(c)** Fixation of the hamate fracture with a percutaneous screw. **(d)** Fixation of the capitate with two percutaneous screws. **(e)** Postoperative PA X-rays. **(f)** Postoperative lateral view.[3]

References

[1] Meals RA, Meuli HC. Carpenter's nails, phonograph needles, piano wires, and safety pins: the history of operative fixation of metacarpal and phalangeal fractures. J Hand Surg Am. 1985; 10(1):144–150

[2] Colton C. Plate fixation. Introduction to the principles of plate fixation. www.aofoundation.org/Structure/education/online-cme/Pages/ eLearning.aspx. Accessed December 22, 2017

[3] Dresing K. The biology of bone healing. AO Principles program. ed. Colton C. https://www.aofoundation.org/Structure/education/online-cme/Pages/eLearning.aspx. Accessed December 22, 2017

[4] Miller DL, Goswami T. A review of locking compression plate biomechanics and their advantages as internal fixators in fracture healing. Clin Biomech (Bristol, Avon). 2007; 22(10):1049–1062

[5] Danis R. Théorie et pratique de l'ostéosynthèse. Paris: Masson & Cie Ed; 1949

[6] Day CS, Stern PJ. Fractures of the metacarpals and phalanges. In: Wolfe SW, Hotchkiss RN, Pederson WC, Kozin SH, eds. Green's Operative Hand Surgery. Vol 1. Philadelphia, PA: Elsevier; 2011:239–290

[7] Saint-Cyr M, Gupta A. Primary internal fixation and bone grafting for open fractures of the hand. Hand Clin. 2006; 22(3):317–327

[8] Egol KA, Kubiak EN, Fulkerson E, Kummer FJ, Koval KJ. Biomechanics of locked plates and screws. J Orthop Trauma. 2004; 18(8):488–493

[9] Yaffe MA, Saucedo JM, Kalainov DM. Non-locked and locked plating technology for hand fractures. J Hand Surg Am. 2011; 36(12):2052–2055

[10] Ruchelsman DE, Mudgal CS, Jupiter JB. The role of locking technology in the hand. Hand Clin. 2010; 26(3):307–319

[11] Doht S, Jansen H, Meffert R, Frey S. Higher stability with locking plates in hand surgery? Biomechanical investigation of the TriLock system in a fracture model. Int Orthop. 2012; 36(8):1641–1646

[12] Barr C, Behn AW, Yao J. Plating of metacarpal fractures with locked or nonlocked screws, a biomechanical study: how many cortices are really necessary? Hand (NY). 2013; 8(4):454–459

[13] Ochman S, Doht S, Paletta J, Langer M, Raschke MJ, Meffert RH. Comparison between locking and non-locking plates for fixation of metacarpal fractures in an animal model. J Hand Surg Am. 2010; 35(4):597–603

[14] Gajendran VK, Szabo RM, Myo GK, Curtiss SB. Biomechanical comparison of double-row locking plates versus single- and double-row non-locking plates in a comminuted metacarpal fracture model. J Hand Surg Am. 2009; 34(10):1851–1858

[15] Dickson JK, Bhat W, Gujral S, Paget J, O'Neill J, Lee SJ. Unicortical fixation of metacarpal fractures: is it strong enough? J Hand Surg Eur Vol. 2016; 41(4):367–372

[16] Afshar R, Fong TS, Latifi MH, Kanthan SR, Kamarul T. A biomechanical study comparing plate fixation using unicortical and bicortical screws in transverse metacarpal fracture models subjected to cyclic loading. J Hand Surg Eur Vol. 2012; 37(5):396–401

[17] Colton C. Screw fixation. Introduction to screw fixation. https://emodules.aoeducation.org/aotdlmat/aot_screws/index.html#page/item_010_en/10/end. Accessed December 27, 2017

[18] Roth JJ, Auerbach DM. Fixation of hand fractures with bicortical screws. J Hand Surg Am. 2005; 30(1):151–153

[19] Freeland AE, Jabaley ME. Open reduction internal fixation: metacarpal fractures. In: Strickland JW, ed. Master Techniques in Orthopaedic Surgery. The Hand. Philadelphia, PA: Lippincott-Raven Publishers; 1998:3–33

[20] Herbert TJ, Fisher WE. Management of the fractured scaphoid using a new bone screw. J Bone Joint Surg Br. 1984; 66(1):114–123

[21] Fowler JR, Ilyas AM. Headless compression screw fixation of scaphoid fractures. Hand Clin. 2010; 26(3):351–361, vi

[22] Moser VL, Krimmer H, Herbert TJ. Minimal invasive treatment for scaphoid fractures using the cannulated Herbert screw system. Tech Hand Up Extrem Surg. 2003; 7(4):141–146

[23] Ruchelsman DE, Puri S, Feinberg-Zadek N, Leibman MI, Belsky MR. Clinical outcomes of limited-open retrograde intramedullary headless screw fixation of metacarpal fractures. J Hand Surg Am. 2014; 39(12):2390–2395

[24] del Piñal F, Moraleda E, Rúas JS, de Piero GH, Cerezal L. Minimally invasive fixation of fractures of the phalanges and metacarpals with intramedullary cannulated headless compression screws. J Hand Surg Am. 2015; 40(4):692–700

[25] Giesen T, Gazzola R, Poggetti A, Giovanoli P, Calcagni M. Intramedullary headless screw fixation for fractures of the proximal and middle phalanges in the digits of the hand: a review of 31 consecutive fractures. J Hand Surg Eur Vol. 2016; 41(7):688–694

[26] Liodaki E, Kisch T, Wenzel E, Mailänder P, Stang F. Percutaneous cannulated compression screw osteosynthesis in phalanx fractures: the surgical technique, the indication and the results. Eplasty. 2017; 17:e8

[27] Sammer DM, Husain T, Ramirez R. Selection of appropriate treatment options for hand fractures. Hand Clin. 2013; 29(4):501–505

[28] Kozin SH, Thoder JJ, Lieberman G. Operative treatment of metacarpal and phalangeal shaft fractures. J Am Acad Orthop Surg. 2000; 8(2):111–121

[29] Weinstein LP, Hanel DP. Metacarpal fractures. J Am Soc Surg Hand. 2002; 2(4):168–180

[30] Jones NF, Jupiter JB, Lalonde DH. Common fractures and dislocations of the hand. Plast Reconstr Surg. 2012; 130(5):722e–736e

[31] Cheah AE-J, Yao J. Hand fractures: indications, the tried and true and new innovations. J Hand Surg Am. 2016; 41(6):712–722

[32] Herbert TJ. Internal fixation of the carpus with the Herbert bone screw system. J Hand Surg Am. 1989; 14(2 pt 2):397–400

[33] Jupiter JB, Winters S. Open reduction internal fixation: phalangeal fractures. In: Strickland JW, ed. Master Techniques in Orthopaedic Surgery. The Hand. Philadelphia, PA: Lippincott-Raven Publishers; 1998:35–51

[34] Hastings IIH. Open reduction internal fixation: intraarticular fractures of the proximal interphalangeal joint. In: Strickland JW, ed. Master Techniques in Orthopaedic Surgery. The Hand. Philadelphia, PA: Lippincott-Raven Publishers; 1998:53–65

[35] Adams JE, Miller T, Rizzo M. The biomechanics of fixation techniques for hand fractures. Hand Clin. 2013; 29(4):493–500

[36] Fricker R, Kastelec M, Nuñez F, Axelrod T. AO Surgery Reference—the hand. Colton C, ed. https://www2.aofoundation.org/wps/portal/surgery?showPage=diagnosis&bone=Hand&segment=Overview. Accessed December 27, 2017

[37] Kang GC, Yam A, Phoon ES, Lee JY, Teoh LC. The hook plate technique for fixation of phalangeal avulsion fractures. J Bone Joint Surg Am. 2012; 94(11):e72

[38] Dabezies EJ, Schutte JP. Fixation of metacarpal and phalangeal fractures with miniature plates and screws. J Hand Surg Am. 1986; 11(2):283–288

[39] Prevel CD, Eppley BL, Jackson JR, Moore K, McCarty M, Wood R. Mini and micro plating of phalangeal and metacarpal fractures: a biomechanical study. J Hand Surg Am. 1995; 20A(1):44–49

[40] Lins RE, Myers BS, Spinner RJ, Levin LS. A comparative mechanical analysis of plate fixation in a proximal phalangeal fracture model. J Hand Surg Am. 1996; 21(6):1059–1064

[41] Robinson LP, Gaspar MP, Strohl AB, et al. Dorsal versus lateral plate fixation of finger proximal phalangeal fractures: a retrospective study. Arch Orthop Trauma Surg. 2017; 137(4):567–572

[42] Zelken JA, Hayes AG, Parks BG, Al Muhit A, Means KR, Jr. Two versus 3 lag screws for fixation of long oblique proximal phalanx fractures of the fingers: a cadaver study. J Hand Surg Am. 2015; 40(6):1124–1129

[43] Kawamura K, Chung KC. Fixation choices for closed simple unstable oblique phalangeal and metacarpal fractures. Hand Clin. 2006; 22(3):287–295

[44] Freeland AE, Sud V. Unicondylar and bicondylar proximal phalangeal fractures. J Am Soc Surg Hand. 2001; 1(1):14–24

[45] Sirota MA, Parks BG, Higgins JP, Means KR, Jr, Means KR. Stability of fixation of proximal phalanx unicondylar fractures of the hand: a biomechanical cadaver study. J Hand Surg Am. 2013; 38(1):77–81

[46] Tan JSW, Foo ATL, Chew WCY, Teoh LC. Articularly placed interfragmentary screw fixation of difficult condylar fractures of the hand. J Hand Surg Am. 2011; 36(4):604–609

[47] Liodaki E, Xing SG, Mailaender P, Stang F. Management of difficult intra-articular fractures or fracture dislocations of the proximal interphalangeal joint. J Hand Surg Eur Vol. 2015; 40(1):16–23

[48] Fusetti C, Della Santa DR. Influence of fracture pattern on consolidation after metacarpal plate fixation. Chir Main. 2004; 23(1):32–36

[49] Boulton CL, Salzler M, Mudgal CS. Intramedullary cannulated headless screw fixation of a comminuted subcapital metacarpal fracture: case report. J Hand Surg Am. 2010; 35(8):1260–1263

[50] Diaconu M, Facca S, Gouzou S, Liverneaux P. Locking plates for fixation of extra-articular fractures of the first metacarpal base: a series of 15 cases. Chir Main. 2011; 30(1):26–30

[51] Carlsen BT, Moran SL. Thumb trauma: Bennett fractures, Rolando fractures, and ulnar collateral ligament injuries. J Hand Surg Am. 2009; 34(5):945–952

[52] Diaz-Garcia R, Waljee JF. Current management of metacarpal fractures. Hand Clin. 2013; 29(4):507–518

[53] Fusetti C, Meyer H, Borisch N, Stern R, Santa DD, Papaloïzos M. Complications of plate fixation in metacarpal fractures. J Trauma. 2002; 52(3):535–539

[54] Pun WK, Chow SP, So YC, et al. Unstable phalangeal fractures: treatment by A.O. screw and plate fixation. J Hand Surg Am. 1991; 16(1):113–117

[55] Page SM, Stern PJ. Complications and range of motion following plate fixation of metacarpal and phalangeal fractures. J Hand Surg Am. 1998; 23(5):827–832

[56] Kurzen P, Fusetti C, Bonaccio M, Nagy L. Complications after plate fixation of phalangeal fractures. J Trauma. 2006; 60(4):841–843

[57] Bannasch H, Heermann AK, Iblher N, Momeni A, Schulte-Mönting J, Stark GB. Ten years stable internal fixation of metacarpal and phalangeal hand fractures-risk factor and outcome analysis show no increase of complications in the treatment of open compared with closed fractures. J Trauma. 2010; 68(3):624–628

[58] Shimizu T, Omokawa S, Akahane M, et al. Predictors of the postoperative range of finger motion for comminuted periarticular metacarpal and phalangeal fractures treated with a titanium plate. Injury. 2012; 43(6):940–945

[59] Soni A, Gulati A, Bassi JL, Singh D, Saini UC. Outcome of closed ipsilateral metacarpal fractures treated with mini fragment plates and screws: a prospective study. J Orthop Traumatol. 2012; 13(1):29–33

[60] Omokawa S, Fujitani R, Dohi Y, Okawa T, Yajima H. Prospective outcomes of comminuted periarticular metacarpal and phalangeal fractures treated using a titanium plate system. J Hand Surg Am. 2008; 33(6):857–863

[61] Desaldeleer-Le Sant AS, Le Sant A, Beauthier-Landauer V, Kerfant N, Le Nen D. Surgical management of closed, isolated proximal phalanx fractures in the long fingers: Functional outcomes and complications of 87 fractures. Hand Surg Rehabil. 2017; 36(2):127–135

7 External Minifixation

Frédéric Schuind, Fabian Moungondo, Wissam El Kazzi

Abstract

External minifixation allows stable bone fixation of hand fractures, allowing early active mobilization, the best way to prevent stiffness and complex regional pain syndrome (CRPS). The problems of internal fixation (infection, local discomfort, tendon impingement) are avoided. External minifixation can be applied in a wide variety of clinical situations, not only to treat open and infected fractures and nonunions, but also to stabilize closed unstable metacarpal and phalangeal fractures, or to perform a corrective osteotomy. Other excellent indications are lengthening and arthrodesis. The main drawbacks are the bone and skin reactions to the pins, not uncommon at the metacarpal level, and the cost of the implant.

Keywords: external fixation, external minifixation, hand fracture, osteotomy, lengthening—arthrodesis, finger stiffness

7.1 Introduction

Stiffness was the rule rather than the exception after nonoperative treatment of hand fractures: after 4 weeks of immobilization of stable hand fractures, only 25% of the 809 patients in the series of Wright regained full active motion, and only 10%, in case of unstable fractures.[1] Similarly, poor fixation using Kirschner's wires, imposing subsequent plaster cast immobilization, leads to stiffness, but, to our surprise, this form of treatment is still widely accepted as standard care of hand fractures. As F. Burny once said, "*la Nature a horreur du plâtre*" ("Nature abhors plaster"), or, according to L. De Smet, "plaster is disaster." The best way to improve the functional results of hand fractures is to allow early or, better, immediate posttraumatic active motion. This is true for stable fractures, which should be managed using minimal functional splints and early remobilization, for example, in buddy taping; a short duration of immobilization in the protective position[2] is, however, sometimes necessary. Unstable fractures should be converted to a stable situation using modern osteosynthesis techniques, allowing early unprotected active mobilization. This principle stands, whether the fracture is isolated, simple, and closed, and also in the case of a severe hand traumatism. Indeed, fracture opening, the presence of multiple fractures, the existence of a segmental bone loss, and/or of associated soft tissue lesions, including tendon lesions, are no reasons to delay postoperative remobilization; on the contrary, the benefits of early active mobilization are especially obvious in complex traumatic situations.

Stable bone fixation can sometimes be achieved by elastic endomedullary nailing, for example, the "bouquet" osteosynthesis of metacarpal neck fractures (see also Chapter 22). Another form of stable osteosynthesis is represented by isolated screws fixing reduced articular fractures; or by miniplates, opposed to bone by conventional or better by locked screws (see also Chapter 6). The latter internal fixation techniques are especially indicated in articular and periarticular fractures and osteotomies, although they can also be used to treat diaphyseal fractures. The use of apposition methods of osteosynthesis imposes, however, an open approach of and around the fracture, a possible cause of adherences and stiffness. Although modern plates are quite thin to prevent soft tissue impingement, these implants may still limit tendon gliding, in particular, of the extensor apparatus. In addition, the use of an internal implant is contraindicated in open, contaminated fractures, particularly in case of poor posttraumatic finger vascularization and/or skin coverage.

Another form of stable osteosynthesis is external minifixation, especially indicated in open, contaminated fractures (▶ Fig. 7.1), and also an excellent technique to treat closed diaphyseal metacarpal and phalangeal fractures (▶ Fig. 7.2). External minifixation is not a new idea, and several authors have already long time ago proposed the use of various small external devices for the osteosynthesis at the hand, foot, and mandible, and for fractures occurring in children.[3–5] These fixators did not gain popularity, because of lack of stability and difficulties in application. Henri Jaquet developed the first modern external minifixator in the years 1975–1976.[6–8] The Brussels school has been using this implant since 1977 and has published a book in 1990 presenting the results of a prospective study of 516 cases.[9] Other publications from our group have followed.[10–13] Since 2004, we use the "Micro Hoffman II Fixator" developed by Stryker following the concept of the Hoffman II.[12,13] The external minifixator is relatively expensive, limiting its widespread use in hand surgery. Recently, various new models of small external fixators have appeared on the market, initiating a regain of interest of the hand surgery community for this method of treatment of hand fractures.

7.2 Surgical Technique

The implantation of an external minifixator, which requires the same rules of sterility as any other form of osteoarticular surgery, is usually performed before the repair of other lesions, allowing the surgeon to perform the soft tissue repairs on a stable skeleton. Rarely, the implantation of a minifixator renders microsurgical repairs difficult, especially in replantation surgery, thus, despite its disadvantages, the use of Kirschner wires in this particular form of open fracture may sometimes be more appropriate.

A C-arm is necessary to check the length of the pins and the quality of fracture reduction. We recommend the use of two 2-mm threaded half-pins, strongly fixed into both

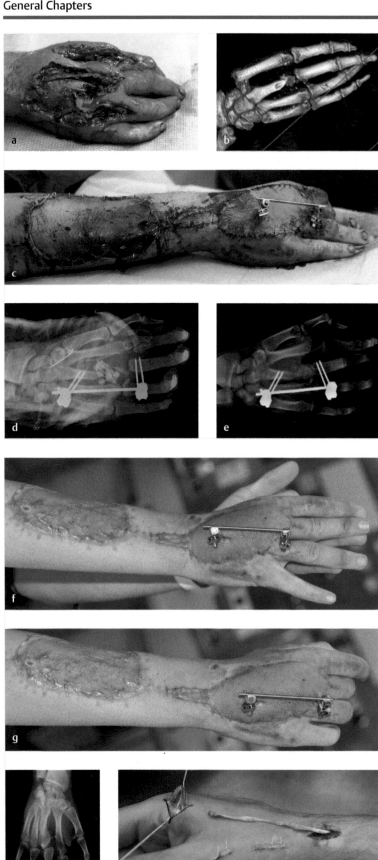

Fig. 7.1 (a) Severe crush open hand fracture in a young man. **(b)** Fracture-dislocation at the base of the second metacarpal, skeletal bone loss at neck and head of third metacarpal. Immediate coverage by posterior interosseous flap with insertion of tendon spacers at the level of the extensor apparatus of the long fingers. **(c)** Osteosynthesis of the second metacarpal by Kirschner's wire and of the third metacarpal by transarticular "bridging" external minifixation. **(d)** Note the insertion at the level of the bone loss of gentabeads—minigentabeads were not available at the time of this trauma. **(e)** After 2 months, replacement of the beads by a cancellous bone autograft. **(f, g)** At the same time, extensor tendon grafts using palmaris longus. **(h)** Good integration of the bone graft and restoration of functional metacarpophalangeal joint motion of third finger. **(i)** The patient regained excellent function but a late operation was needed to restore the index finger abduction (isolated palsy of first dorsal interosseous muscle related to the carpometacarpal dislocation of the base of the second ray).

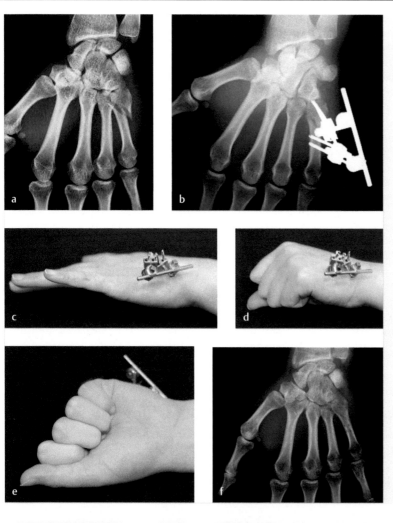

Fig. 7.2 (a) Closed fracture of the fifth metacarpal bone in a young woman. (b) Closed reduction and external minifixation. (c–e) Immediate postoperative active mobilization. (f) Solid bone union, 4 weeks later.

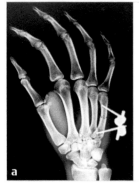
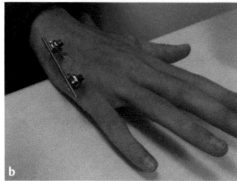

Fig. 7.3 (a, b) Use of one single pin in each fracture fragment.

cortices of intact parts of the bone on each side of the fracture, as close as possible to the fracture. The pins should not protrude more than 2 mm on the opposite site of insertion, to avoid soft tissue lesions, particularly of the flexor tendons and neurovascular bundles (in some rare cases we have used only one pin on either side of the fracture, relying on the good hold of this isolated pin in cortical bone, ▶ Fig. 7.3). One incision of 6 to 10 mm is used for the insertion of each group of parallel half-pins. The tendons and neurovascular structures are protected and the bone must be clearly visualized. Pilot holes of 1.5 mm are created with a power drill. The pins are then manually inserted. In the metacarpal bones of the long fingers, the pins are implanted in a 45-degree posteromedial or posterolateral direction, avoiding the extensor tendons and the superficial terminal sensory branches of the radial or ulnar nerves. In the first metacarpal, the pins should be implanted in the posteroradial aspect of the bone, radial to the extensor pollicis brevis tendon. In the proximal phalanx of the long bones, the pins are implanted on either side of the finger, in a posterolateral or posteromedial direction, through a small incision in the extensor apparatus. In the middle phalanx of the long bones or in the proximal phalanx of the thumb, the pins are implanted in the lateromedial or laterolateral aspect of the bone, if necessary through the oblique retinacular ligament, palmar to the extensor apparatus. In the distal phalanx, the pins must be inserted in the lateral or medial aspect of the bone, to avoid injury to the finger pulp or to the nail matrix. In the distal phalanx, the use of transfixing pins with a triangular frame is another choice.

Each cluster of two pins is fixed in a pin holder, positioned 5 mm away from the skin to allow postoperative care at the pin exit sites. In most cases, a single half-frame is constructed, connecting the pin holders by a single connecting rod. Before locking the clamps, the fracture is closely manually reduced, by manipulating the bone fragments through the pins, and the quality of reduction checked using the C-arm. It is particularly important to also visually check the rotational alignment. In rare circumstances, a limited open approach of the fracture is necessary to obtain a perfect reduction, but this can be avoided in most cases. In periarticular fractures, a transarticular "bridging" configuration may be applied, if the fracture is too close to the joint or extends up to the articular space, or to apply transarticular distraction with a ligamentotaxis effect to reduce a comminuted articular fracture (▶Fig. 7.1). At the end of the procedure, a light dressing is used, in closed fractures covering only the pin skin exit sites. No plaster or other form of hand immobilization is used. Elevation of the hand is recommended in the first postoperative days. Active motion of all joints is immediately permitted, initially under the control and encouragements of a physiotherapist. Pin tract care is done by the patient himself. After bone healing, the external minifixator is removed on an outpatient basis, usually without anesthesia.

7.3 Indications

The undisputed indication of external minifixation is the open metacarpal or phalangeal fracture, usually in association with various soft tissue injuries (▶Fig. 7.1). After initial debridement, irrigation, and assessment of the lesions, the external minifixator is first implanted and an anatomical reduction is obtained. In case of a bone loss, a temporary cement spacer or mini gentabeads are disposed at the fracture site.[14] Then all soft tissue lesions are repaired, including tendon, vessels, and nerve, using when necessary microsurgical technique. For the skin, a local or regional flap is frequently indicated. All efforts should be done to make it possible for the patient to shortly or immediately after the operation to be able to actively move the affected fingers. Sometimes, after a severe crush, an external minifixator is used to maintain the first web space open, to prevent a posttraumatic contracture.[15]

Infected nonunions are similarly treated by resecting all infected bone, stabilizing the finger by external minifixation—also useful to keep skeletal length, by inserting at the bone defect a cement antibiotic spacer, if necessary

by flap coverage, and by general antibiotherapy; after local healing and disappearance of all signs of infection, a cancellous bone autograft is applied, keeping the external minifixator until final healing.

External minifixation is as well a good technique to treat closed unstable metacarpal[11] or phalangeal fractures. Closed reduction and stable osteosynthesis by external minifixation allows immediate postoperative motion, the best way to prevent stiffness (▶Fig. 7.2). The alternative is plate fixation, not well tolerated in the phalanges under the extensor tendons, despite many artifices proposed by the proponents of internal fixation to prevent postoperative adherences. Some long oblique or spiral metacarpal fractures may be treated by isolated screws, but, after this form of osteosynthesis, the stability is not always sufficient to avoid some form of postoperative immobilization.

Comminuted articular or periarticular fractures may be treated by transarticular distraction, maintained by external fixation (▶Fig. 7.1). Because the ligaments are kept into tension, the affected joint may be fixed in extension, including at metacarpophalangeal level, a position usually contraindicated following the classical principles of protective position.[2] An alternative is the use of an articulated bridging minifixator, allowing early active motion.[16] However, it has been our experience that, at the hand, the quality of reduction obtained by "ligamentotaxis"[17] is not as good as at the distal radius[17] or at the base of the first metacarpal[18]: small articular fragments are not well pulled in place by transarticular distraction. This is especially true at the proximal interphalangeal joint level. Closed displaced articular hand fractures are indeed best treated by stable internal fixation with anatomical reduction and early motion (see also Chapter 18).

Because damage to the growth plate in children or adolescents easily can be avoided with this technique, external minifixation is also applicable in selected fractures in children, although Kirschner wires are more usually used at this age, as stiffness is less a concern in pediatrics.[12]

Corrective osteotomies for angular or rotation deformities can be fixed by external minifixation. The angle between the preimplanted pins may provide an easy reference for the final position of the corrected bone.

A classical indication of external fixation at the hand is finger lengthening, either after traumatic loss or in the context of a congenital deformity. Progressive distraction in the range of 1 mm per day allows spontaneous osteogenesis at the finger corticotomy site (▶Fig. 7.4). External minifixation may be used in selected cases of Kienböck's disease, to lengthen the capitate after lunarectomy.[19,20]

There are many other indications of external minifixation at the hand: treatment of a neglected joint dislocation, arthrodesis, maintenance of the length of the thumb and the space between the scaphoid and the base of the first metacarpal after trapeziectomy,[21] management of an infected trapeziometacarpal prosthesis (▶Fig. 7.5), soft tissue lengthening (burn, Dupuytren),[22–24] to cite some examples. Indeed, the possibilities of external fixation

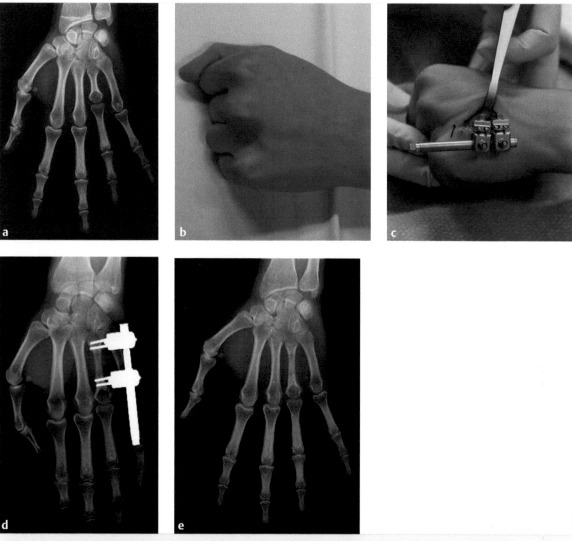

Fig. 7.4 (a, b) Congenital shortening of the fourth metacarpal. **(c, d)** Lengthening by external minifixation. **(e)** Final result.

are almost unlimited and the technique can be adapted to many different clinical situations.

7.4 Results

Fractures constituted 77.2% of the indications of external minifixation in our prospective study of 516 cases (closed fractures 55.6%, open fractures 21.6%). A transarticular bridging configuration was applied in 47.8%. Pin tract reactions were present in 9.8% of metacarpal pins and 2.5% of phalangeal pins. Overall, the average duration of external minifixation was 40.4 days. Primary bone healing was obtained in 95.3%, and there was no single case of a refracture. The rate of late CRPS was 5.5%.[9]

Selecting in the series 63 closed diaphyseal metacarpal fractures, closed reduction was possible in 74.2%; the median duration of fixation was 29 days; all fractures were united; an anatomical reduction was obtained in 86.1%; there was no case of CRPS, and the functional results were excellent or good in 96.6%.[9,11] The results were almost as excellent at the finger level: in 54 closed diaphyseal phalangeal fractures, a closed reduction could be performed in 81.1%; after a median duration of fixation of 30.3 days, all fractures were healed, and the reduction was anatomical in 90.5%; the rate of CRPS was 3.8%, and excellent or good functional results were obtained in 94.1%.[9]

7.5 Discussion

External minifixation is a KISS technique ("Keep It Safe and Simple"). The problems of internal fixation of infection, local discomfort, and tendon impingement are avoided. The natural bone healing processes are respected. The preservation of the gliding surfaces, and the stability provided by the mounting allow immediate mobilization of the injured finger, even in case of

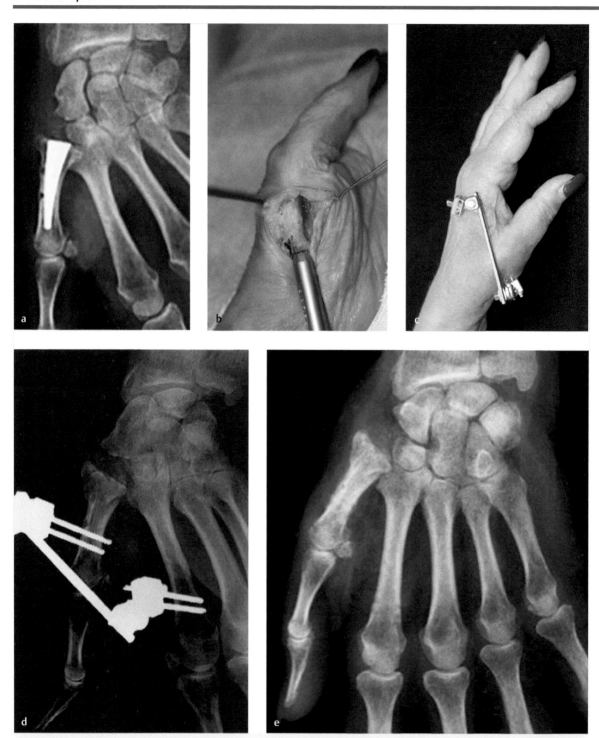

Fig. 7.5 (a) Infected trapeziometacarpal prosthetic arthroplasty, persistence of the infected metacarpal stem. The patient had earlier a trapeziectomy removing the trapezial cup, which did not resolve the infection. **(b)** A corticotomy was necessary to remove the well-integrated stem, despite the existence of lytic granulomas. **(c, d)** The first metacarpal bone was stabilized by an external minifixator, also maintaining the length of the thumb and preventing scaphometacarpal impingement. **(e)** Final result.

severe comminution or bone loss. Early active motion is the best way to prevent stiffness and CRPS.[25] In the first weeks after implantation, it is possible to readjust the frame to correct an insufficient reduction or a secondary displacement—the reduction errors, in particular in rotation, seen after internal fixation are impossible to correct without another surgical operation. Retrieval of the external minifixator is done on an outpatient basis, making a second operative procedure for hardware removal unnecessary.

A wide variety of clinical situations, including complex open fractures and fractures occurring in ischemic digits, and pediatric fractures, can be managed using external minifixation. Open and infected fractures and nonunions are of course classical indications. In case of bone loss, the length of the injured finger can easily be maintained, which is more difficult with other techniques. External minifixation is also an excellent technique to treat closed unstable metacarpal or phalangeal fractures, or to perform a corrective osteotomy. The possibility to apply progressive distraction allows the use of external minifixation to treat congenital or acquired hypoplasia.

External minifixation has drawbacks. The external frame can get caught in clothing. Some patients may find the presence of an external device unpleasant, especially if their surgeon is not at ease with it. If given a choice, immediate mobilization and early use of the hand with a minifixator, versus having their hand imprisoned in a bulky plaster cast, most patients vote in favor of external minifixation. Bone and skin reactions to the pins are not uncommon, especially in metacarpal bones. Most infections are superficial and successfully treated by local pin disinfection and/or oral antibiotherapy. In the fingers, the transfixion of the extensor apparatus may cause some limitation of active motion. Full mobility is usually regained after retrieval of the device, after a couple of weeks. This problem is usually worse if Kirschner's wires are used, as the wires, usually implanted obliquely, restrain a larger tendon area. Adhesions of the extensor apparatus are also seen after dorsal plate osteosynthesis, the plate staying longer time in place. The main disadvantage of external minifixation is that it remains an expensive implant. Hopefully the industry will soon make this excellent technique more affordable. We reuse the clamps and the rods, the Belgian social security allowing renting this material. Of course, the pins are single use.

References

[1] Wright TA. Early mobilization in fractures of the metacarpals and phalanges. Can J Surg. 1968; 11(4):491–498

[2] James JIP. The assessment and management of the injured hand. Hand. 1970; 2(2):97–105

[3] Stellbrink G. Ausseres Fixationsgerät für Fingerarthrodesen. Chirurg. 1969; 40(9):422–423

[4] Dickson RA. Rigid fixation of unstable metacarpal fractures using transverse K-wires bonded with acrylic resin. Hand. 1975; 7(3):284–286

[5] Volkov MV, Oganesian OV. The Volkov-Oganesian apparatus for interphalangeal joint movement restitution. Model V Moscow 1976:1–6

[6] Asche G, Haas HG, Klemm K. Erste Erfahrungen mit dem Minifixateur externe nach Jaquet. Aktuelle Traumatol. 1979; 9(5):261–268

[7] Burny F, Moermans JP, Quintin J. Utilisation du minifixateur en chirurgie de la main. Acta Orthop Belg. 1980; 46(3):251–261

[8] Asche G, Burny F. Indikation für die Andwendung des Minifixateur externe. Eine statistische Analyse. Akt Traumatol.. 1982; 12:103–110

[9] Schuind F, Burny F. New techniques of osteosynthesis of the hand. Principles, clinical applications and biomechanics with special reference to external minifixation. In: Eberle H, ed. Reconstruction Surgery and Traumatology. Basel, Switzerland: Karger; 1990:1–159

[10] Schuind FA, Burny F, Chao EY. Biomechanical properties and design considerations in upper extremity external fixation. Hand Clin. 1993; 9(4):543–553

[11] Schuind F, Donkerwolcke M, Burny F. External minifixation for treatment of closed fractures of the metacarpal bones. J Orthop Trauma. 1991; 5(2):146–152

[12] De Kesel R, Burny F, Schuind F. Mini external fixation for hand fractures and dislocations: The current state of the art. Hand Clin. 2006; 22(3):307–315

[13] Schuind F, El Kazzi W, Cermak K, Donkerwolcke M, Burny F. Fixation externe au poignet et à la main. Rev Med Brux. 2011; 32 suppl:71–75

[14] Schuind F, Potaznik A, Burny F. A technique for finger reconstruction after open injury with skeletal defect. In: Kasdan ML, Amadio PC, Bowers WH, eds. Technical Tips on Hand Surgery. Philadelphia, PA: Mosby, St Louis, MO: Hanley & Belfus; 1994:37–38

[15] Lees VC, Wren C, Elliot D. Internal splints for prevention of first web contracture following severe disruption of the first web space. J Hand Surg [Br]. 1994; 19(5):560–562

[16] Leloup T, De Greef A, Bantuelle S, et al. Design of an articulated mini-fixation device for proximal interphalangeal joint finger fractures. Proceedings of the annual conference of the IEEE/ Engineering in Medicine and Biology Society. 2007;100–103

[17] Schuind F, Donkerwolcke M, Rasquin C, Burny F. External fixation of fractures of the distal radius: a study of 225 cases. J Hand Surg Am. 1989; 14(2 pt 2):404–407

[18] Schuind F, Noorbergen M, Andrianne Y, Burny F. Comminuted fractures of the base of the first metacarpal treated by distraction-external fixation. J Orthop Trauma. 1988; 2(4):314–321

[19] Schuind F, Eslami S, Ledoux P. Kienbock's disease. J Bone Joint Surg Br. 2008; 90(2):133–139

[20] Schuind F, Moungondo F. Lunarectomy and progressive capitate lengthening (modified Graner-Wilhelm procedure). In: Lichtman DM, Bain GI, eds. Kienböck's Disease. Advances in Diagnosis and Treatment. Switzerland: Springer; 2016:249–254

[21] Putterie G, Créteur V, Mouraux D, Robert C, El-Kazzi W, Schuind F. Trapeziometacarpal osteoarthrosis: clinical results and sonographic evaluation of the interposed tissue after trapeziectomy and first metacarpal suspension by external minifixation at a minimal two-year follow-up. Chir Main. 2014; 33(1):29–37

[22] Gulati S, Joshi BB, Milner SM. Use of Joshi External Stabilizing System in postburn contractures of the hand and wrist: a 20-year experience. J Burn Care Rehabil. 2004; 25(5):416–420

[23] Hodgkinson PD. The use of skeletal traction to correct the flexed PIP joint in Dupuytren's disease. A pilot study to assess the use of the Pipster. J Hand Surg [Br]. 1994; 19(4):534–537

[24] Agee JM, Goss BC. The use of skeletal extension torque in reversing Dupuytren contractures of the proximal interphalangeal joint. J Hand Surg Am. 2012; 37(7):1467–1474

[25] Schuind F, Burny F. Can algodystrophy be prevented after hand surgery? Hand Clin. 1997; 13(3):455–476

8 Role of Arthroscopy in the Treatment of Carpal Fractures and Nonunion

Peter Jørgsholm

Abstract

Arthroscopy has resulted in a new three-dimensional (3D) and dynamic understanding of the wrist joint and carpal joints and a better comprehension of the pathomechanism of carpal fractures and ligament injuries. MRI and CT scans have added better diagnosis of carpal fractures and injuries and combined with arthroscopy a possibility of a tailored treatment plan for these often complex injuries. This new knowledge can benefit the patients and give them a faster return of wrist function.

Keywords: arthroscopy, scaphoid fracture, carpal fracture, scapholunate (SL) ligament injury, lunotriquetral (LT) ligament injury, scaphoid nonunion, cannulated screw fixation, bone grafting

8.1 Introduction

The most common carpal fracture is scaphoid fracture followed by capitate and triquetral fracture[1,2] (▶ Fig. 8.1). Combined carpal fractures are not uncommon (12%) and often seen after high-energy trauma—probably as part of a greater arc injury presenting as a perilunate injury nondislocated (PLIND).[3] The most frequent carpal fracture combination is that of a scaphoid and capitate fracture (8% of scaphoid fractures). The sensitivity of radiography is low in diagnosing carpal fractures especially in children and MRI or CT is often necessary to get the diagnosis and should always be considered when adequate trauma is involved.[1,2]

After the introduction of wrist arthroscopy in the 1980s, the technical advances of scopes, cameras, instruments, and traction devices as well as fluoroscopes and cannulated screws have made arthroscopic reduction and internal fixation (ARIF) possible. The stability of fractures and ligament injuries is visualized in a live 3D fashion and the surgeon can tailor a treatment and postoperative mobilization for each individual injury. In the case of late presentation and bone deficit, techniques for percutaneous bone grafting are increasingly used particularly in scaphoid nonunions.

8.2 Indications

It is generally accepted that proximal pole fractures of the scaphoid have a poor prognosis when treated conservatively with one-third going into nonunion.[4] Many therefore offer surgery to patients with fracture in the

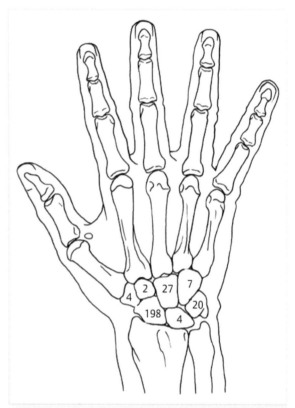

Fig. 8.1 Two hundred and sixty-two carpal fractures diagnosed by MRI in 403 patients presenting with posttraumatic radial-sided wrist pain: 75% scaphoid fractures, 10% capitate fractures, 8% triquetral fractures, and 3% hamate fractures.

proximal third of the scaphoid. Proximal pole fractures are easily approached from dorsal when using a traction tower and often quite stable and nondisplaced.

Displaced (> 1 mm) fractures have a nonunion rate of 27% and require twice as long to unite as nondisplaced (13 weeks).[5] Comminuted fractures have a nonunion rate of 11% with 60% longer time to union (10 weeks).[5] Displaced and comminuted scaphoid fractures are more difficult to treat by ARIF as the reduction can be challenging. Greater arc injuries need reduction and stability to unite[6] and several reports on arthroscopic approach to these injuries are reported in recent years.[7,8]

The current recommendations for surgical treatment of scaphoid fractures are listed in ▶ Table 8.1.

Other carpal fractures and intercarpal ligament injuries will reveal during MRI, CT, and the arthroscopic procedure.

Table 8.1 Indication for surgical treatment of scaphoid fractures (ORIF or ARIF)

1. Displaced fractures (> 1 mm/15-degree palmar)[a]

2. Comminuted fractures[a]

3. Proximal pole fractures (proximal third)[b]

4. Transscaphoid perilunate dislocation

5. More than one fracture (PLIND?)

6. Late diagnosed fractures (> 4 weeks)[b]

7. Bilateral fractures

8. Multitrauma

Abbreviations: ARIF, arthroscopic reduction and internal fixation; ORIF, open reduction internal fixation; PLIND, perilunate injury nondislocated.
[a] Significant higher risk of nonunion (Grewal 2013[5]).
[b] Significant higher risk of delayed union (Grewal 2013,[5] 2016[9]).

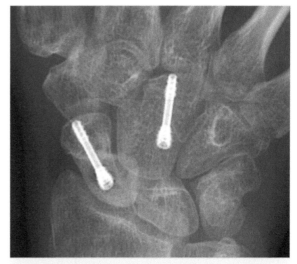

Fig. 8.3 Posteroanterior radiograph of ARIF with cannulated screws of simultaneous scaphoid and capitate fracture by dorsal approach.

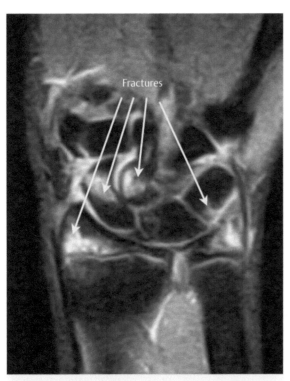

Fractures

Fig. 8.2 STIR coronal of an ice hockey player's wrist after a high-energy trauma. Nondisplaced scaphoid fracture found on CT. MRI reveals further nondisplaced fractures in radius, capitate, and triquetrum as indicated by *arrows*.

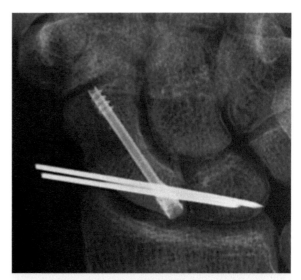

Fig. 8.4 PA radiograph of ARIF with cannulated screw and temporary K-wire fixation of simultaneous scaphoid and SL ligament injury.

At arthroscopy, the carpal and fracture stability can be tested by probing carpal bones and fractures fragments, respectively. A tailored treatment can then be implemented accordingly. In some cases, multiple fractures are diagnosed by MRI (▶Fig. 8.2) and found stable at arthroscopy and consequently treated with a cast. These patients are checked at 6 weeks and union estimated by CT scans. In other instances, both unstable scaphoid fractures and capitate fractures need ARIF (▶Fig. 8.3). In some cases, a combination of ARIF and percutaneous pinning is necessary, for example, in the simultaneous scaphoid waist

fracture and complete SL ligament injury which is seen in 24%[10] (▶Fig. 8.4). Even carpal fractures other than scaphoid are sometimes found unstable and therefor suitable for ARIF (▶Fig. 8.5).

In the case of late presentation, particularly scaphoid delayed union and nonunion, a CT scan will give a hint of whether cleaning of fracture area and bone grafting will be necessary. This can be done with cancellous bone from radius in case of smaller defects and/or cysts, but if a larger defect or deformity is encountered, cancellous bone graft from the iliac crest is needed (▶Fig. 8.6). The union rate after arthroscopic scaphoid nonunion procedures are similar or better than with open procedures.[11–15]

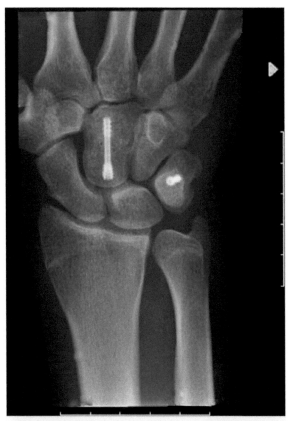

Fig. 8.5 PA radiograph of ARIF with cannulated screws in simultaneous capitate and triquetral fractures by dorsal approach.

8.3 Method

8.3.1 Diagnosis

At least four radiographic views of the wrist and the scaphoid are recommended as initial investigation. If no fracture is found but clinical suspicion persists, MRI is indicated. MRI with a low-field scanner (> 0.23 T) is sufficient for diagnosis of carpal fractures and has a high sensitivity.[1,2] If a carpal fracture is found on radiographs, CT scans are indicated to evaluate if any displacement or comminution exist. If a fracture reveal on MRI and any displacement is suspected, CT scan is indicated. CT scanning with axial sections of less than 0.6 mm and reconstructions in the coronal and sagittal planes defined by the long axis of the scaphoid and a 3D reconstruction will give detailed information of comminution or any displacement such as translation (step-off), gapping (diastasis), or angulation (humpback deformity). All this information enables the treating surgeon to decide on operation and provide him/her with a better 3D understanding of the injury.

8.3.2 Surgical Procedures

For arthroscopic procedures in the radiocarpal and the midcarpal joint, a small arthroscope (< 3 mm) and small joint instruments are needed. A traction device will help the surgeon to keep a constant distraction for easy joint access and support from the tower will minimize the need for an assistant surgeon (▶Fig. 8.7). For reduction, a steady probe is important and 1.25-mm K-wires as joysticks or for temporary arthrodesis in intercarpal ligament injuries are needed. For internal fixation, cannulated screws in different dimensions and length should be available (▶Fig. 8.8). A fluoroscope is a must for viewing and documenting fracture reduction and hardware position (▶Fig. 8.9).

A dorsal approach is possible for most of the carpal fractures (▶Fig. 8.10). In scaphoid fractures, flexion of the wrist will present the proximal pole for insertion of a guidewire through portal 3–4 with the scope inserted in portal 4–5 or 5–6 (▶Fig. 8.11). Cleaning of debris, blood, and synovitis gives a better view and facilitates correct placement of a guidewire as palmar as possible and just adjacent to the SL ligament (▶Fig. 8.12). The guidewire is directed toward the thumb base blindly and then controlled on fluoroscope. By introducing the guidewire into the trapezium, the wire is secured during drilling (▶Fig. 8.13). Reduction is often obtained by traction and controlled by midcarpal arthroscopy. If not reduced, the guidewire is retracted to the fracture gap and by manipulating fragments eventually using probe, the blunt trocar, or K-wires as joysticks, the fracture can gently be reduced. In smaller wrists a 1.9-mm scope can be used for the midcarpal arthroscopy. The SL and LT intervals are controlled for any instability. Most capitate, lunate, triquetral, and some hamate fractures are seen by midcarpal arthroscopy. SL and LT ligament injuries are visualized by both radiocarpal and midcarpal arthroscopy. The triangular fibrocartilage complex (TFCC) injuries are viewed from radiocarpal ulnar portals. All joint surfaces in radiocarpal and midcarpal joint are carefully inspected for any lesions and eventually loose bodies removed. In case of simultaneous fracture and ligament injury, it is advisable to start with the fracture as the screws are more bulky and difficult to insert if several K-wires cross the joints. The combination of an unstable scaphoid waist fracture and a complete SL ligament injury creates a floating proximal scaphoid pole (▶Fig. 8.14).

When bone grafting is indicated, standard instrumentations can be used for arthroscopic bone grafting (▶Fig. 8.15). The bone is taken from the distal radius or iliac crest depending on the amount needed for filling the defect. A minimal invasive motorized drill system for taking morselized bone facilitates this procedure (Acumed, Oregon, United States) (▶Fig. 8.16). If a humpback deformity has been reduced, plenty of packed cancellous bone graft will be able to fill and support the reconstruction. Tissue glue is sometimes added to protect the graft. The fragments are stabilized with screw(s) and/or K-wires.

If the fractures, delayed unions, or nonunions are considered arthroscopically stable after screw fixation, the patient is mobilized. If the fracture is not stable,

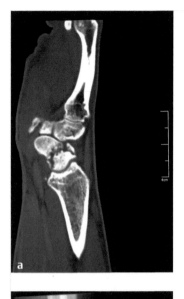
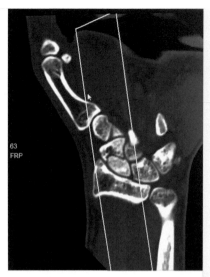

Fig. 8.6 (a) Lateral and PA CT scans of scaphoid nonunion with large defect. (b) PA and lateral radiographs at 5 months showing united nonunion (confirmed by CT at 3 months).

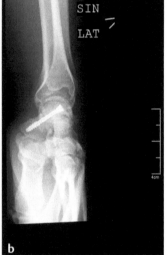
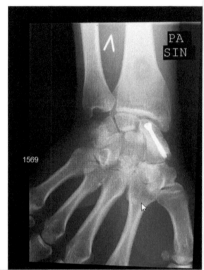

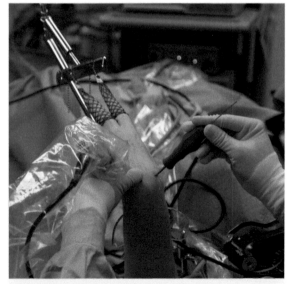

Fig. 8.7 Dorsal approach with wrist in traction tower.

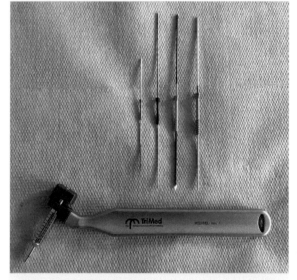

Fig. 8.8 Cannulated screws from left 1.7, 2.3, 3, and 3.5-mm. Guidewire sleeve and drill sleeve for 2.3-mm screw. (Trimed, California, United States)

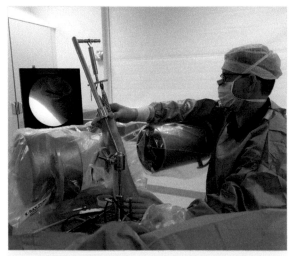

Fig. 8.9 Intraoperative fluoroscopy during ARIF of scaphoid fracture.

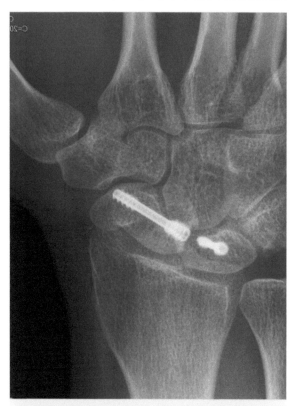

Fig. 8.10 ARIF with cannulated screws of simultaneous scaphoid and lunate fracture approached from dorsal.

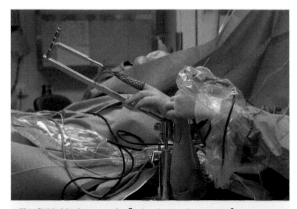

Fig. 8.11 Maximum wrist flexion in traction tower for easy access to proximal pole of the scaphoid.

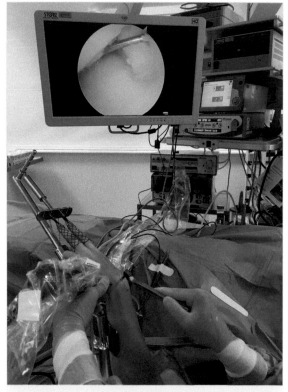

Fig. 8.12 Entrance point of guidewire as palmar as possible and just adjacent to the SL ligament.

the patient is immobilized in a below-elbow cast until union is greater than 50% as seen by CT scan.[16] When any temporary intercarpal fixation is used, a protective plaster is applied until removal of K-wires usually around 6 weeks. The patient is not allowed to take part in any heavy lifting, contact sport, or risky activity before at least 50% union is seen on CT scan and 80% of contralateral grip force is regained.

8.3.3 Clinical Example

An 18-year-old right-hand dominant man, toolmaker crashed on his mountain bike. Following the injury, he visited the emergency room complaining of radial-sided pain in his left wrist. According to the treating doctor and the radiologist, no sign of fracture was seen on initial X-rays (▶Fig. 8.17). He was treated with a dorsal splint and planned for orthopedic follow-up, but he never received any appointment and removed his splint after 2 weeks. Because of persistent pain, he was referred to a hand surgeon by his general practitioner 3 weeks following the initial injury.

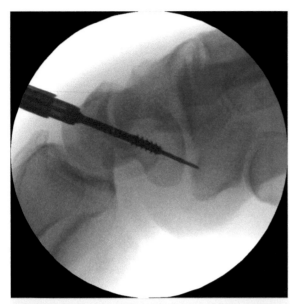

Fig. 8.13 By driving K-wire through the scaphoid into the trapezium, it is secured during drilling.

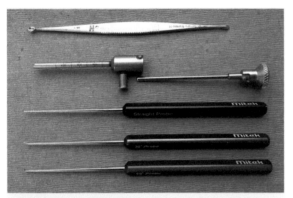

Fig. 8.15 Bone grafting instruments: mini curette, 2.7-mm cannula, and blunt troachar for inserting cancellous bone into nonunion defect. Different study probes for reduction and bone packing.

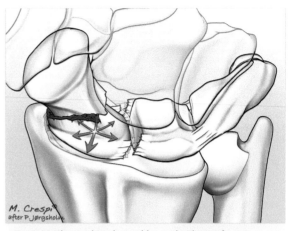

Fig. 8.14 The combined unstable scaphoid waist fracture and complete SL ligament rupture. The "floating" proximal scaphoid fracture fragment with minimal vascular supply. (Copyright Peter Jørgsholm and Massimiliano Crespi.)

Pearls

- In young male patients, with high-energy trauma combined injuries can be expected and MRI and/or CT scans are indicated.
- If a fracture is displaced, manipulation in the traction tower, probing, and eventually use of K-wires as joysticks will reduce the displacement in most cases.
- To avoid withdrawal of the guidewire after drilling, it could be inserted through the scaphoid into the trapezium.
- Intra-articular capitate, lunate, triquetral, and hamate fractures can be approached from a dorsal proximal direction. Proximal capitate fractures can be reached from a distal dorsal direction.

Pitfalls

- When using a cannulated screw, the screw used should allow for a guidewire of at least 1 mm. A thinner guidewire is difficult to drill through the bone as you might lose control of the direction while drilling.
- In the case of a small proximal pole fragment, a standard headless cannulated screw is too large in diameter and often too long in the threaded part to be able to have a compression function. In these cases, a mini cannulated screw or eventually a set of two will be convenient. The guidewire then often has a diameter of less than 1 mm, but guidewire insertion in proximal pole fractures are straightforward with a 0.8-mm guidewire since the screws have to penetrate the distal fragment for a short distance only.

Fluoroscan showed a scaphoid waist fracture and CT revealed a translunate arc injury[17] (▶ Fig. 8.18): a comminuted transverse scaphoid waist fracture, a palmar chip fracture in the lunate, and a transverse fracture in the triquetrum (▶ Fig. 8.19).

As comminution in the scaphoid was observed and instability, therefore likely arthroscopy was offered and revealed an unstable scaphoid and lunate fracture (palmar chip too small for osteosynthesis) and a stable triquetrum fracture. The scaphoid fracture was stabilized with an antegrade cannulated screw and the lunate and triquetrum fractures were treated conservatively with a below-elbow thumb spica. At 9 weeks, CT scans showed the fractures united and the patient was able to start pzart time on his job at 12 weeks.

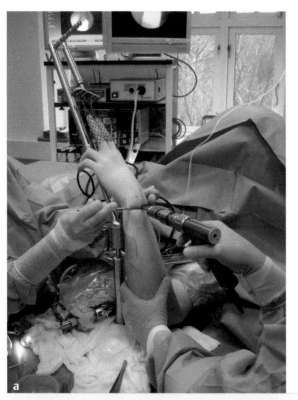
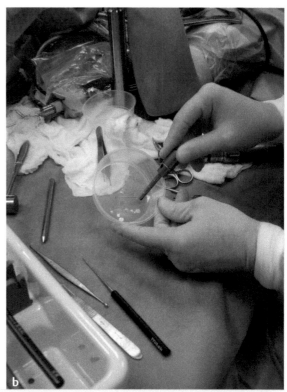

Fig. 8.16 **(a)** Motorized bone drill for bone harvest. **(b)** Cancellous bone to be introduced into the wrist through a cannula.

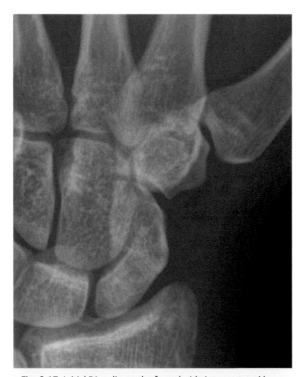

Fig. 8.17 Initial PA radiograph of scaphoid—interpretated by treating doctor and radiologist as normal.

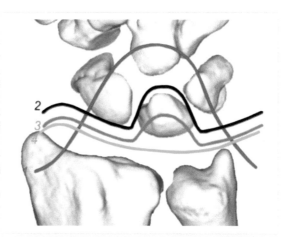

Fig. 8.18 Arc injuries, coronal plane. 1: greater arc; 2: lesser arc; 3: translunate arc; 4: inferior arc.

8.4 Conclusion

Arthroscopic-assisted evaluation, reduction, and percutaneous fixation of carpal fractures is challenging for the surgeon, but combined with preoperative MRI and CT scans with 3D reconstruction, it allows for a tailored treatment ranging from simple plaster treatment to advanced arthroscopic pinning and screw fixation

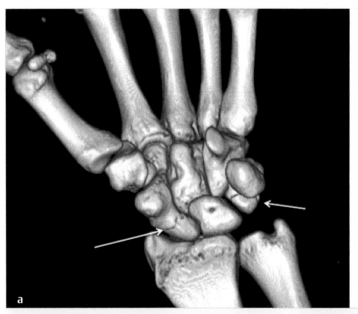
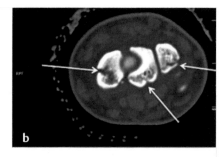
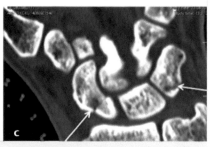

Fig. 8.19 (a) Three-dimensional CT with the scaphoid and triquetral fractures visible. (b) Transverse view showing all three fractures (scaphoid, lunate, and triquetral fractures). (c) Coronal view showing scaphoid and triquetral fractures.

Table 8.2 Advantages of arthroscopic carpal fracture treatment

- Minimal invasive
- Direct vision of fracture stability
- Diagnosis and treatment of ligament injuries
- Cleaning of interposed soft tissue
- Reduction of displacement
- Control of hardware
- Information on cartilage injuries
- Viability of fracture fragments by releasing tourniquet
- A better 3D understanding of fracture morphology

depending on injury pattern (e.g., lesser arc and greater arc injuries,[18] translunate and inferior arc injuries,[17] and PLIND injuries[3]). The advantages of arthroscopic techniques in fracture treatment are listed in ▶Table 8.2.

References

[1] Jørgsholm P, Thomsen NO, Besjakov J, Abrahamsson SO, Björkman A. The benefit of magnetic resonance imaging for patients with posttraumatic radial wrist tenderness. J Hand Surg Am. 2013; 38(1):29–33

[2] Jørgsholm P, Thomsen NO, Besjakov J, Abrahamsson SO, Björkman A. MRI shows a high incidence of carpal fractures in children with posttraumatic radial-sided wrist tenderness. Acta Orthop. 2016; 87(5):533–537

[3] Herzberg G. Perilunate injuries, not dislocated (PLIND). J Wrist Surg. 2013; 2(4):337–345

[4] Eastley N, Singh H, Dias JJ, Taub N. Union rates after proximal scaphoid fractures; meta-analyses and review of available evidence. J Hand Surg Eur Vol. 2013; 38(8):888–897

[5] Grewal R, Suh N, Macdermid JC. Use of computed tomography to predict union and time to union in acute scaphoid fractures treated nonoperatively. J Hand Surg Am. 2013; 38(5):872–877

[6] Herzberg G, Comtet JJ, Linscheid RL, Amadio PC, Cooney WP, Stalder J. Perilunate dislocations and fracture-dislocations: a multicenter study. J Hand Surg Am. 1993; 18(5):768–779

[7] Kim JP, Lee JS, Park MJ. Arthroscopic treatment of perilunate dislocations and fracture dislocations. J Wrist Surg. 2015; 4(2):81–87

[8] Liu B, Chen SL, Zhu J, Tian GL. Arthroscopic management of perilunate injuries. Hand Clin. 2017; 33(4):709–715

[9] Grewal R, Lutz K, MacDermid JC, Suh N. Proximal pole scaphoid fractures: a computed tomographic assessment of outcomes. J Hand Surg Am. 2016; 41(1):54–58

[10] Jørgsholm P, Thomsen NO, Björkman A, Besjakov J, Abrahamsson SO. The incidence of intrinsic and extrinsic ligament injuries in scaphoid waist fractures. J Hand Surg Am. 2010; 35(3):368–374

[11] Slade JF, III, Gillon T. Retrospective review of 234 scaphoid fractures and nonunions treated with arthroscopy for union and complications. Scand J Surg. 2008; 97(4):280–289

[12] Wong WY, Ho PC. Minimal invasive management of scaphoid fractures: from fresh to nonunion. Hand Clin. 2011; 27(3):291–307

[13] Kim JP, Seo JB, Yoo JY, Lee JY. Arthroscopic management of chronic unstable scaphoid nonunions: effects on restoration of carpal alignment and recovery of wrist function. Arthroscopy. 2015; 31(3):460–469

[14] Kang HJ, Chun YM, Koh IH, Park JH, Choi YR. Is arthroscopic bone graft and fixation for scaphoid nonunions effective? Clin Orthop Relat Res. 2016; 474(1):204–212

[15] Delgado-Serrano PJ, Jiménez-Jiménez I, Nikolaev M, Figueredo-Ojeda FA, Rozas-López MG. Arthroscopic reconstruction for unstable scaphoid non-union. Rev Esp Cir Ortop Traumatol. 2017; 61(4):216–223

[16] Singh HP, Forward D, Davis TR, Dawson JS, Oni JA, Downing ND. Partial union of acute scaphoid fractures. J Hand Surg [Br]. 2005; 30(5):440–445

[17] Bain GI, Pallapati S, Eng K. Translunate perilunate injuries-a spectrum of this uncommon injury. J Wrist Surg. 2013; 2(1):63–68

[18] Mayfield JK, Johnson RP, Kilcoyne RK. Carpal dislocations: pathomechanics and progressive perilunar instability. J Hand Surg Am. 1980; 5(3):226–241

9 Strategies in Compound Hand Injuries

Thomas Giesen, Olga Politikou, Maurizio Calcagni

Abstract

Compound fractures of the hand are one of the ultimate challenges for the surgeon and probably these contribute to define a hand surgeon. Complex open fractures with soft tissue destruction should be treated by someone with a solid knowledge about the diagnosis and treatment of all structures of the hand (and a great confidence in microsurgical reconstruction). These injuries need a precise strategy from the very beginning in order to achieve a reasonable good outcome, saving surgical time and useless procedures. It is in the interest of the patient, of the surgeon, and the community that a dedicated surgeon with all those competencies will deal with such devastating injuries. In this field, it is of paramount difficulty to provide evidence-based solutions and strategies. The authors offer their point of view about general strategies for the compound hand and some advices about how to deal with the different structures.

Keywords: compound injuries of the hand, open fracture, bone reconstruction, nerve tissue reconstruction, tendon repair, hand flaps, soft tissue reconstruction

9.1 Introduction

Decision making in compound hand injuries is one of the most complicated fields in hand surgery. The treatment of these complex injuries requires highly skilled hand surgeons, with great technical confidence in dealing with complex patterns of fractures, multiple soft tissue injuries and defects, reconstructive procedures, and high-level microsurgery. A complex compound injury to the hand should never be treated by different specialties in different surgical sessions; this would jeopardize a good functional result by delaying rehabilitation, while implying multiple operations for the patient, a longer hospitalization time, and higher costs for the community.[1] Every injury is significantly different and a systematic classification is a paramount challenge. "Evidence-based" medicine is far from being available.

On top of this, social and cultural differences among different countries in the world, and also among different regions in the same country, as well as the social and cultural status of the patient, are elements heavily influencing the decision making.

Finally, yet important, it should be clear that a concomitant open fracture of a phalanx and a metacarpal with skin loss is not comparable with an open tibia fracture with skin loss; the principles of limbs traumatology do not apply necessarily to the hand, and in many cases are counterproductive.

9.2 Patient Expectation

We often take our hands for granted and only realize how functionally and aesthetically important they are when they are injured.

The goal of management of hand trauma is to restore anatomy and function while avoiding prolonged immobilization. No other part of our extremities is susceptible to stiffness as the hand; this fact is easily acknowledged when considering that the hand is the part of our skeleton that is most constantly moving.

Restoration of the aesthetic element is also a goal of the management.

In severe hand traumas, this task is even more difficult due to its anatomical and functional complexity. Reconstructive procedures have to address all damaged structures and tissues in order to achieve a good recovery.

Unfortunately, very often the expectation of patients is not realistic. In the compound hand, it should be made clear from the very beginning to the patient that a return to normality is a rare exception. The first contact with the patient should be done by an experienced hand surgeon who realistically can advise the patient about the expected outcome.

9.3 Clinical Examination

A complete medical history of the patient might be difficult to obtain in an emergency situation. Nevertheless, the mechanism of injury, the occupation of the patient, and potential pathologies that can jeopardize the result of a microsurgical procedure should be clarified before surgery.

In an ideal setup, the examination of the severely mangled hand should be performed by a most experienced hand surgeon in the operating theater. The main goal of the first examination is to assess the following:

The vitality of the soft tissue of the injured areas, including the perfusion of the digital extremities; the stability of the skeleton; the contamination of the injury; a primary balance of the structures that need to be reconstructed. As in traumatology in general, the most obvious lesion should be the latest to examine. Amputated parts, also from other extremities like the lower extremities, should never be discarded (▶ Fig. 9.1), as they may be used as tissue banks.

9.4 Imaging

Radiographs are the mandatory first-level examination. If available as an emergency examination, a computed tomography (CT) scan completes the radiographs for a better evaluation especially of the joints and adds

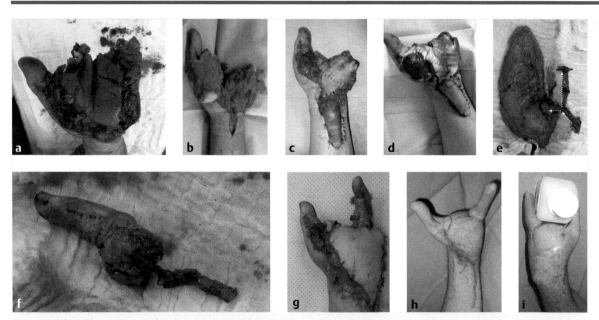

Fig. 9.1 **(a)** Highly contaminated explosion trauma to the nondominant hand of a 52-year-old male patient. In the first surgical time, an aggressive debridement was performed and dorsal and palmar skin to the midcarpal hand temporarily readapted. **(b, c)** The only replantable middle finger was temporarily etherotopically replanted to the wrist on the ulnar artery. **(d)** In a second surgical time, when the extension of the necrosis to the palmar and dorsal skin became evident, a second debridement was performed, the palmar and dorsal skin of the hand restored with an ALT flow-through flap. **(e, f, g)** The previously replanted finger at the distal forearm was reamputated and replanted on the top of the fourth metacarpal through the vessels of the flow-through ALT flap. **(h, i)** The final functional result.

valuable information about bone and joint status in concomitant closed injuries (e.g., adjacent fingers). Magnetic resonance imaging (MRI) is very rarely indicated, if ever. Angiograms might be indicated in injuries involving macrosegments.

9.5 Classification

The fracture classification of Gustilo and Anderson,[2] originally developed from experience with tibial fractures and frequently applied to long bones, has rarely been applied to injuries of the hand and current classification schemas for open fractures are insufficient to describe and indicate treatment of fractures of the hand. For example, the laceration size cutoffs for Gustilo–Anderson types (1 and 10 cm) are not realistic for a limb as small as the hand and its fingers.[3] A specialized classification has been introduced[3] that could take into account risk factors for infection specific to the hand when determining the best treatment of open fractures. This classification, summarized in ▶Table 9.1, also introduced the concept that not all open fractures to the hand should be treated as emergency cases.

9.6 Timing

"Current guidelines suggest early surgical treatment of open fractures. This rule in open hand fractures is not well supported and may be practically difficult to observe."[4]

Table 9.1 Classification of compound hand lesions (adapted from Tulipan and Ilyas)[3]

Location		Modifiers	
Type I	Phalanx	A	Primary soft tissue coverage not possible
Type II	Metacarpal	B	Frank contamination
Type III	Carpus	C	Avascularity requiring revascularization

The classification proposed by Tulipan and Ilyas is more reasonable for use in hand traumas, even if some mixed complex injuries involving metacarpal and digits or multiple fingers might be difficult to classify.

The treatment of open fractures in the hand has not been well established. The above-mentioned study did not support the necessity of immediate operation (within 6–8 hours) on all compound lesion to the hands as the infection rate did not correlate to the timing of the definitive intervention.

However, the lesion should be immediately rinsed and antibiotic treatment started. Especially in compound lesion to the digits, a more complex reconstructive surgery can be delayed if we are able to adequately rinse the fracture, adapt the skin over the bone, and stabilize it with a splint or with an external fixator.

On the other hand, devascularizing injuries or instability of the skeleton, putting the survival of the segments at risk, must be treated without delay.

9.7 Surgery

In our practice, surgery of the compound hand is performed in several steps, but following few principles:

- **Simplify:** In a very complex injury, restoring a digit or hand with all its structures to perfect anatomy increases the complexity of the procedure and may be far too time and resource consuming and not going to improve the functional outcome. Focus on the important structures. A typical example is the priority that flexors have above the extensors. Or, the management of complex phalanx fractures with a small shortening of the bone resulting in an easy and more stable fixation and a more straightforward approximation of tendons, vessels, and nerves, avoiding the need of multiple grafts.

  Another example is in case of multiple finger injuries. The thumb has always the highest priority. Then it is important to "ulnarize" the hand giving priority to the middle finger, for example, over the index finger, possibly using the index finger to reconstruct a better middle finger than spend time to reconstruct a bad index and a bad middle finger.

- **Do everything in a single session:** As largely reported in Europe[1] and United States,[5] we tend to repair or reconstruct as much as we can in one session in order to start the mobilization of the hand as soon as possible. This principle is only apparently in contrast with the principle of simplification. In reality, it means that once a plan is made for the repair or reconstruction of the injured segments, most of the steps should be performed during primary surgery in order to permit early mobilization.

- **Work systematically:** When repairing or reconstructing, we prefer to do it structure by structure rather than segment by segment in case of multiple segment injuries.[6] This has an important practical value; for example, finish the work needing an image intensifier before proceeding to the microscope, rather than alternating several times. Or, in the case of revascularization of multiple segments, avoid delaying revascularization of the last segment, when, for example, being happy with the reestablished vascularity of the first two segments.

9.8 Surgical Steps

9.8.1 Debridement

Debridement is the most difficult moment in the reconstructive process. Not because of the required technical skills, but because of the expertise required to make a judgement of the lesion, to decide whether tissues are viable or not, and to decide what shall be reconstructed and what shall not be reconstructed. The most experienced surgeon at hand with the highest confidence in the reconstructive possibilities should perform the debridement. As stated by Lister and Scheker, "... much discipline is necessary when debriding because the luxury of a second look is surrendered."[7]

In simple words, debridement should be performed by someone who is not afraid of excising tissue of dubious viability, thanks to her or his solid experience. Tissue without potential viability must be excised in order to make a proper reconstruction and not preserved in the hope that it may possibly to survive.

9.8.2 Bone Fixation

Bone fixation is probably the field where the principles of orthopaedic traumatology that apply to the long bones strongly diverge from the principles for the reconstruction of the hand.

In compound lesions, and especially in devascularizing injuries, bone fixation needs to be quick. In multiple replantation or in severe trauma, the use of longitudinal K-wires or K-wires and intramedullary screws[8] saves time for the microsurgical procedures as in the example in ▶ Fig. 9.2. Intramedullary fixation with screws is preferred to plates as it is a quick way for fixation without applying fixation material on the outer surface of the bone, giving a better functional result.

Bone grafting, contrary to what is believed by many, can be performed in primary surgery after adequate debridement if viable soft tissue coverage can be provided immediately, using a local, distant, or free flap.[9,10]

Likewise, in case of joint destruction, the use of silastic implants or spacers simplifies the procedure, providing mobile joints. There is no evidence whatsoever of an increased risk of infection.[11] Also in this case, well-vascularized soft tissue coverage is mandatory as shown in ▶ Fig. 9.3.

9.8.3 Revascularization

If any terminal segment is devascularized, the next surgical step is to restore vascularity. If an additional venous drainage is needed, the first author of this chapter prefers to perform the vein anastomosis first. In case of vein defect, very rarely a graft is needed; a vein can be harvested in some cases from an adjacent finger or a dorsal V–Y flap or hatchet flap[12] can be harvested in order to reapproximate the vein ends. In injuries to the midcarpal hand, the wrist and the forearm, a proximal vein can be rerouted to fulfill the length requirements.

In avulsion injuries, even after significant bone shortening, a vein graft may be needed. Vein grafts can be harvested from the distal forearm for the fingers, including a skin pad as an antegrade free venous flap if there is skin shortage.[13] In case of large skin defects to the midcarpal hand or more proximal part of the upper extremity, a flow through flap can carry the vessel for the segment to be revascularized (▶ Fig. 9.1).

9.8.4 Flexor Tendon Reconstruction

Flexor tendon repair should be the next step. In our study on simple flexor tendon injuries in zone 2,[14] we refrained in some cases from repairing the flexor digitorum superficialis (FDS) tendon. In the case of compound fractures in zone 2, we usually do not repair the FDS tendon. This is also the case in lesions at the level of the carpal tunnel. The bulky repair of both the FDS and the flexor profundus (FDP) tendons together will unavoidably cause adhesion in the restricted space of the carpal tunnel. In our opinion, the technique of suture in itself is not as relevant as commonly believed. We prefer a six-strand core suture known as the M modification of the Tang technique,[15] as it has been demonstrated that there is no need for a circumferential suture with this technique.[16] Saving time by avoiding, for example, six or seven circumferential sutures may be crucial in extensively lacerated hands.

In the fingers, we do not reconstruct pulleys primarily, provided that there is no concomitant lesion of the A1 and the A2 pulleys, and there is no concomitant lesion of the A4 and A2 pulleys. In cases with concomitant lesion of the A1 and A2 pulleys or A2 and A4 pulleys, we usually use the resected FDS to reconstruct a diagonal pulley at the A2 level.

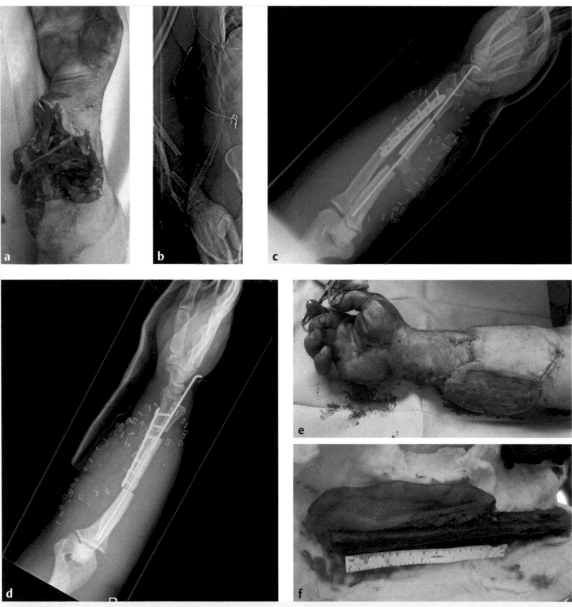

Fig. 9.2 (a, b) Explosion trauma with a devascularized hand, open fracture to the radius and ulna with a segmental loss of the ulna bone, skin defect, loss of the FDS and FDP muscles, and median nerve defect. Primary debridement and radius fixation with a plate. (c, d) The ulna was fixed with an intramedullary nail for ischemia time reasons leaving the bone reconstruction for a secondary procedure). The median nerve was immediately reconstructed with a sural nerve cable graft, the flexor carpi radialis transferred to the FDP, and the palmaris longus to the FPL. (e) The wound was closed primarily with a skin graft.

(Continued)

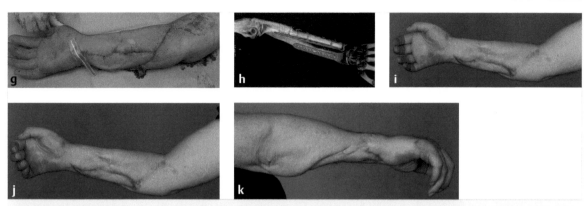

Fig. 9.2 *(Continued)* **(f, g)** In a second surgical time, the ulna was reconstructed with an osteocutaneous free fibula anastomosed end to side to the brachial artery at the elbow with a vein graft and fixed with a plate. **(h, i, j, k)** The results at 6 months.

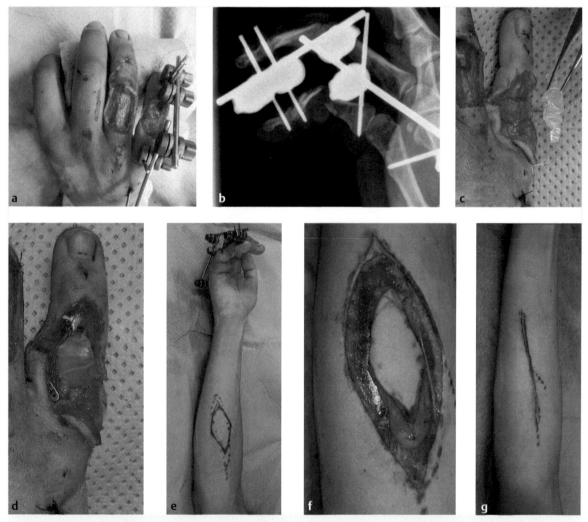

Fig. 9.3 A 32-year-old female patient, professional motor biker, following a friction burn injury to the right ring and little finger, with a skin defect and a large bone defect at the PIP joint of the little finger. **(a, b)** The patient was referred to our service few days after debridement and a temporary fixation was done with an external fixateur. **(c, d)** After further debridement, we reconstruct the PIP joint and the missing bone with a spacer carved out from an implantable silastic block **(c)** that was secured with an artificial ligament **(d)**. **(e, f, g, h)** We did not reconstruct the extensor tendon and covered the two fingers, put in syndactyly, with a retrograde free venous flap from the ipsilateral forearm.

(Continued)

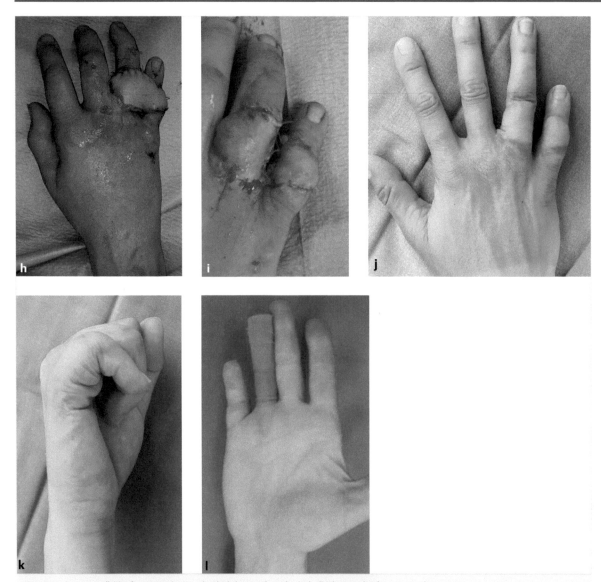

Fig. 9.3 *(Continued)* **(i)** After 3 weeks, we divided the syndactyly. **(j, k, l)** The result after 4 months.

Historically, the thumb suffered from bad outcomes even in simple lesions.[16] In compound fractures of the thumb, we repair the flexor pollicis longus (FPL), but we do not perform any pulley reconstruction as the tendon will most likely adhere to the scar tissue.

In severe explosion, trauma, or severe compound trauma to the forearm, we perform straightforward tendon transfers, using the available muscle tendon complexes for the reconstruction of the FDP group as a common tendon and of the FPL (▶Fig. 9.2).

9.8.5 Extensor Tendon Reconstruction

In severe compound fractures with extensive soft tissue loss, we do not reconstruct the extensor tendon distally to the metacarpophalangeal (MCP) joint. Even if the

defect is covered with a fasciocutaneous flap, the scarring will be so aggressive that the finger ultimately will extend by simple recoil of the scar tissue. This is true in our experience with mainly Caucasian patients. It might be that in Asian patients this indication is not be valid. If the intrinsics are severely damaged, we prefer to perform tendon transfer later (as an exception to the principle of repairing everything in one session[1]).

9.8.6 Nerve Reconstruction

The management of nerves in severe trauma cases does not differ from simple lacerations; we repair all the nerves that can be repaired using nerve grafts from the lower extremities in the forearm,[2] and the lateral antebrachial cutaneous nerve in case of digital nerve defects.[17] The choice of the lateral antebrachial cutaneous nerve is more practical since the nerve is consistent and does not divide in many small branches like the medial cutaneous nerve. Furthermore, skin sensation on the medial side of the forearm is far more important than on the lateral as we normally rest on a table with the ulnar side of the forearm (Elliot D, after private conversation). We sometimes use the muscle in vein technique[18] for small defects in the finger. We recently started to use allograft but we do realize that it may not be affordable.

9.8.7 Skin Coverage

A comprehensive review of skin coverage in compound hand fractures would require a book on itself. Furthermore, it is impossible to give universally valid guidelines, since strategies nowadays mostly depend on the surgeon's experience, skills, and preferences.

With the steadily increasing use of microsurgery in hand units around the world, plastic as well as orthopaedic, the surgeon should not be afraid to imagine a free flap even in the case of relatively small defects, and even in emergency if indicated.[7] Even though local flaps and distant pedicled flaps still find an indication in our practice, the indications for free flaps are still widening. We specifically are very keen to use retrograde free venous flaps from the forearm even for relatively large defects, especially on the dorsum of the hand and the fingers.[19] The elasticity of the skin of the forearm in Caucasian patient gives a much better quality than the skin of the thigh,[19] while the length and caliber of the feeding artery of the groin flap often is disappointing and aesthetically not very satisfactory except in very thin patients. Moreover, free venous flaps can be customized with regard to the diameter of the required vessels, and the necessity of including nerves and tendons (▶Fig. 9.4). We still use the anterolateral thigh flap (ALT) for very large defects of the hand with underlying terminal bone stumps (phalanges, metacarpals); we observed that the bones have the tendency to protrude through muscular flaps, even if the bone ends are rounded sufficiently.

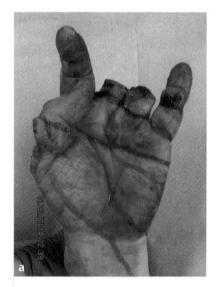
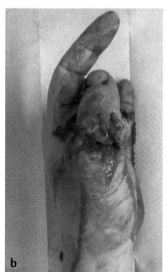
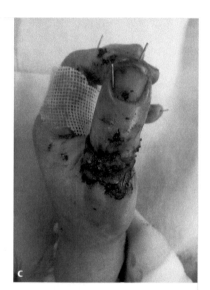
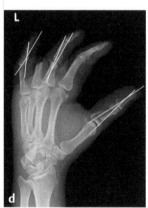
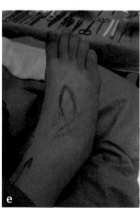
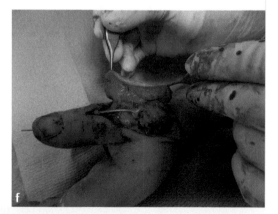

Fig. 9.4 A 42-year-old male patient with a burr injury to the left nondominant hand. **(a, b)** Amputation of the middle and ring finger and severe open fracture to the thumb with bone loss. Initial debridement, replantation of the middle finger, as it was the only available finger, and acute reconstruction of the bone to the thumb with an iliac crest bone graft. **(c, d)** The skin showed a secondary total necrosis. Immediate cover with a composite free venous flap including the extensor digitorum longus from the foot to cover the bone graft and reconstruct the extensor pollicis longus (EPL). **(e, f, g)** The foot was chosen as a donor site as the patient was obese.

(Continued)

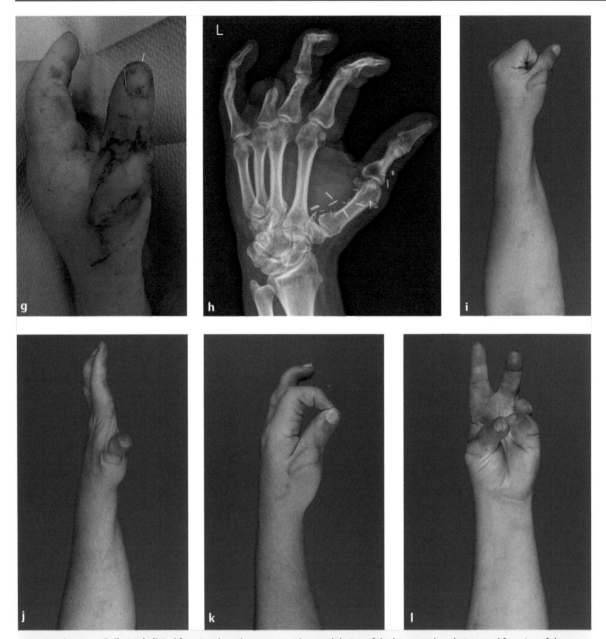

Fig. 9.4 *(Continued)* **(h, i, j, k, l)** End functional result at 1 year with consolidation of the bones and a relative good function of the hand.

In complex compound injuries of the forearm, the use of free tissue transfer is almost the rule as shown in ▶ Fig. 9.2, both for bone and for soft tissue reconstruction, sometimes with composite flaps. We tend to use fascial or fasciocutaneous flaps for the hand, for a better gliding of the tendons, even though we observed that muscular flaps tend to give good long term aesthetic results in some large defects in the dorsum of the wrist and the forearm as well as in the palm, sometimes better than fasciocutaneous flaps. Nevertheless, reopening a muscular flap for a secondary procedure is way more complex and time consuming than reopening a fasciocutaneous flap.

The right timing in our practice for covering a compound fracture would be ideally within 48 hours form injury,[7] and sometimes we perform emergency flaps. In practice, because of the limitation of manpower, operating spaces and general resources, this rule is not always applicable, even in our setup.

Acknowledgments: We specially thank Dr. M Scaglioni for having performed the initial replantation in case of ▶ Fig. 9.1. We would like to thank the therapists of the Hand Therapy Department at the University Hospital Zurich for their engagement and invaluable help.

Disclosures: No disclosures.

References

[1] Foucher G, Merle M, Michon J. [Treatment in one stage of complex injuries of the hand with early mobilisation (author's transl)] Ann Chir. 1977; 31(12):1059–1063

[2] Anderson JT, Gustilo RB. Immediate internal fixation in open fractures. Orthop Clin North Am. 1980; 11(3):569–578

[3] Tulipan JE, Ilyas AM. Open fractures of the hand: review of pathogenesis and introduction of a new classification system. Orthop Clin North Am. 2016; 47(1):245–251

[4] Ng T, Unadkat J, Bilonick RA, Wollstein R. The importance of early operative treatment in open fractures of the fingers. Ann Plast Surg. 2014; 72(4):408–410

[5] Sundine M, Scheker LR. A comparison of immediate and staged reconstruction of the dorsum of the hand. J Hand Surg [Br]. 1996; 21(2):216–221

[6] Sabapathy SR, Venkatramani H, Bharathi RR, Bhardwaj P. Replantation surgery. J Hand Surg Am. 2011; 36(6):1104–1110

[7] Lister G, Scheker L. Emergency free flaps to the upper extremity. J Hand Surg Am. 1988; 13(1):22–28

[8] Giesen T, Gazzola R, Poggetti A, Giovanoli P, Calcagni M. Intramedullary headless screw fixation for fractures of the proximal and middle phalanges in the digits of the hand: a review of 31 consecutive fractures. J Hand Surg Eur Vol. 2016; 41(7):688–694

[9] Saint-Cyr M, Miranda D, Gonzalez R, Gupta A. Immediate corticocancellous bone autografting in segmental bone defects of the hand. J Hand Surg [Br]. 2006; 31(2):168–177

[10] Sabapathy SR, Venkatramani H, Giesen T, Ullah AS. Primary bone grafting with pedicled flap cover for dorsal combined injuries of the digits. J Hand Surg Eur Vol. 2008; 33(1):65–70

[11] Mantero R, Grandis C, Rota F, Meloni P. Considerazioni sull'impiego in urgenza delle endoprotesi di Swanson in alcune lesioni traumatiche esposte della mano. Riv Chir Mano. 1979; 16:79–89

[12] Emmett AJ. The closure of defects by using adjacent triangular flaps with subcutaneous pedicles. Plast Reconstr Surg. 1977; 59(1):45–52

[13] Tsai TM, Matiko JD, Breidenbach W, Kutz JE. Venous flaps in digital revascularization and replantation. J Reconstr Microsurg. 1987; 3(2):113–119

[14] Giesen T, Calcagni M, Elliot D. Primary flexor tendon repair with early active motion: experience in Europe. Hand Clin. 2017; 33(3):465–472

[15] Wang B, Xie RG, Tang JB. Biomechanical analysis of a modification of Tang method of tendon repair. J Hand Surg [Br]. 2003; 28(4):347–350

[16] Giesen T, Sirotakova M, Copsey AJ, Elliot D. Flexor pollicis longus primary repair: further experience with the tang technique and controlled active mobilization. J Hand Surg Eur Vol. 2009; 34(6):758–761

[17] Pilanci O, Ozel A, Basaran K, et al. Is there a profit to use the lateral antebrachial cutaneous nerve as a graft source in digital nerve reconstruction? Microsurgery. 2014; 34(5):367–371

[18] Tos P, Battiston B, Ciclamini D, Geuna S, Artiaco S. Primary repair of crush nerve injuries by means of biological tubulization with muscle-vein-combined grafts. Microsurgery. 2012; 32(5):358–363

[19] Giesen T, Forster N, Künzi W, Giovanoli P, Calcagni M. Retrograde arterialized free venous flaps for the reconstruction of the hand: review of 14 cases. J Hand Surg Am. 2014; 39(3):511–523

10 Pediatric Hand Fractures

Pernille Leicht

Abstract

The hand is the most frequently injured part of the body in the pediatric population and an injury will often result in a fracture. The treatment of pediatric hand fractures is in some way different from the treatment of fractures in the adult population. Pediatric hand fractures often involves the growth plate and in the treatment of the pediatric hand fractures it is essential to be aware of the growing potential of the bones in children. Most of the fractures can be treated conservatively, but some special fractures should be operated. The special fractures which requires early operative treatment include fractures of the neck of the proximal and medial phalanx and dislocation of the nail combined with an epiphyseal fracture of the distal phalanx.

Keywords: pediatric hand fracture, Seymour's fracture, distal tuft fracture, phalangeal neck fracture, proximal phalanx fracture, metacarpal fracture, scaphoid fracture

10.1 Introduction

Pediatric hand fractures are fractures in children who still have open physes and therefore have special considerations regarding immobilization, remodelling potential, and surgical indications. The fractures in children heal more quickly than in adults and the short healing time makes early diagnosis and fracture reduction essential. Especially if the fracture involves the physes, where 5 days are the limit for safe reduction.

The frequency of hand fractures in children is in some studies shown to be the second most frequent fracture in children following distal forearm fractures.[1,2]

Several studies have shown that the frequency of fractures increases from 11 years of age and peaks at 14 to 15 years of age[1-5] since the children at that age begin to participate in sport activities. The fractures are frequently seen in boys with a ratio of 3 boys to 1 girl except in the age group younger than 2 years where four out of six fractures are seen in girls.

The fracture type and the injury pattern are different in different age groups. The most commonly involved ray is the fifth ray where the metacarpal is the most commonly fractured bone followed by the proximal phalanx.[3,5]

The injury pattern varies with age and in most of the children between 0 and 5 years of age it is a crush injury at the fingertip and in the children between 10 and 17 years of age it is sports-related trauma.[6] Children aged 0 to 4 years mostly get tuft fractures, 5- to 8-year-olds get fracture of the distal phalanx (tuft and transverse fractures), 9- to 12-year-olds get fracture of the proximal phalanx in the small finger, and children between 13 and 16 years of age get metacarpal neck fractures.[7]

Many of the hand fractures in children can involve the physes and can be classified in relation to the Salter–Harris classification types 1 to 5 (►Table 10.1) (see also Fig. 1.5). In the hand, the physes are in the proximal part of the phalangeal bones, in the proximal part of the first metacarpal bone, and in the distal part of the second to fifth metacarpal bone. The proximal phalangeal epiphyses ossify between 10 and 24 months of age and the epiphyses of the middle and distal phalanges will ossify 6 to 8 months later. The closure of the physeal goes from distal to proximal direction and the physes are closed in boys when they are 16.5 years old and in girls when they are 14.5 years old. Until the closure, the physes are not mineralized and are therefore weaker than the surrounding mature bone, and hence the physes are more often involved in fractures in children. The periosteum that surrounds the pediatric bone is highly vascularized and serves as the source for cell differentiation during fracture healing. Following a fracture in a pediatric bone, the growth in the physes and remodeling in the diaphysis can correct an initial fracture deformity. This correction is more effective in the sagittal plane and near the physes, and better in younger children, while the remodeling is less good in the coronal plane. Rotational deformities cannot be remodeled and will therefore always require treatment with reduction and possibly closed reduction and percutaneous pinning (CRPP) or open reduction and internal fixation (ORIF). Even though one-third of all bone damage in the child's hand involves the physes, epiphysiodesis is a rare consequence.[8] However, in younger children, the physes are very sensitive and therefore multiple attempts to reduce physeal fractures may destroy the physeal plate thus resulting in an iatrogenic physeal arrest. If reduction is impossible in one or two trials, it is recommended to consider an open reposition to avoid growth arrest.[9]

It is often a challenge to examine an injured child. Observation of the child and a gentle maneuver are mandatory to get the correct information needed for the diagnosis. Try to talk about other things and give the child something to play with. And then look for swelling, hematoma, and active motion. The tenodesis effect or a gentle pressure to the muscle bellies proximal for the injury can be helpful to evaluate a rotational deformity. A careful examination of the nail plate is also useful. Rotation greater than 10 degrees out of the plane of adjacent nail plates should alert the examiner of

Table 10.1 Classification of types of Salter–Harris fractures

Type 1 Widening of the epiphyseal plate

Type 2 Fracture through the metaphysis

Type 3 Fracture through the growth plate

Type 4 Fracture through the epiphysis and metaphysis

Type 5 Compression of epiphysis

a rotational deformity. Nevertheless, the best way to examine for malrotation is, if it is possible, to get the child to make a fist and always compare with the not-injured hand.

The diagnosis of fractures in children can usually be determined from clinical examination and radiographs. It is essential to carry out the radiographs examination in two planes. A true lateral radiograph of the injured finger without overlap from the other fingers is important. It is rarely necessary to do further examinations, except for scaphoid fractures (see later).

The treatment of pediatric hand fractures is in some areas different from the treatment of hand fractures in adults. About 80% of hand fractures in children can be treated nonoperatively with a normal functional and aesthetic result.[6] The nonoperative treatment consists of plaster, splint, or buddy taping (▶ Fig. 10.1a,b). These treatments can be used for stable fractures, without dislocation or fractures reduced to an acceptable position. The use of tape requires that the children are cooperative and can therefore only be used when the children are from 7 to 8 years of age. In children who are noncompliant or younger than 7 to 8 years, a splint or a plaster cast should be used. Unstable fractures and irreducible fractures require CRPP or ORIF with K-wires or screws. In small children (< 5 years), it may often be necessary to use an above-elbow circular soft cast (▶ Fig. 10.2) or plaster cast bandage to prevent them from removing the bandage. Immobilization time is 3 to 4 weeks. After this, the child can start using the hand without restrictions. There is usually no need for occupational therapy. The children do their own occupational therapy by using their hand and fingers in the daily play and sporting activities.

The operative treatment is usually CRPP or, if not possible, ORIF. Closed reduction is impossible later than 1 to 2 weeks after the trauma due to the initial bone healing.

Internal fixation must be protected by a splint or a cast, since children are not compliant to early mobilization and since they will quickly regain mobility after immobilization.

There are specific pediatric fractures that require special attention.

10.2 Special Children Fractures

10.2.1 Seymour's Fracture

A Seymour's fracture is a juxta-epiphyseal fracture or a Salter–Harris types 1 to 2 fracture in the distal phalanx with nail bed laceration (▶ Fig. 10.3), flexion deformity on the fracture site, and often nail plate subluxation.[10–13] It is an open fracture and should be treated as such. The fracture often occurs when the finger is crushed in a door and is therefore a frequent fracture in smaller children. Clinically, it looks like a mallet finger and often the proximal part of the nail lays superficially to the proximal nail fold (▶ Fig. 10.4).

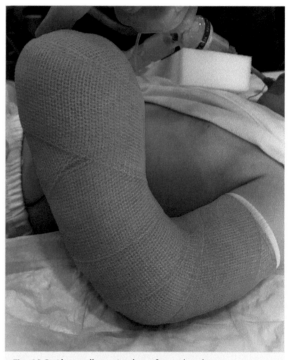

Fig. 10.2 Above-elbow circular soft cast bandage.

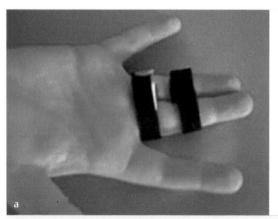
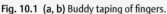
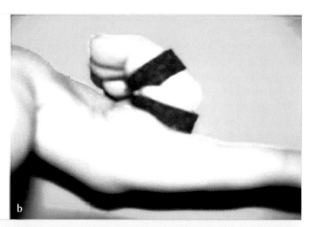

Fig. 10.1 (a, b) Buddy taping of fingers.

The extensor tendon and the palmar plate inserts onto the epiphysis of the distal phalanx, while the flexor tendon inserts onto the palmar part of the metaphysis. This

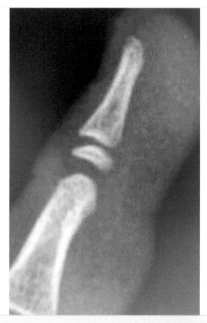

Fig. 10.3 Salter–Harris type 1 fracture in distal phalanx.

results in a dorsal displacement of the proximal fragment and a palmar displacement of the distal fragment. The bone between the metaphysis and the epiphysis is the weakest part of the bone because of the nonmineralized physes. The surgical treatment of a Seymour fracture consists of debridement, removal of any interposed soft tissue from the fracture line, reposition of fracture/epiphysiolysis, nailbed repair, and nail plate fixation. It may be necessary to remove the nail, suture the nailbed with absorbable sutures, and reattach the nail to give support for the fracture/epiphysiolysis. When the proximal part of the nail lays superficially to the proximal nail fold, it must be repositioned under the proximal nail fold. It is also advisable to transfix the distal interphalangeal (DIP) joint with a 0.8-mm K-wire. The K-wire is cut outside the skin, so it easily can be removed after 3 weeks without anesthesia. In the case of small children younger than 4 to 5 years, it is advisable to bandage them with an above-elbow circular plaster cast including the entire hand (►Fig. 10.2) to prevent them from removing the bandage. Children older than 5 years can often be immobilized in a finger splint depending on the child's compliance. After removal of the bandage and K-wire, the children can use the hand and fingers freely.

Seymour's fracture is a relatively serious injury and very important to diagnose and treat properly.

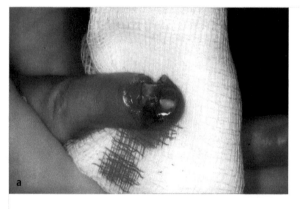
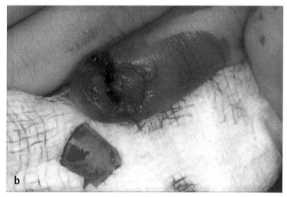
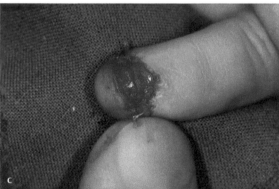
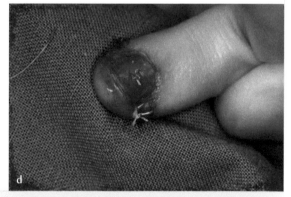

Fig. 10.4 Nail bed lesion in connection with Seymour fracture. **(a)** The proximal part of the nail lays superficially to the proximal nail fold. **(b)** After removal of the nail the lacerated nail bed is revealed. **(c)** After reposition of the fracture and debridement the wound in the nail bed is adapted with absorbable sutures. **(d)** The nail is replaced and stabilized with absorbable sutures. If unstable, the fracture may be stabilized with a longitudinal K-wire. (These images are provided courtesy of Michel E.H. Boeckstyns.)

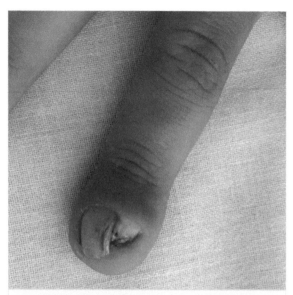

Fig. 10.5 Deformed nail grows after a Seymour fracture.

If not treated properly, a Seymour's fracture carries a risk of growth disturbance due to premature physeal closure, bony deformity, nail deformity (▶Fig. 10.5), and infection. Even if treated properly, nail deformity may occur due to destruction of the germinal nail matrix.

10.2.2 Tuft Fractures

In case of trauma, where children have crushed the distal part of a finger, there may be a fracture of the distal phalanx or an epiphysiolysis. Radiographs should be taken in two planes. The sagittal view may reveal a fracture that cannot be seen in the posteroanterior (PA) view. Fractures or epiphysiolyses without nailbed laceration and/ or subluxation of the nail plate can be treated with a closed reposition and a palmar splint for 3 weeks in children older than 3 to 4 years. If reduction is insufficient or the child younger than 3 to 4 years, closed reposition and transfixation of the DIP joint with K-wire is advised. It is important to obtain a control radiograph after 1 week, because of the risk of redislocation needing ORIF.

10.2.3 Phalangeal Neck Fractures

Phalangeal neck fractures include several different types of fractures located to the distal part of proximal or medial phalanx, distally to the collateral ligament recess (▶Table 10.2). These fractures are relatively rare[14] but occur 10 times more frequently in children than in adults and may cause problems. Phalangeal neck fractures often occur when a finger is trapped in a door and at the same time retracted. The fractures can be difficult to recognize and are therefore often found late and with malunion. Despite the relatively large distance to the growth plate, it has been shown in several studies that the remodeling potential, especially in the sagittal plane is acceptable. Thus, it is recommended to treat late discovered phalangeal neck fractures conservatively in children younger than 9 years[15-17] if there is no rotational deformity or coronal angulation. Else, an osteotomy may be required.

The fractures may be classified in three types according to Al Qattan's classification[18] (▶Table 10.3).

Type 1 fractures are undisplaced fractures and can be treated with a cast or a splint for 3 to 4 weeks, but

Table 10.2 Phalangeal neck fractures

Subcondylar fracture

Subcapital fracture

Cartilage cap fracture

Distal condylar phalangeal fracture

Supracondylar fracture

Unicondylar phalangeal fracture

Bicondylar phalangeal fracture

Transcondylar phalangeal fracture

Avulsion phalangeal fracture

Table 10.3 Al Quattan's classification of phalangeal neck fractures

Type 1 Undisplaced fracture

Type 2 Displaced fracture with some bone-to-bone contact

Type 3 Displaced fracture without bone-to-bone contact

control radiographs in two planes are important after 1 week due to the risk of displacement. Types 2 and 3 are displaced fractures (▶ Fig. 10.6) and the cartilaginous cap of the condyle is often rotated in a dorsal direction because of the lack of tendon attachment at the distal

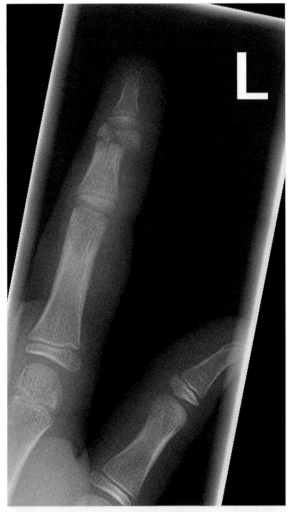

Fig. 10.6 Bicondylar phalangeal neck fracture.

fragment. They require reduction and fixation with a K-wire or a screw, either percutaneously or by open reduction (▶ Fig. 10.7a).[18,19] Open reduction can be performed through a dorsal or a midlateral approach. Care must be taken to preserve the collateral ligament attachments to the condylar head. This is essential because of the blood supply to the condyles comes from the collateral ligaments and the soft tissue around them. If this blood supply is destroyed, there is a risk of avascular necrosis of the condyles.

If the child is seen more than 2 weeks after the injury and there is no tenderness at the fracture site, healing of the fracture is likely and closed reduction is impossible. If there is no rotational or angulatory deformity in the coronal plane, it is recommended to start mobilization and await remodeling. In case of unacceptable deformity, open osteotomy is required, despite the risk of avascular necrosis and joint stiffness.

10.2.4 Proximal Phalanx Fractures

In children, these fractures are most frequently located to the epiphysis as a Salter–Harris type 2 (▶ Fig. 10.8a) (see also Chapter 1). The fifth finger is most commonly involved finger and a fracture in the proximal phalanx of the fifth finger often results in the so-called "extra octave fracture" (▶ Fig. 10.8a), as the finger at the trauma is maximally abducted. The fractures can be treated with a splint or a circular bandage if they are undisplaced. Children older than 7 to 8 years can be treated with buddy taping with the neighbouring finger (▶ Fig. 10.8b), encouraging early mobilization. In case of more than 10 degrees of angulation in the coronal plane or if a rotational deformity is present, reduction is required. A larger angulation in the sagittal plane can be accepted. Closed reduction is usually possible and a cast or a splint involving at least two fingers can be applied for 3 to 4 weeks. Radiographical control after 1 week is important. Unstable fractures must be treated by closed reduction and percutaneous with a 0.8-mm

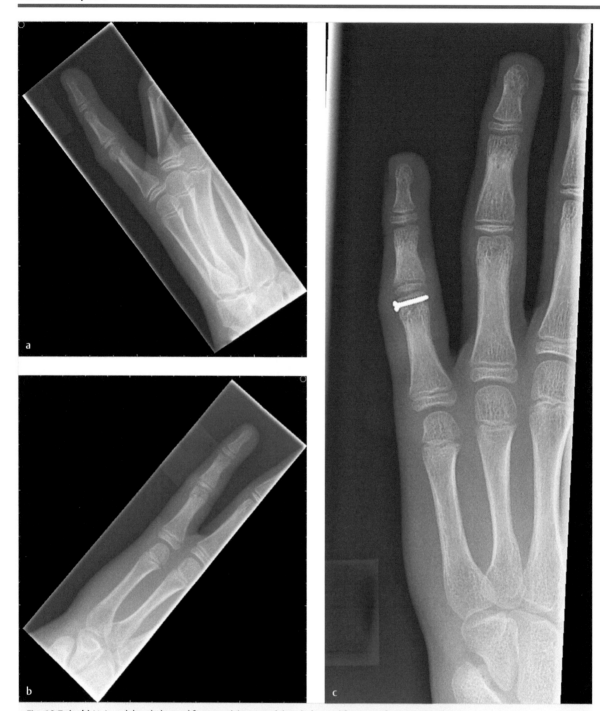

Fig. 10.7 (a, b) Unicondylar phalangeal fracture. **(c)** Unicondylar phalangeal fracture after osteosynthesis.

K-wire. Irreducible fractures require ORIF with K-wires. It is recommended to leave the K-wires outside the skin as this usually will permit removal in the outpatient clinic without anesthesia. This requires an above-elbow cast in children younger than 5 to 6 years to prevent them removing the dressings.

10.2.5 Metacarpal Fractures

Metacarpal fractures account for 10 to 30% of all pediatric hand fractures (see also Chapter 1). They are rare in young children and occur most often in children aged 13 to 16 years due to sport activities.

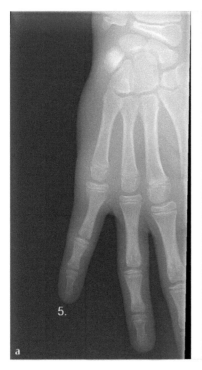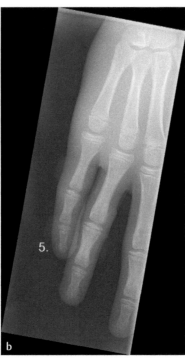

Fig. 10.8 (a, b) "Extra octave fracture" treated with reduction and buddy taping with the ring finger.

The fractures can be divided into fractures located to the metacarpal head, neck, shaft, or base, the neck and shaft fractures being the most common.

Treatment is similar as in adults with reposition and immobilization in a plaster cast or a splint. Sometimes K-wire fixation is necessary.

Fractures of the metacarpal head are usually of the Salter–Harris type 2, typically in the fifth metacarpal bone. These fractures can result in avascular necrosis and growth arrest. Too many attempts at closed reduction should be avoided as this can affect the growth zone, and lead to growth arrest. Thus open reduction and K-wire fixation may be required.

Because of the potential of remodeling, an angulation in the sagittal plane up to 15 degrees is acceptable in the second and third metacarpal neck up to 30 degrees in the fourth and fifth metacarpal neck. In shaft fractures, a palmar angulation of 10 degrees can be accepted in the second and third metacarpal and 20 degrees in the fourth and fifth metacarpal. It is important to have a straight sagittal radiograph to evaluate the angulation. As in adults, a clinical examination for malrotation is essential. This requires the child to try to make a fist to assess the rotation. Even a small malrotation will result in scissoring of the fingers when making a fist. A malrotation of 5 degrees can result in a finger overlap of 1.5 cm.

Shaft fractures of the first metacarpal are common and remodel rapidly. Up to 30 degrees of lateral angulation can be accepted.

Fractures of the base of the first metacarpal often involve the physes as a Salter–Harris type 3 or 4. These are pediatric Bennett's fractures and are unstable. CRPP is usually required.

10.2.6 Carpal Fractures

Carpal fractures as well as carpal ligament injuries are rare in children. In the early childhood, the carpal bones are resistant to injury because they are largely cartilaginous. On radiographs the scapholunate gap appears to be wide in the normal child's wrist because of the incomplete ossification of the carpal bones.[20]

As in adults, the most frequent carpal bone fractures occurs in the scaphoid, but it only represents 3% of all fractures of the hand in children. Scaphoid fractures can be caused by a fall with the wrist in maximal extension. They are very rare in children younger than 6 years, since the scaphoid consists primarily of cartilage until that age. The ossification starts in the distal pole when the child is 4 to 5 years old, progresses in a proximal direction, and is completed around the age of 12. This may explain a greater frequency of fractures in the distal pole of younger children.

Traditionally, scaphoid fractures have predominantly been considered to be located at the distal pole in children and adolescents. In the later years, the distribution has shifted toward the same pattern as in adults and the waist fracture is now the most common injury of the scaphoid in children too. This may be explained by the increase of high-energy sports activities in children as well as an increase in body mass index (BMI).[21]

A clinical suspicion of scaphoid fracture is present when there is tenderness in the anatomical snuffbox and/or at the scaphoid tubercle and indirect tenderness when applying a longitudinal force to the thumb. In this case, PA and lateral radiograph of the wrist should be supplemented with special radiographs of the scaphoid bone (▶Fig. 10.9a). If the radiographs reveal no fracture, the patient should be treated with a splint for 2 weeks and reexamined radiographically or with a computed tomography (CT) scan or magnetic resonance imaging (MRI) (▶Fig. 10.9b).

Some studies recommend primary MRI of all children who have scaphoid-related pain and negative radiographs.[22,23] In some cases, MRI can reveal other carpal fractures, but their clinical relevance is unknown.[24]

Most of the scaphoid fractures in children can be treated with a plaster cast. Fractures in the distal pole are treated with a below-elbow circular plaster cast for 4 to 6 weeks. Undisplaced fractures in the waist of scaphoid are treated with a below-elbow circular plaster cast until radiographical healing typically 6 to 8 weeks possibly up to 12 weeks. Dislocated fractures in waist or proximal pole are treated wizth ORIF with a compression screw or K-wires. Nonunion of scaphoid fractures are seen in children typically due to late recognition of the fracture or insufficient immobilization. The treatment principles for nonunion scaphoid fractures are the same as in the adult (see Chapter 25).

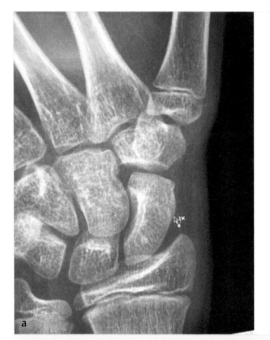
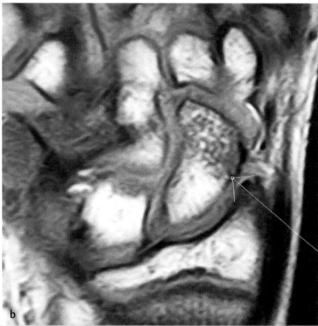

Fig. 10.9 (a) Undisplaced scaphoid fracture. (b) MRI showing scaphoid fracture.

References

[1] Landin LA. Fracture patterns in children. Analysis of 8,682 fractures with special reference to incidence, etiology and secular changes in a Swedish urban population 1950–1979. Acta Orthop Scand Suppl. 1983; 202(54):1–109

[2] Naranje SM, Erali RA, Warner WC, Jr, Sawyer JR, Kelly DM. Epidemiology of pediatric fractures presenting to emergency departments in the United States. J Pediatr Orthop. 2016; 36(4):e45–e48

[3] Bhende MS, Dandrea LA, Davis HW. Hand injuries in children presenting to a pediatric emergency department. Ann Emerg Med. 1993; 22(10):1519–1523

[4] Chew EM, Chong AK. Hand fractures in children: epidemiology and misdiagnosis in a tertiary referral hospital. J Hand Surg Am. 2012; 37(8):1684–1688

[5] Vadivelu R, Dias JJ, Burke FD, Stanton J. Hand injuries in children: a prospective study. J Pediatr Orthop. 2006; 26(1):29–35

[6] Liu EH, Alqahtani S, Alsaaran RN, Ho ES, Zuker RM, Borschel GH. A prospective study of pediatric hand fractures and review of the literature. Pediatr Emerg Care. 2014; 30(5):299–304

[7] Rajesh A, Basu AK, Vaidhyanath R, Finlay D. Hand fractures: a study of their site and type in childhood. Clin Radiol. 2001; 56(8):667–669

[8] Hastings H, II, Simmons BP. Hand fractures in children. A statistical analysis. Clin Orthop Relat Res. 1984(188):120–130

[9] Nellans KW, Chung KC. Pediatric hand fractures. Hand Clin. 2013; 29(4):569–578

[10] Seymour N. Juxta-epiphysial fracture of the terminal phalanx of the finger. J Bone Joint Surg Br. 1966; 48(2):347–349

[11] Al-Qattan MM. Extra-articular transverse fractures of the base of the distal phalanx (Seymour's fracture) in children and adults. J Hand Surg [Br]. 2001; 26(3):201–206

[12] Krusche-Mandl I, Köttstorfer J. Thalhammer, Aldrian S, Erhart J, Platzer P. Seymore fractures: retrospective analysis and therapeutic considerations. J Hand Surg Am. 2013; 38A:258–264

[13] Goodell PB, Bauer A. Problematic pediatric hand and wrist fractures. JBJS Rev. 2016; 4(5):1–9

[14] Al-Qattan MM, Al-Qattan AM. A review of phalangeal neck fractures in children. Injury. 2015; 46(6):935–944

[15] Puckett BN, Gaston RG, Peljovich AE, Lourie GM, Floyd WE, III. Remodeling potential of phalangeal distal condylar malunions in children. J Hand Surg Am. 2012; 37(1):34–41

[16] Mintzer CM, Waters PM, Brown DJ. Remodelling of a displaced phalangeal neck fracture. J Hand Surg [Br]. 1994; 19(5):594–596

[17] Hennrikus WL, Cohen MR. Complete remodelling of displaced fractures of the neck of the phalanx. J Bone Joint Surg Br. 2003; 85(2):273–274

[18] Al-Qattan MM. Phalangeal neck fractures in children: classification and outcome in 66 cases. J Hand Surg [Br]. 2001; 26(2):112–121

[19] Matzon JL, Cornwall R. A stepwise algorithm for surgical treatment of type II displaced pediatric phalangeal neck fractures. J Hand Surg Am. 2014; 39(3):467–473

[20] Leicht P, Mikkelsen JB, Larsen CF. Scapholunate distance in children. Acta Radiol. 1996; 37(5):625–626

[21] Gholson JJ, Bae DS, Zurakowski D, Waters PM. Scaphoid fractures in children and adolescents: contemporary injury patterns and factors influencing time to union. J Bone Joint Surg Am. 2011; 93(13):1210–1219

[22] Johnson KJ, Haigh SF, Symonds KE. MRI in the management of scaphoid fractures in skeletally immature patients. Pediatr Radiol. 2000; 30(10):685–688

[23] Dorsay TA, Major NM, Helms CA. Cost-effectiveness of immediate MR imaging versus traditional follow-up for revealing radiographically occult scaphoid fractures. AJR Am J Roentgenol. 2001; 177(6):1257–1263

[24] Jørgsholm P, Thomsen N, Besjakov J, Abrahamsson S, Björkman A. MRI shows a high incidence of carpal fractures in children with posttraumatic radial-sided wrist tenderness. Acta Orthop. 2016; 87(5):533–537

11 Fractures in the Paralytic Extremity

Gürsel Leblebicioğlu, Egemen Ayhan, Tüzün Fırat

Abstract

Muscle function is an important part of preserving bone structure and function. Many studies suggest bone loss in different paralytic conditions including spinal cord injury, stroke, peripheral nerve injuries, and even botulinum toxin injections. Paralysis leads bone mineral loss and fractures in addition to the systemic adverse effects of the pathological condition. Even minor loadings may result with fractures in paralytic disorders. The preceding long-lasting limited mobility contributes to higher morbidity and mortality following fractures in paralytic patients. Therefore, knowledge of paralytic bone mineral loss and fractures may help to prevent bone mineral loss–related fractures and morbidities. This chapter provides extensive knowledge on the causes of bone mineral loss and fracture in different paralysis models. Also, prevention and management methods in fractures are mentioned. Nevertheless, this field requires more research especially in lower motor neuron lesions.

Keywords: paralysis, fracture, spinal cord injury, stroke, botulinum toxin

11.1 Introduction

Loss of musculoskeletal functions secondary to dysfunction of the central and peripheral nervous system is mostly a devastating injury. Many patients are young, and treatment possibilities are usually limited to improve their quality of life, to regain self-ambulation, and to prolong survival. Neural involvement, as well as its secondary consequences such as decreased mobility and diminished sensation related to primary disease can be excruciating. Treatment of primary neural problems and prevention of secondary complications may help improve the quality of life.

Patients with central and peripheral nervous system disorders may have an increased risk of sustaining serious fractures of spine and extremities. Fractures may develop at the time of the neural injury, such as fractures of clavicle at birth in babies with brachial plexus birth palsy, or later in the course of the disease such as hip fractures in patients with paraplegia.

Loss of bone mineral density (BMD) which can be related to muscle paralysis and metabolic changes decreases mechanical resistance of bone. Consequently, fractures are possible even under physiological loads or during physical therapy. Depending on neural involvement, limbs may have different levels of muscle paralysis and loss of sensation. Pattern of muscle weakness and dystonia, duration of immobilization, altered metabolic and hormonal conditions, and duration of the disease affect the bone density in various ways.[1] The risk of fracture may vary depending on the underlying condition and duration. The majority of these fractures occurs during chronic conditions. Fracture in a paralytic extremity causes severe functional limitation, even if it was not used functionally before the fracture.

The most common sites of fracture in paralytic disorders are the diaphysis and supracondylar region of femur. The involvement of upper extremity and hand are relatively rare. In this section, etiology, pathogenesis, diagnosis, and possible treatment modalities in the fractures of paralytic upper extremity are reviewed.

11.2 Basic Science

11.2.1 Changes in Bone

Spinal Cord Injury

Complete spinal cord injury (SCI) causes an instant paralysis of muscles and disuse atrophy of the paralyzed extremities. This is followed by connective tissue invasion, vascular system disruption, cartilage degeneration, and bone mass loss.[2–5] Osteoporosis is also a common finding in individuals with SCI.[6,7] This is due to unloading of extremity similar to those observed with aging, bed rest, or disuse atrophy.[8,9] Loss of bone mass is associated with deterioration of trabecular microarchitecture.[7,10,11] The imbalance of bone turnover favoring resorption occurs after injury, peaks at third to fifth months, reaches to a steady state at 2 years, and possibly continues beyond that.[12–20] Bone loss occurs more rapidly in trabecular bone, and continues steadily in cortical bone.[19] In the study by Garland et al,[15] the rapid decline in bone mass for the first 4 months was attributed to metabolic changes after SCI. The exact etiology of bone weakening is not known.[7,17] It is suggested that, besides the loss of normal biomechanical stress and the neurotrophic failure, insufficient nutritional support, disordered vasoregulation, hypercorticoidism, alterations in gonadal function, and other endocrine disorders are other possible causes of the changes in the bone.[7,15–17,21]

The severity of injury, the extent of functional impairment, the duration of injury, and aging influence bone mass in SCI patients.[17] Many studies have highlighted the osteoporosis below the level of injury.[15,16,22] Mechanical loading and active muscle forces may affect the composition of the bone.[7] In their cross-sectional study, Tsuzuku et al[23] compared the BMD of 10 tetraplegic and 10 paraplegic patients. The authors found that lumbar spine, upper extremity, and trochanter region BMD of tetraplegic patients were significantly less than those of paraplegic patients. Similarly, other authors had reported more bone loss in arms of tetraplegic patients than those of paraplegic patients.[15,19,24–26] The extent of SCI is also another important factor for bone metabolic response. In an early, but a still worthy, study of Comarr et al,[27] the authors suggested that the more incomplete a lesion was, the more muscles preserved, the less atrophy would result and the less osteoporosis would develop. Supporting this, some authors reported greater BMD loss in their complete SCI patients than in incomplete SCI patients.[24,28–30] In complete SCI patients, it is postulated that the lack of reflex contractions possibly increases demineralization.[31] Several authors reported that the bone mass reduce with increasing time postinjury and age in patients with SCI.[7,17,20,32]

Lower motor lesion patients were found to be relatively more prone to fractures than the upper motor neuron lesion patients.[27] Lower motor neuron lesions result in flaccid paralysis and muscle atrophy, however, upper motor neuron lesions results with spastic paralysis and muscle spasms. The muscle atrophy causes reduced or absent mechanical forces on bone and may initiate osteoporosis. Supporting this theory, Demirel et al[24] reported lesser BMD loss in their patients with spasticity compared with their flaccid patients. Similarly, Eser et al[33] found that bone loss in the femur after SCI was reduced in subjects with stronger spasticity, compared with subjects with weaker or absent spasticity. However, Wilmet et al[34] claimed that spasticity and flaccidity had no effect on BMD loss. It is probable that spasticity is effective at preserving bone mass and reducing fracture risk.[5] On the other hand, in a recent study of Kostovski et al,[30] the authors found that higher frequency and severity of spasticity correlated with lower BMD 12 months after the SCI. They reported that SCI men with incomplete injuries have less spasticity and are more ambulant, and hence spasticity correlates negatively with BMD. Although mild spasticity may have beneficial effects for preserving bone mass, the severe forms of spasticity would cause ambulation or rehabilitation problems that would make patients prone to fractures.

The most common site of SCI is the cervical region, causing upper extremity dysfunction and accounting for 50 to 64% of traumatic spinal cord injuries.[35] In regard to severity of permanent neurological dysfunction, SCI may be complete or incomplete. Since 2010, the most frequent neurological categories have been incomplete tetraplegia (41%), incomplete paraplegia (19%), complete paraplegia (18%), and complete tetraplegia (12%).[36]

Tetraplegia occurs due to injury in one of cervical one to eight spinal cord segments. The area of injured spinal cord—which is called *injured metamere*—determines the type of paralysis.[36,37] The muscles that are innervated above the level of injury have normal strength (nerve function above the injured metamere is normal). The muscles in *injured metamere* will be flaccid but may improve by time (nerve function is absent). The muscles below the *injured metamere* may be flaccid or may have some spasticity. If the lower motor neuron is intact below the *injured metamere*, stimulation of the muscle is possible.

Other common causes of loss of neural functions are stroke, cerebral palsy, traumatic brain injury, infectious or metabolic diseases, genetic diseases, multiple sclerosis, Guillain–Barre syndrome, brain or spinal tumors. Whatever the cause, the bone is affected in a nonworking extremity.

Calcium homeostasis changes within the first months after injury in SCI. These changes involve hypercalcemia and hypercalciuria that lead renal calculi and changes in calciotropic hormonal profile. According to the histomorphometric data, the main cause of bone loss is increase in bone resorption due to increased number of eroded surfaces and osteoclasts.[17] Bone resorption increases constantly from the first week after injury and peaks between weeks 10 and 16. In the first few months after SCI, BMD decreases 2 to 4% a month. This rate is 5 to 20 times greater than a metabolic factor. Bone mass loss is greater in trabecular than cortical regions.[38] After 1 year of injury, hydroxyproline and deoxyproline, the markers of bone resorption, remain elevated, while the bone markers show a minor rise. This imbalance begins immediately after injury and peaks between 3 and 5 months. Around 2 years after injury, bone metabolic process reaches steady-state level. However, depending on the lesion level, gender, age, and accompanying systemic problems, even after 2 years from injury, bone tissue turnover can be seen up to 8 years. Bone loss at the lower extremity is independent of the lesion level while loss at upper extremity is mostly seen tetraplegic patients. Trauma level determines the extent but not the degree of bone loss.[39,40]

Some magnetic resonance imaging (MRI) studies showed that reduced bone volume and trabecular number resulting with increased trabecular space in long-standing complete SCI. Similar changes have also been shown with computed tomography (CT). After all process, BMD values of the patients with SCI are 50 to 60% lower than healthy peers.[38]

Bone changes in SCI also have been supported in mouse studies. Increment in bone marrow cavity by 24% and thinning in cortical width by around 30% have been shown.[38] Moreover, SCI resulted in more severe BMD loss and disruption in trabecular microarchitecture and cortical bone geometry than hind limb cast immobilization (HCI) model in mouse.[41]

Hammond et al[42] stated prevalence of osteoporosis in SCI as 34.9%. Duration of injury more than 1 year was associated with a threefold increased osteoporosis.[20,42] As a consequence, fractures are common in SCI. In chronic SCI, the most common fracture causes were falling from wheel chair (51%), twisting the lower extremity during transferring (14%), and hitting the lower extremity on doorframe during using wheelchair.[43] Bone impairments occur almost 75% of patients of SCI due to BMD decrease. Fracture rates were found 1.8% in men and 2.5 in women who had SCI over 5 years.[44] In the United States, fracture rate in 5 years after injury were given 14%. This rate increases to 28% after 10 years and 39% after 15 years. Besides, fracture rate increases with age and is higher in complete lesions, in paraplegics and in women.[41] Additionally, rate of fractures other than the spine were 28% in SCI. Of those fractures, 52% were in chest, 25% were in lower extremity, 24% were in upper extremity, 17% were in head, and 9% were in pelvis.[45]

Stroke

Osteoporosis is accepted as one of the major complications in stroke.[46] Fractures in stroke are also common due to bone loss in paretic extremities. BMD loss, functional level, and risk of fall increase fracture risk in stroke. Disuse is defined as main causative factor BMD loss in stroke.[47] Ramnemark et al[48] stated that 1 year after stroke there was no significant BMD loss in head or spine. However, after 4 months from stroke, distal radius and proximal femur showed BMD loss compared to nonparetic side. Moreover, total arm showed BMD loss even 1 month after stroke. Similarly, de Brito et al[46] suggested lower BMD values in paretic forearms in proportion to unaffected forearms very recently to the stroke. Within the first year after stroke, BMD loss of femur neck in paretic extremity was 14% in nonambulatory patients, while it was 8% in ambulatory patients. Similarly, BMD loss in proximal humerus was higher than nonparetic arm 1 year after stroke.[46] The effect of immobilization duration on BMD loss also has been showed in SCI.[47]

Cerebral Palsy

Fracture rates are relatively high in cerebral palsy (CP). In children with CP, diminished linear growth with defined risk factors, including weight bearing, muscle mass insufficiency, calcium and phosphate homeostasis, nutrition, medications, and immobilization lead to poor mineralization of bone and nontraumatic fractures. Additionally, severity of motor impairment was correlated with BMD loss.[49–52]

In the study of Leet et al,[53] 50 of 418 children had fractures. Thirty-six patients were quadriplegic, 10 were diplegic, and 4 were hemiplegic. Mean age for fracture was 8.6 ± 4.0. Lower extremity rate was 70%, while upper was 25%. Most common fractures were in femur and in humerus. Children using standing equipment in physical therapy were more prone to having fracture.[53]

Obstetrical Brachial Plexus Palsy

Obstetrical brachial plexus palsy (OBPP) is one of the lower motor neuron models that lead to paralysis. Several studies showed BMD loss in OBPP. The Z-score is a comparison with the bone density of people of the same age and gender as the patient and helpful in diagnosing secondary osteoporosis. Ibrahim et al[54] stated severe BMD loss in axonometric type brachial plexus injury and Z-scores in 30 of 45 children indicated increased risk in their study. BMD loss was associated with severity of paralysis. Lack of muscle contraction and mechanical loading were suggested as main causes of BMD loss.[54,55]

In a series of 1,576 cases with OBPP, we observed three cases with fractures of the surgical neck of humerus (▶Fig. 11.1). Two of these fractures developed during physical therapy, and one was after a fall during cycling. In two cases, fractures were observed in the middle third of radius at the level of the bone anchor, which

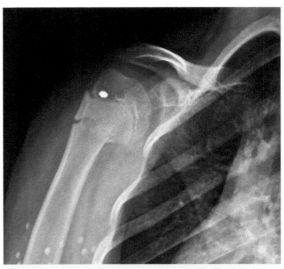

Fig. 11.1 Fracture of the surgical neck of right humerus in a 10-year-old girl with obstetrical brachial plexus palsy. She had subscapularis muscle release and latissimus dorsi muscle transfer 4 years before.

was used in the supinator transfer of the brachioradialis muscle.

Lower Motor Neuron Lesions

Patients with Charcot–Marie–Tooth (CMT) have increased fracture risk. The patients are prone to fall. Pouwels et al[56] showed that CMT patients had 1.5-fold increased risk for nonosteoporotic fracture in the hand, foot, and ankle in line with clinical feature of the disease. However, BMD with diabetic CMT patients were found unaffected while lower limbs and femur neck were highly affected. Moreover, lower limb BMD was found correlated with peroneal nerve conduction velocity.[57]

Isolated peripheral nerve injury leads similar bone degradation. Suyama et al[58] showed bone mineral content decrease and TRAP-positive multinucleated osteoclast increase following sciatic nerve constriction injury in rats since the second week.

Botulinum Toxin

Botulinum toxin causes artificial paralysis. It interferes with presynaptic release of the vesicle-bound neurotransmitter acetylcholine.[1] However, it affects bone structure as well as muscle as Warner showed that trabecular degradation and trabecular thinning in femur following botulinum toxin injection to mice quadriceps muscle after 21 days, despite nonrestricted mobility. Cortical shell bone volume was found diminished as well.[59]

Similar results have been shown in the study of Grimston et al.[60] Twelve weeks after a single-dose botulinum toxin injection, 14% loss was observed in the injected limb in mice. Moreover, cortical bone thickness was lower in the injected limb. This rapid and significant bone loss was not fully recovered even if muscle recovered.[60]

11.3 Epidemiology

It is not surprising that bone loss in paralytic extremity leads to increased risk of low-impact fractures. However, several studies reported an increased low-energy fracture rate for the lower limbs but not for the upper limbs.[14,27,32,61–63] Fractures have been reported to occur during transfer from bed to chair or due to wheelchair accidents.[43,64] Vestergaard et al[61] evaluated 438 patients and 654 controls to find out fracture rates and risk factors for fractures in patients with various types and levels of SCI. The authors reported that while fractures of the lower extremity were more prominent in patients than controls, the upper extremity fracture rates did not differ between groups. They suggested that upper extremity fractures were rare because paraplegic patients using manual wheelchairs were protected from bone loss of upper extremity and tetraplegic patients were unable to use their upper extremity to prevent falls. In the same study, women were found to have more fracture frequency than men.[61] The authors related this finding with higher frequency of osteoporosis in women.

To assess fracture risk in SCI patients is a difficult subject. Heterotopic ossification or neuropathic changes may erroneously increase the BMD.[65,66] The most appropriate method (dual-energy X-ray absorptiometry, peripheral quantitative CT), measurement site (proximal femur, distal femur, proximal tibia), variable (BMD, bone area, bone geometry), or threshold that should be used to define fracture risk in the SCI population has yet to be defined.[67,68]

11.4 Prevention

The prevention of bone loss is a meaningful way to impede fractures. However, there is generally no standardized treatment guidelines for management of osteoporosis in patients with SCI.[69,70]

To regulate diet to increase calcium and vitamin D uptake may be the easiest first step.[71] Also, it is known that alcohol intake and cigarette smoking have toxic effects on bone. Moreover, alcohol consumption, on its own, arises as a risk factor for low-impact fractures in SCI patients. In a prospective study, Morse et al[43] found that low-impact fractures are more common in motor-complete SCI and are associated with greater alcohol use after injury.

Nonpharmacological treatment methods such as standing up, orthotically aided walking, weight-bearing physical exercises, functional electrical stimulation, low-intensity pulsed ultrasound, and pulsed electromagnetic fields have been studied in the literature. Passive mechanical loading may have a beneficial effect to preserve bone mass.[72,73] Goemaere et al[72] reported a better-preserved BMD in their paraplegic patients who perform standing. Saltzstein et al[28] demonstrated a strong correlation between the mobility of their patients and BMD. However, Biering-Sørensen et al[6]

reported that the spasticity and passive mechanical loading did not influence BMD significantly. Likewise, Dauty et al[31] reported that there is no effect of biomechanical stress (i.e., standing, walking, sitting) on the increase of sublesional BMD in SCI patients.

The effects of functional electrical stimulation exercise on bone in SCI patients are inconclusive.[67] Some studies have reported the functional electrical stimulation exercise to be ineffective for increasing bone mass.[74–76] Several studies suggest that functional electrical stimulation may enhance BMD.[77–80] In the study of Warden et al,[81] no benefit from low-intensity pulsed ultrasound was reported. Although reports about impact vibration and pulsed electromagnetic fields were promising, the studies were of poor quality.[82,83]

To prevent osteoporosis, pharmacological treatment on reversing bone resorption is another option. The bisphosphonates found to be efficient to reduce bone resorption in patients with SCI.[43,84,85] However, the treatment cannot stop the demineralization process.[17] The pathophysiological process of bone resorption in paralytic extremities is quite different from those of postmenopausal women. Therefore, a pharmacological treatment guideline for SCI patients needs to be developed.[17] Reviewing the literature gives many clues for preventing paralytic fractures. Keeping the patient as far as mobile is the key approach regardless of etiology. Supportive regimes should be kept in mind during all the process.

- Weight bearing: Extremity should be loaded in axial direction for preventing trabecular degradation. Keeping patient standing especially in SCI and stroke is essential as early as possible to preserve BMD of long bones including femur and tibia.[72,86] Similarly, weight bearing of arm in lower motor neurons should be implemented to all rehabilitation methods.
- Early mobilization: Shortening the immobilization duration especially in upper motor neuron lesions is essential. Higher BMD loss values have been showed in SCI and stroke.
- Neuromuscular electrical stimulation (NMES): NMES can be applied in either upper or lower extremity paralytic conditions to support preserving BMD. Its effectiveness has been showed together with weight-bearing and rehabilitation approaches.[87]
- Low-intensity vibration: The effectiveness of low-intensity vibration on BMD has been showed in several studies. Mechanical signals generated from vibration seem a safe and effective approach especially in SCI.[88]
- Dietary supplements: Menatetrenone (MK-4) is a vitamin K_2 homologue has been used especially in Japan for preventing BMD. Its effectiveness can be investigated in paralytic conditions.[89,90]
- Environmental adjustment: Environmental adjustments including home and outside should be considered in all paralytic patients. Falling due to stumbling is very common in stroke patients. Lightning of the environment is also beneficial.

11.5 Diagnosis

Diagnosis may be challenging in paralytic extremity. In many patients, pain can be insignificant. A close examination for crepitus, hematomas, or deformity is essential. Caregivers must be instructed to be watchful for these signs.

11.6 Management of Fractures

The management of upper extremity fractures is mostly surgeon's choice. Spasticity in an extremity is usually associated with heterotopic ossification, aberrant callus formation, and angular deformities.[91] Although conservative methods are promising, some surgeons prefer internal fixation to facilitate self-care or transfer of the patient.[27,62,91]

11.7 Evidence

Randomized controlled studies are difficult in patients with fractures of paralytic upper extremity. This population is quite small and interindividual variability such as age, sex, level of lesion, and time after injury are great.[67] It is difficult to establish adequate matching between control and intervention groups.

11.8 Future

Lack of evidence-based studies led to empirical methods for following the patients having paralysis. Suggestions mentioned involve nonstandard parameters and there is no consensus for any paralytic condition. Although pertinent literature offers detailed basic science aspects, treatment and prevention strategies are still obscure.

References

[1] Laurent MR, Dubois V, Claessens F, et al. Muscle-bone interactions: from experimental models to the clinic? A critical update. Mol Cell Endocrinol. 2016; 432:14–36
[2] Järvinen TA, Józsa L, Kannus P, Järvinen TL, Järvinen M. Organization and distribution of intramuscular connective tissue in normal and immobilized skeletal muscles. An immunohistochemical, polarization and scanning electron microscopic study. J Muscle Res Cell Motil. 2002; 23(3):245–254
[3] Olive JL, Dudley GA, McCully KK. Vascular remodeling after spinal cord injury. Med Sci Sports Exerc. 2003; 35(6):901–907
[4] Vanwanseele B, Eckstein F, Knecht H, Stüssi E, Spaepen A. Knee cartilage of spinal cord-injured patients displays progressive thinning in the absence of normal joint loading and movement. Arthritis Rheum. 2002; 46(8):2073–2078
[5] Eser P, Frotzler A, Zehnder Y, Denoth J. Fracture threshold in the femur and tibia of people with spinal cord injury as determined by peripheral quantitative computed tomography. Arch Phys Med Rehabil. 2005; 86(3):498–504
[6] Biering-Sørensen F, Bohr H, Schaadt O. Bone mineral content of the lumbar spine and lower extremities years after spinal cord lesion. Paraplegia. 1988; 26(5):293–301
[7] Jiang SD, Dai LY, Jiang LS. Osteoporosis after spinal cord injury. Osteoporos Int. 2006; 17(2):180–192

[8] Giangregorio L, Blimkie CJ. Skeletal adaptations to alterations in weight-bearing activity: a comparison of models of disuse osteoporosis. Sports Med. 2002; 32(7):459–476
[9] Vandenborne K, Elliott MA, Walter GA, et al. Longitudinal study of skeletal muscle adaptations during immobilization and rehabilitation. Muscle Nerve. 1998; 21(8):1006–1012
[10] Slade JM, Bickel CS, Modlesky CM, Majumdar S, Dudley GA. Trabecular bone is more deteriorated in spinal cord injured versus estrogen-free postmenopausal women. Osteoporos Int. 2005; 16(3):263–272
[11] Modlesky CM, Majumdar S, Narasimhan A, Dudley GA. Trabecular bone microarchitecture is deteriorated in men with spinal cord injury. J Bone Miner Res. 2004; 19(1):48–55
[12] Szollar SM, Martin EM, Parthemore JG, Sartoris DJ, Deftos LJ. Densitometric patterns of spinal cord injury associated bone loss. Spinal Cord. 1997; 35(6):374–382
[13] de Bruin ED, Vanwanseele B, Dambacher MA, Dietz V, Stüssi E. Long-term changes in the tibia and radius bone mineral density following spinal cord injury. Spinal Cord. 2005; 43(2):96–101
[14] Zehnder Y, Lüthi M, Michel D, et al. Long-term changes in bone metabolism, bone mineral density, quantitative ultrasound parameters, and fracture incidence after spinal cord injury: a cross-sectional observational study in 100 paraplegic men. Osteoporos Int. 2004; 15(3):180–189
[15] Garland DE, Stewart CA, Adkins RH, et al. Osteoporosis after spinal cord injury. J Orthop Res. 1992; 10(3):371–378
[16] Chantraine A, Nusgens B, Lapiere CM. Bone remodeling during the development of osteoporosis in paraplegia. Calcif Tissue Int. 1986; 38(6):323–327
[17] Maïmoun L, Fattal C, Micallef JP, Peruchon E, Rabischong P. Bone loss in spinal cord-injured patients: from physiopathology to therapy. Spinal Cord. 2006; 44(4):203–210
[18] Roberts D, Lee W, Cuneo RC, et al. Longitudinal study of bone turnover after acute spinal cord injury. J Clin Endocrinol Metab. 1998; 83(2):415–422
[19] Biering-Sørensen F, Bohr HH, Schaadt OP. Longitudinal study of bone mineral content in the lumbar spine, the forearm and the lower extremities after spinal cord injury. Eur J Clin Invest. 1990; 20(3):330–335
[20] Eser P, Frotzler A, Zehnder Y, et al. Relationship between the duration of paralysis and bone structure: a pQCT study of spinal cord injured individuals. Bone. 2004; 34(5):869–880
[21] Uebelhart D, Demiaux-Domenech B, Roth M, Chantraine A. Bone metabolism in spinal cord injured individuals and in others who have prolonged immobilisation. A review. Paraplegia. 1995; 33(11):669–673
[22] Chantraine A. Clinical investigation of bone metabolism in spinal cord lesions. Paraplegia. 1971; 8(4):253–259
[23] Tsuzuku S, Ikegami Y, Yabe K. Bone mineral density differences between paraplegic and quadriplegic patients: a cross-sectional study. Spinal Cord. 1999; 37(5):358–361
[24] Demirel G, Yilmaz H, Paker N, Onel S. Osteoporosis after spinal cord injury. Spinal Cord. 1998; 36(12):822–825
[25] Frey-Rindova P, de Bruin ED, Stüssi E, Dambacher MA, Dietz V. Bone mineral density in upper and lower extremities during 12 months after spinal cord injury measured by peripheral quantitative computed tomography. Spinal Cord. 2000; 38(1):26–32
[26] Finsen V, Indredavik B, Fougner KJ. Bone mineral and hormone status in paraplegics. Paraplegia. 1992; 30(5):343–347
[27] Comarr AE, Hutchinson RH, Bors E. Extremity fractures of patients with spinal cord injuries. Am J Surg. 1962; 103:732–739
[28] Saltzstein RJ, Hardin S, Hastings J. Osteoporosis in spinal cord injury: using an index of mobility and its relationship to bone density. J Am Paraplegia Soc. 1992; 15(4):232–234
[29] Sabo D, Blaich S, Wenz W, Hohmann M, Loew M, Gerner HJ. Osteoporosis in patients with paralysis after spinal cord injury. A cross sectional study in 46 male patients with dual-energy X-ray absorptiometry. Arch Orthop Trauma Surg. 2001; 121(1–2):75–78
[30] Kostovski E, Hjeltnes N, Eriksen EF, Kolset SO, Iversen PO. Differences in bone mineral density, markers of bone turnover and extracellular matrix and daily life muscular activity among patients with recent motor-incomplete versus motor-complete spinal cord injury. Calcif Tissue Int. 2015; 96(2):145–154

[31] Dauty M, Perrouin Verbe B, Maugars Y, Dubois C, Mathe JF. Supralesional and sublesional bone mineral density in spinal cord-injured patients. Bone. 2000; 27(2):305–309

[32] Lazo MG, Shirazi P, Sam M, Giobbie-Hurder A, Blacconiere MJ, Muppidi M. Osteoporosis and risk of fracture in men with spinal cord injury. Spinal Cord. 2001; 39(4):208–214

[33] Eser P, Frotzler A, Zehnder Y, Schiessl H, Denoth J. Assessment of anthropometric, systemic, and lifestyle factors influencing bone status in the legs of spinal cord injured individuals. Osteoporos Int. 2005; 16(1):26–34

[34] Wilmet E, Ismail AA, Heilporn A, Welraeds D, Bergmann P. Longitudinal study of the bone mineral content and of soft tissue composition after spinal cord section. Paraplegia. 1995; 33(11):674–677

[35] Tator CH, Duncan EG, Edmonds VE, Lapczak LI, Andrews DF. Neurological recovery, mortality and length of stay after acute spinal cord injury associated with changes in management. Paraplegia. 1995; 33(5):254–262

[36] Van Heest AE. Tetraplegia. In: Wolfe SW, Hotchkiss RN, Pederson WC, Kozin SH, Cohen MS, eds. Green's Operative Hand Surgery. 7th ed. Philadelphia, PA: Elsevier; 2017:1122–1145

[37] Coulet B, Allieu Y, Chammas M. Injured metamere and functional surgery of the tetraplegic upper limb. Hand Clin. 2002; 18(3):399–412, vi

[38] Gross TS, Poliachik SL, Prasad J, Bain SD. The effect of muscle dysfunction on bone mass and morphology. J Musculoskelet Neuronal Interact. 2010; 10(1):25–34

[39] Marteau P, Nelet F, Le Lu M, Devaux C. Adverse events in patients treated with 5-aminosalicyclic acid: 1993–1994 pharmacovigilance report for Pentasa in France. Aliment Pharmacol Ther. 1996; 10(6):949–956

[40] Cirnigliaro CM, Myslinski MJ, La Fountaine MF, Kirshblum SC, Forrest GF, Bauman WA. Bone loss at the distal femur and proximal tibia in persons with spinal cord injury: imaging approaches, risk of fracture, and potential treatment options. Osteoporos Int. 2017; 28(3):747–765

[41] Dionyssiotis Y. Spinal cord injury-related bone impairment and fractures: an update on epidemiology and physiopathological mechanisms. J Musculoskelet Neuronal Interact. 2011; 11(3):257–265

[42] Hammond ER, Metcalf HM, McDonald JW, Sadowsky CL. Bone mass in individuals with chronic spinal cord injury: associations with activity-based therapy, neurologic and functional status, a retrospective study. Arch Phys Med Rehabil. 2014; 95(12):2342–2349

[43] Morse LR, Battaglino RA, Stolzmann KL, et al. Osteoporotic fractures and hospitalization risk in chronic spinal cord injury. Osteoporos Int. 2009; 20(3):385–392

[44] Ragnarsson KT, Sell GH. Lower extremity fractures after spinal cord injury: a retrospective study. Arch Phys Med Rehabil. 1981; 62(9):418–423

[45] Wang CM, Chen Y, DeVivo MJ, Huang CT. Epidemiology of extraspinal fractures associated with acute spinal cord injury. Spinal Cord. 2001; 39(11):589–594

[46] de Brito CM, Garcia AC, Takayama L, Fregni F, Battistella LR, Pereira RM. Bone loss in chronic hemiplegia: a longitudinal cohort study. J Clin Densitom. 2013; 16(2):160–167

[47] del Puente A, Pappone N, Mandes MG, Mantova D, Scarpa R, Oriente P. Determinants of bone mineral density in immobilization: a study on hemiplegic patients. Osteoporos Int. 1996; 6(1):50–54

[48] Ramnemark A, Nyberg L, Lorentzon R, Englund U, Gustafson Y. Progressive hemiosteoporosis on the paretic side and increased bone mineral density in the nonparetic arm the first year after severe stroke. Osteoporos Int. 1999; 9(3):269–275

[49] Houlihan CM. Bone health in cerebral palsy: who's at risk and what to do about it? J Pediatr Rehabil Med. 2014; 7(2):143–153

[50] Marciniak C, Gabet J, Lee J, Ma M, Brander K, Wysocki N. Osteoporosis in adults with cerebral palsy: feasibility of DXA screening and risk factors for low bone density. Osteoporos Int. 2016; 27(4):1477–1484

[51] Lingam S, Joester J. Spontaneous fractures in children and adolescents with cerebral palsy. BMJ. 1994; 309(6949):265

[52] Mughal MZ. Fractures in children with cerebral palsy. Curr Osteoporos Rep. 2014; 12(3):313–318

[53] Leet AI, Mesfin A, Pichard C, et al. Fractures in children with cerebral palsy. J Pediatr Orthop. 2006; 26(5):624–627

[54] Ibrahim AI, Hawamdeh ZM, Alsharif AA. Evaluation of bone mineral density in children with perinatal brachial plexus palsy: effectiveness of weight bearing and traditional exercises. Bone. 2011; 49(3):499–505

[55] Heinrich CH, Going SB, Pamenter RW, Perry CD, Boyden TW, Lohman TG. Bone mineral content of cyclically menstruating female resistance and endurance trained athletes. Med Sci Sports Exerc. 1990; 22(5):558–563

[56] Pouwels S, de Boer A, Leufkens HG, Weber WE, Cooper C, de Vries F. Risk of fracture in patients with Charcot-Marie-Tooth disease. Muscle Nerve. 2014; 50(6):919–924

[57] Young MJ, Marshall A, Adams JE, Selby PL, Boulton AJ. Osteopenia, neurological dysfunction, and the development of Charcot neuroarthropathy. Diabetes Care. 1995; 18(1):34–38

[58] Suyama H, Moriwaki K, Niida S, Maehara Y, Kawamoto M, Yuge O. Osteoporosis following chronic constriction injury of sciatic nerve in rats. J Bone Miner Metab. 2002; 20(2):91–97

[59] Warner SE, Sanford DA, Becker BA, Bain SD, Srinivasan S, Gross TS. Botox induced muscle paralysis rapidly degrades bone. Bone. 2006; 38(2):257–264

[60] Grimston SK, Silva MJ, Civitelli R. Bone loss after temporarily induced muscle paralysis by Botox is not fully recovered after 12 weeks. Ann N Y Acad Sci. 2007; 1116:444–460

[61] Vestergaard P, Krogh K, Rejnmark L, Mosekilde L. Fracture rates and risk factors for fractures in patients with spinal cord injury. Spinal Cord. 1998; 36(11):790–796

[62] Nottage WM. A review of long-bone fractures in patients with spinal cord injuries. Clin Orthop Relat Res. 1981(155):65–70

[63] Gifre L, Vidal J, Carrasco J, et al. Incidence of skeletal fractures after traumatic spinal cord injury: a 10-year follow-up study. Clin Rehabil. 2014; 28(4):361–369

[64] Kirby RL, Ackroyd-Stolarz SA, Brown MG, Kirkland SA, MacLeod DA. Wheelchair-related accidents caused by tips and falls among noninstitutionalized users of manually propelled wheelchairs in Nova Scotia. Am J Phys Med Rehabil. 1994; 73(5):319–330

[65] Liu CC, Theodorou DJ, Theodorou SJ, et al. Quantitative computed tomography in the evaluation of spinal osteoporosis following spinal cord injury. Osteoporos Int. 2000; 11(10):889–896

[66] Jaovisidha S, Sartoris DJ, Martin EM, Foldes K, Szollar SM, Deftos LJ. Influence of heterotopic ossification of the hip on bone densitometry: a study in spinal cord injured patients. Spinal Cord. 1998; 36(9):647–653

[67] Giangregorio L, McCartney N. Bone loss and muscle atrophy in spinal cord injury: epidemiology, fracture prediction, and rehabilitation strategies. J Spinal Cord Med. 2006; 29(5):489–500

[68] Bauman WA. Risk factors for osteoporosis in persons with spinal cord injury: what we should know and what we should be doing. J Spinal Cord Med. 2004; 27(3):212–213

[69] Morse LR, Giangregorio L, Battaglino RA, et al. VA-based survey of osteoporosis management in spinal cord injury. PM R. 2009; 1(3):240–244

[70] Phaner V, Charmetant C, Condemine A, Fayolle-Minon I, Lafage-Proust MH, Calmels P; groupe de travail Sofmer-AFIGAP. [Osteoporosis in spinal cord injury. Screening and treatment. Results of a survey of physical medicine and rehabilitation physician practices in France. Proposals for action to be taken towards the screening and the treatment] Ann Phys Rehabil Med. 2010; 53(10):615–620

[71] Bauman WA, Zhong YG, Schwartz E. Vitamin D deficiency in veterans with chronic spinal cord injury. Metabolism. 1995; 44(12):1612–1616

[72] Goemaere S, Van Laere M, De Neve P, Kaufman JM. Bone mineral status in paraplegic patients who do or do not perform standing. Osteoporos Int. 1994; 4(3):138–143

[73] Kaplan PE, Roden W, Gilbert E, Richards L, Goldschmidt JW. Reduction of hypercalciuria in tetraplegia after weight-bearing and strengthening exercises. Paraplegia. 1981; 19(5):289–293

[74] Leeds EM, Klose KJ, Ganz W, Serafini A, Green BA. Bone mineral density after bicycle ergometry training. Arch Phys Med Rehabil. 1990; 71(3):207–209

[75] Pacy PJ, Hesp R, Halliday DA, Katz D, Cameron G, Reeve J. Muscle and bone in paraplegic patients, and the effect of functional electrical stimulation. Clin Sci (Lond). 1988; 75(5):481–487

[76] Eser P, de Bruin ED, Telley I, Lechner HE, Knecht H, Stüssi E. Effect of electrical stimulation-induced cycling on bone mineral density in spinal cord-injured patients. Eur J Clin Invest. 2003; 33(5):412–419

[77] Castello F, Louis B, Cheng J, Armento M, Santos AM. The use of functional electrical stimulation cycles in children and adolescents with spinal cord dysfunction: a pilot study. J Pediatr Rehabil Med. 2012; 5(4):261–273

[78] Bélanger M, Stein RB, Wheeler GD, Gordon T, Leduc B. Electrical stimulation: can it increase muscle strength and reverse osteopenia in spinal cord injured individuals? Arch Phys Med Rehabil. 2000; 81(8):1090–1098

[79] Mohr T, Podenphant J, Biering-Sorensen F, Galbo H, Thamsborg G, Kjaer M. Increased bone mineral density after prolonged electrically induced cycle training of paralyzed limbs in spinal cord injured man. Calcif Tissue Int. 1997; 61(1):22–25

[80] Chen SC, Lai CH, Chan WP, Huang MH, Tsai HW, Chen JJ. Increases in bone mineral density after functional electrical stimulation cycling exercises in spinal cord injured patients. Disabil Rehabil. 2005; 27(22):1337–1341

[81] Warden SJ, Bennell KL, Matthews B, Brown DJ, McMeeken JM, Wark JD. Efficacy of low-intensity pulsed ultrasound in the prevention of osteoporosis following spinal cord injury. Bone. 2001; 29(5):431–436

[82] Petrofsky JS, Phillips CA. The use of functional electrical stimulation for rehabilitation of spinal cord injured patients. Cent Nerv Syst Trauma. 1984; 1(1):57–74

[83] Garland DE, Adkins RH, Matsuno NN, Stewart CA. The effect of pulsed electromagnetic fields on osteoporosis at the knee in individuals with spinal cord injury. J Spinal Cord Med. 1999; 22(4):239–245

[84] Gilchrist NL, Frampton CM, Acland RH, et al. Alendronate prevents bone loss in patients with acute spinal cord injury: a randomized, double-blind, placebo-controlled study. J Clin Endocrinol Metab. 2007; 92(4):1385–1390

[85] Bubbear JS, Gall A, Middleton FR, Ferguson-Pell M, Swaminathan R, Keen RW. Early treatment with zoledronic acid prevents bone loss at the hip following acute spinal cord injury. Osteoporos Int. 2011; 22(1):271–279

[86] Lanyon LE. Using functional loading to influence bone mass and architecture: objectives, mechanisms, and relationship with estrogen of the mechanically adaptive process in bone. Bone. 1996; 18 suppl (1):37S–43S

[87] Elnaggar RK. Shoulder function and bone mineralization in children with obstetric brachial plexus injury after neuromuscular electrical stimulation during weight-bearing exercises. Am J Phys Med Rehabil. 2016; 95(4):239–247

[88] Asselin P, Spungen AM, Muir JW, Rubin CT, Bauman WA. Transmission of low-intensity vibration through the axial skeleton of persons with spinal cord injury as a potential intervention for preservation of bone quantity and quality. J Spinal Cord Med. 2011; 34(1):52–59

[89] Iwasaki-Ishizuka Y, Yamato H, Murayama H, et al. Menatetrenone ameliorates reduction in bone mineral density and bone strength in sciatic neurectomized rats. J Nutr Sci Vitaminol (Tokyo). 2003; 49(4):256–261

[90] Iwasaki-Ishizuka Y, Yamato H, Murayama H, Ezawa I, Kurokawa K, Fukagawa M. Menatetrenone rescues bone loss by improving osteoblast dysfunction in rats immobilized by sciatic neurectomy. Life Sci. 2005; 76(15):1721–1734

[91] Garland DE. Clinical observations on fractures and heterotopic ossification in the spinal cord and traumatic brain injured populations. Clin Orthop Relat Res. 1988(233):86–101

12 Hand Injuries in the Athlete

William Geissler, David Alvarez

Abstract

The pursuit of excellence drives the athletes to expose their body to relentless physical punishment. Consequently, the high severity injuries that may result and unforgiving recovery time frames present unique treatment challenges. Fortunately, the athlete is a highly motivated patient with vast rehabilitation resources at his or her disposal. As a result, they are often candidates for more aggressive procedures that may otherwise plague the typical patient with stiffness or weakness. The team physician will constantly find themselves walking the line between early return to play and avoiding potentially career ending reinjury. The successful management of a sports-related injury requires involving the athlete, family, coach, and physician in the decision-making process. Special considerations in the decision-making process include recognizing when surgery can safely be delayed to the post season, identifying when surgery should be accelerated, and ensuring early return to play will not result irreparable damage. This chapter explores evaluation and management of scapholunate instability, phalangeal, metacarpal, and carpal fractures.

Keywords: athlete, hand fractures, carpal fractures, scapholunate ligament injury

12.1 Metacarpal and Phalangeal Fractures

Metacarpal and phalangeal fractures are the most common injuries in the upper extremity both in athletes and the general population alike.[1] Although fracture patterns may not differ from those seen in the general population, time to recovery and functional expectations are much greater for the athlete. Stable anatomical fixation is key to initiating early active range of motion (ROM). Recent advancements in instrumentation allow for percutaneous techniques that are rigidly stable and minimally invasive.

12.1.1 Intra-articular Phalangeal Fractures

Unicondylar fractures are common among athletes. Unfortunately, these injuries are frequently misdiagnosed as a sprain and, consequently, often present in a subacute fashion.[2] Weiss et al[3] reported on their series on 30 consecutive patients with unicondylar fractures of the proximal phalanx. Their findings indicated that 19 of their 38 fractures occurred at sporting events and identified four predominant fracture patterns. Class 1 was a volar oblique, class 2 a long sagittal, class 3 dorsal coronal, and class 4 volar coronal. Types 1 and 2 failed under tension applied across the collateral ligaments, whereas types 3

and 4 failed in compressions due to hyperflexion or hyperextension, respectively. Class 1 volar oblique type fractures were the most common (n = 22). The mechanism of injury is thought to occur due to a force, which produces lateral angulation and rotation on a slightly flexed digit. Additionally, the volar oblique fracture pattern affected the inner condyle of the outermost digits. Lastly, fractures treated with a single K-wire were most likely to undergo late displace and have the worst outcomes.[3]

Authors' Favored Surgical Technique

Percutaneous techniques are attempted when patients present within 7 to 10 days of injury. If a closed or percutaneous reduction cannot be obtained, a mini-open midlateral approach is used to expose the fracture site. The skin is divided sharply, the lateral bands are identified and retracted dorsally. A pointed reduction clamp is used for provisional fixation, and reduction is confirmed with fluoroscopy. A guidewire for a cannulated headless compression screw is then advanced parallel to the articular surface as perpendicular to a fracture plane as possible. A second K-wire is placed into the fracture fragment to prevent rotation on screw insertion. Screw size is estimated using the cannulated depth gauge. The near cortex is then reamed and an appropriately sized screw is advanced over the guidewire and across fracture. A typical screw measures 8 to 10 mm. If there is a large metaphyseal extension, the derotational guidewire can be used to insert an additional screw. If the insertion of two screws is anticipated, the second guidewire should be inserted from the phalanx into the condylar fragment from the opposite side of the digit. The trajectory of the second K-wire typically takes a dorsal proximal to volar distal orientation to traverse the fracture plane in a perpendicular fashion. The skin is nicked with a 11 blade and blunt dissection is carried down to the bone with hemostats. The length of the screw is estimated with a depth gauge and the appropriate-sized screws are then inserted as previously described.

Post-op Care and Outcomes

Active ROM exercises are initiated immediately post-op and strengthening exercises are started 4 to 6 weeks following surgery. Athletes can return to competitive athletics a week after surgery with the injured finger buddy taped to an adjacent digit.

Geissler et al[4] reported on 25 patients with intra-articular fractures of the phalanges stabilized percutaneously with cannulated headless compression screws. Eighteen patients had unicondylar fractures of the proximal phalanx, three had intra-articular fractures of the base of the proximal phalanx, and four had intra-articular fractures of the base of the distal phalanx of the thumb. All fractures healed without displacement or malunion. No patient required hardware removal. Average ROM for unicondylar phalangeal fractures was 5 degrees of flexion to 85 degrees of flexion. Average ROM for fractures of the thumb distal phalanx base was 15 degrees of extension to 60 degrees of flexion. Geissler[4] concluded that percutaneous cannulated headless compression screw fixation was superior to K-wires as it affords stable fixation without the risk of pin tract infection or hardware irritation. We apply this fixation principles to other coronally unstable intra-articular phalangeal fractures (▶Fig. 12.1, ▶Fig. 12.2, ▶Fig. 12.3, ▶Fig. 12.4, ▶Fig. 12.5, ▶Fig. 12.6).

12.1.2 Phalangeal Shaft Fractures

Phalangeal shaft fractures occur in various morphologies, including transverse, oblique, spiral, and comminuted patterns, all of which are amendable to various fixation

techniques. However, the athlete has the added burden of early return to play. Low-profile locked plating provides the most ridged fixation at our disposal. The increased

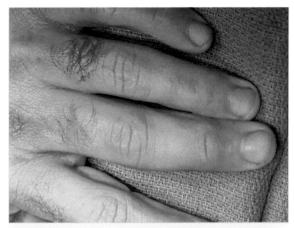

Fig. 12.2 Middle phalanx fracture with clinically evident ulnar angulation.

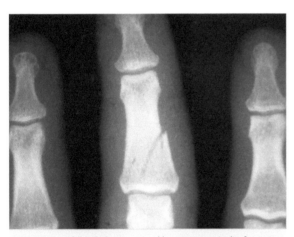

Fig. 12.1 Middle phalanx proximal base intra-articular fracture with ulnar angulation.

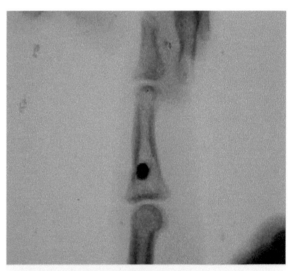

Fig. 12.4 Lateral P2 base fracture with intra-articular extension. Single cannulated screw provides rotational stability by applying compression across the fracture.

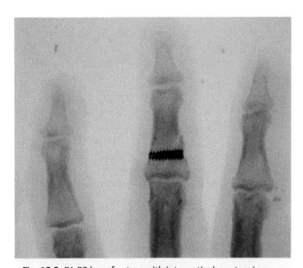

Fig. 12.3 PA P2 base fracture with intra-articular extension. Single cannulated screw provides rotational stability by applying compression across the fracture.

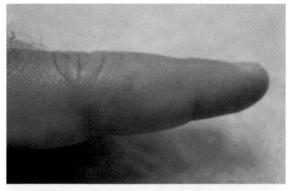

Fig. 12.5 Eight weeks' status postpercutaneous cannulated screw fixation.

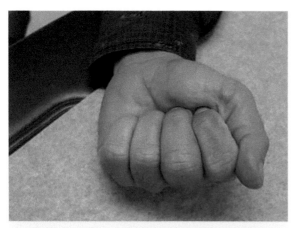

Fig. 12.6 Eight weeks' status postpercutaneous cannulated screw fixation.

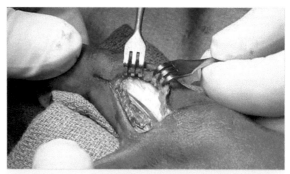

Fig. 12.7 Midlateral approach on the ulnar aspect of the digit.

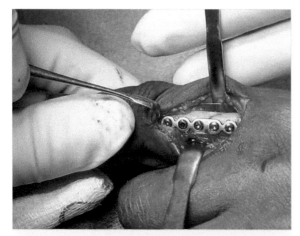

Fig. 12.8 2-mm locking plate. Medartis. (Basel, Switzerland)

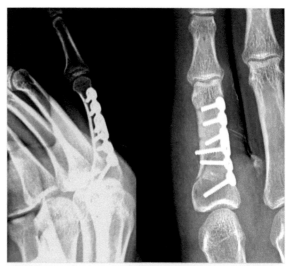

Fig. 12.9 2-mm locking plate. Medartis. (Basel, Switzerland)

dissection required for application plate have been associated with increased stiffness and prolonged time to union. The increased risk of stiffness occurs because of the intimate relationship between the extensor and flexor mechanisms of the digit to the phalanges. Consequently, there is no optimal surface available for plate placement that would avoid insult to the tendon apparatus of the digits. The risk of scaring and stiffness may be somewhat mitigated in the collegiate athlete due to the abundant physical therapy resources at their disposal. Kodama and colleagues[5] retrospectively reviewed 105 metacarpal and phalangeal fractures. They identified 20 athletes who required early return to sport within 1 month from injury. This subgroup was treated with ORIF. Mean follow-up was 27 months and average total active ROM was 263 degrees. Conclusions are somewhat limited due to sample size of 20 and heterogeneity in fracture morphology treated.

Authors' Favored Surgical Technique

A midaxial approach is centered over the fracture as previously described (▶ Fig. 12.7, ▶ Fig. 12.8). If access to the base of the phalanx is required, a portion of the lateral band can be divided to improve exposure. When practical, we prefer to approach the fracture on the ulnar aspect of the digit to avoid injury to the insertions of the lumbricals on the lateral bands. The fracture is identified and fracture hematoma is cleared and the fracture is provisionally fixed with K-wire and clamps as necessary. Rotational alignment is checked clinically and fracture reduction is confirmed under fluoroscopy. A 1.5-mm plate is precontoured and placed along the side of the phalanx. Nonlocking screws are used to secure the plate to the bone followed by locking screws to create a fixed angle construct. We typically attempt to place three screws on the other side of the fracture (▶ Fig. 12.9).

If early return to sports is not necessary, less invasive percutaneous techniques may be implemented as previously described. Long oblique fractures, where the length of greater than twice the diameter of the diaphysis and spiral fractures are well suited for cannulated headless compression screw fixation. When using headless screws in the shaft, it is important to predrill both the near and far cortex to avoid cortical blowout on screw insertion.

Post-op Care and Outcomes

Dabezies[6] reported on 22 patients who attained average total active ROM 247 degrees open reduction and

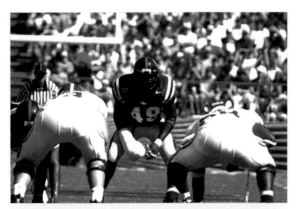

Fig. 12.10 Ole Miss linebacker 1 week's status post-ORIF of proximal phalanx.

internal fixation (ORIF) of proximal phalangeal fractures. Skilled athletes return to sport as soon as wound heals with injured digit buddy tapped to the adjacent digit. Contact players may return to play with club cast to avoid forceful gripping of an opponent's jersey (▶Fig. 12.10).

12.1.3 Metacarpal Fractures

Metacarpal (MC) fractures occur commonly among contact sport players. The most frequently affected metacarpals are those of the small and ring finger. Of note, MC neck fractures (aka boxer's fracture), is rarely seen in actual boxers and is more characteristic in amateur brawlers. The major deforming force acting on the MC are the intrinsic musculature. The volar axis of pull produces the typical apex dorsal angulation seen with these fractures. The border metacarpals are more susceptible to shortening than the central metacarpals which are tethered by the deep transverse intermetacarpal ligaments. Malalignment of the metacarpals is known to produce to unique complications in the hand. Every 2 mm of fracture shortening produces 7 degrees of extensor lag. There is measureable loss of grip strength with greater than 30 degrees of volar angulation.[7] Any amount of malrotation produces digit scissoring and clinically noticeable overlap.[8]

Conceptually, MC shaft malalignment tolerances increase as you move distally and ulnarly in the hand. The increased motion at the carpometacarpal (CMC) joints of the ulnar metacarpals allows them to compensate for greater angulation than their radial counterparts. Fractures that occur more distally produce less shortening and less volar displacement of the MC joint for a given amount of flexion angulation than a more proximal fracture with the same amount of angulation. As a result, a distal small finger MC neck fractures may tolerate as much as 70 degrees of flexion, where as an index finger midshaft fracture should not be allowed to heal with greater than 5 to 10 degrees of malalignment. Fractures within alignment tolerances after reduction typically heal with excellent outcomes after cast immobilization for 8 to 12 weeks. As with phalangeal fractures, if immediate return to play is necessary, ORIF of even well-aligned fractures should be discussed with the player and their family.

Authors' Favored Surgical Technique

We usually prefer 2-mm plates with 1.5- or 2-mm screws for MC fracture fixation. We aim to place a minimum of four bicortical locking screws on either side of the fracture. Locking cage plates with staggered screw holes allow for placement of screws over a broader surface area. Oblique fractures are provisionally reduced with clamps and fixed with lag screws. Fixation is then protected with a 2.0 mm plate in the standard neutralization fashion. Maximizing the construct's working length and contact foot print minimizes stress risers and the potential for refracture in the athlete (▶Fig. 12.11, ▶Fig. 12.12).

Post-op Care and Outcomes

Active ROM in initiated immediately post-op. Athlete returns to play 1 to 2 weeks postoperatively after wound has healed. Geissler[9] reported on retrospective cohort of 10 patients with MC shaft fractures treated with ORIF. Eight patients were treated with plates and screws, two with simple lag screws. All patients returned to play within 2 weeks from surgery. All fractures healed within 8 weeks postoperatively.

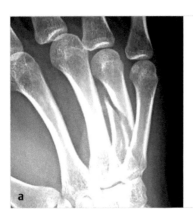
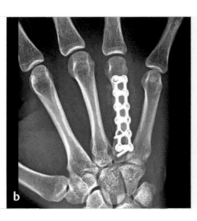

Fig. 12.11 Unstable ring finger spiral metacarpal shaft fracture **(a)** in a collegiate football player stabilized with 2-mm Medartis (Basel, Switzerland) locking cage plate **(b)**.

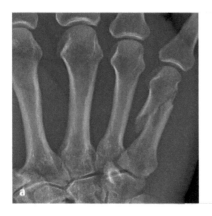
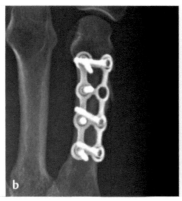

Fig. 12.12 Unstable small finger spiral metacarpal shaft fracture (**a**) in a collegiate football player stabilized with 2-mm Medartis (Basel, Switzerland) locking cage plate (**b**).

12.2 Carpal Fractures

Hand and wrist injuries constitute 3 to 9% of all sports injuries.[10] Carpal fractures typically result from a direct axial load or a direct blow from a solid object such as a ball or a bat. Eliciting the sport and position of the athlete plays a critical part of the medical history as certain injuries are characteristics of specific sports. Scaphoid fractures, for example, can occur in an instance of 1 in a 100 of college football players.[10] Hook of the hamate and trapezial ridge fractures often occur in stick handling sports such as golf, baseball, and tennis.

12.2.1 Scaphoid Fractures

Scaphoid fractures are the most common carpal fractures accounting for 6 to 7% of all carpal fractures.[11] Scaphoid fractures are not unique to the athlete and are commonly seen after a fall of outstretched hand and forcible hyperextension when catching a ball. Scaphoid fractures, in general, have gained notoriety for their propensity to progress to nonunion. The irregular anatomy of the bone makes it difficult to identify fractures on plain films. As a result, these fractures classically present in a delayed fashion. Tenuous blood supply and strong deforming forces further contribute difficulties achieving union. The primary blood supply of the scaphoid enters along its dorsal ridge and perfuses the proximal 80% of the bone in a retrograde fashion.[12] Consequently, the more proximal of the fracture line, the longer time to union and the higher the incident of avascular necrosis (AVN). The prevalence of AVN of the proximal pole has been reported to be as high as 30% after scaphoid waist fracture and nearly 100% with proximal fifth fractures.[13] Time to union can be as fast as 6 weeks in scaphoid tubercle fractures and greater than 4 months for proximal pole fractures. Scaphoid waist fractures can be expected to heal by 3 months when treated conservatively with cast immobilization. Prolonged healing time frames can have serious implications on an athlete's career and should be discussed in depth at initial presentation.

Evaluation

The athlete will present in an acute or subacute fashion with radial-sided wrist pain after falling onto outstretched hand. Symptoms may be relatively mild and the injury may have been misdiagnosed as a wrist sprain. On physical examination, the patient will demonstrate snuff box tenderness or tenderness directly over the scaphoid tubercle. A scaphoid view should be obtained in addition to the three standard projections of the wrist. This view is obtained by placing the palm flat on the cassette, the shoulder and elbow at 90 degrees, and the wrist in ulnar deviation. If radiographs are negative but there is high clinical suspicion of a fracture, the patient can be placed in short arm cast and repeat images are obtained in 2 weeks out of plaster. If immediate identification of the fracture is required, an MRI can be performed within the first 48 hours or a scintigraphy maybe performed after 72 hours to identify an occult fracture.[14-16] Computed tomography (CT) scan has been used to characterize fracture pattern and malalignment, but has been less effective in identifying an occult fracture compared to magnetic resonance imaging (MRI) and scintigraphy.[17] When return to play is not necessary, nondisplaced fractures of the scaphoid waist can be managed with casting immobilization with union rates of 90 to 95%. Fractures of the middle and proximal third have been shown to have shorter time to union when immobilized with long arm thumb spicas. Fractures of the scaphoid tubercle or the distal third healed quickly regardless of type of cast.[18]

Absolute indications for acute fixation are displacement and fractures associated with carpal instability. Scaphoid displacement is characterized by 1-mm translation, 1-mm gap, or 15 degrees of angulation.[19,20] Angulation of the scaphoid can be estimated on a lateral projection by measuring the scapholunate or radiolunate angles. Values greater than 60 for scapholunate or 15 degrees for radiolunate are considered abnormal and are correlated with nonunion rates as high as 50%.[13,21,22] Proximal third scaphoid fractures, unstable fracture patterns, and delayed presentation are considered relative indications for fixation. Delayed presentation beyond 4 to 6 weeks increases incidence of nonunion in conservative management. Vertical oblique fracture patterns are inherently unstable, are unlikely to remain nondisplaced throughout their period of mobilization. Although fractures of the proximal third have been treated conservatively with cast mobilization, they typically require 4 to 5 months of casting. Consequently, some authors recommend early internal fixation for these troublesome fractures to minimize the complications associated with prolonged immobilization. Established scaphoid nonunions are known to progress to scaphoid nonunion advance collapse (SNAC).[23] Accordingly, it is generally recommended that nonunions be addressed surgically even if asymptomatic. However, in the athlete, once an asymptomatic nonunion has been established, it should be addressed after the end of the season.

Surgical Treatment

Several surgical techniques have been described in the literature for the treatment of scaphoid fractures. Examples include dorsal and volar percutaneous techniques, arthroscopic-assisted techniques, and dorsal and volar open techniques. The palmar open exposure provides access to middle and distal third of the scaphoid, allows correction of the humpback deformity, and provides an opportunity for vascularized bone grafting. Additionally, it leaves the main dorsal blood supply undisturbed. The dorsal approach provides access to the proximal pole of the scaphoid. However, exposure and reduction maneuvers are limited by the dorsal blood supply.[24] The palmar approach extends from the scaphoid tubercle proximally along the radial aspect of the flexor carpi radialis (FCR). The superficial branch of the radial artery is identified and retracted. Alternatively, it may be ligated if more exposure is necessary. The FCR tendon sheath is then incised and the FCR is retracted ulnarly to expose the volar wrist capsule. The capsule is divided and in line with the incision. The scaphotrapeziotrapezoidal (STT) joint is identified and the volar tubercle of the trapezium is excised to gain access for the starting point of the guidewire of the Acutrak screw.[25] K-wires are inserted into the proximal and distal fragments and used as joysticks to reduce the fracture. A third K-wire can be advanced across the fracture site to hold the provisional reduction and protect against rotational displacement during screw insertion. Next, the guidewire for the cannulated screw may be driven in a retrograde fashion across the fracture along the axis of the scaphoid. Confirm with fluoroscopy that the far end of the guidewire has not been driven past the dense subchondral bone of the proximal pole. At this point, if there is a residual bony deficit at the fracture site, it may be filled with cancellous autograft harvested from the distal radius. Choose a screw that is 4-mm shorter than the estimated screw size predicted by the depth gauge. Appropriately countersinking the screw avoids prominent hardware proximally and distally. Confirm hardware position and fracture reduction on orthogonal fluoroscopic views. Remove the derotational K-wire and close the capsule. Hemostasis confirmed prior to skin closure.

The proximal pole of the scaphoid is exposed via a dorsal approach. A longitudinal incision is centered over the proximal pole of the scaphoid and made in line with the radial aspect of the long finger. Subcutaneous tissue is bluntly dissected to avoid injury to the dorsal cutaneous branches of the superficial radial sensory nerve. Identify and develop the interval between the third and fourth dorsal compartments and incise the capsule in line with the incision. Take care to avoid injury to the scapholunate ligament during the capsulotomy. Once the proximal pole of the scaphoid is identified, avoid excessive dissection over the dorsal scaphoid to prevent injury to its blood supply. Flex the wrist to gain access to the volar most aspect of the proximal scaphoid. The starting point for the guidewire will be immediately radial to the insertion of the scapholunate ligament on the proximal pole. Aim the trajectory of the guidewire down to the axis of the scaphoid and bury wire into the far subchondral bone. Confirm position of the wire with fluoroscopy taking care not to bend the guidewire during manipulation of the wrist. A second K-wire may be passed across the fracture site to protect against rotational displacement during screw insertion. Screw length is measured and inserted as previously described. Confirm hardware placement and fracture reduction on orthogonal fluoroscopic views (▶ Fig. 12.13).

Arthroscopic techniques are best suited for nondisplaced scaphoid fractures. Given that nondisplaced fractures are typically treated nonoperatively, clear indications for implementation of these surgical techniques remain somewhat controversial. Benefits include percutaneous insertion of hardware, direct visualization of fracture reduction, and limited postoperative immobilization.

Authors' Favored Surgical Technique

A standard diagnostic wrist arthroscopy is performed with the scope inserted through the 3–4 portal. After

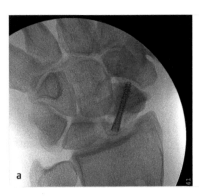
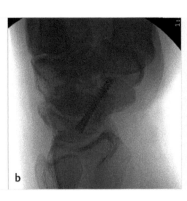

Fig. 12.13 (a, b) Cannulated screw fixation via a dorsal approach.

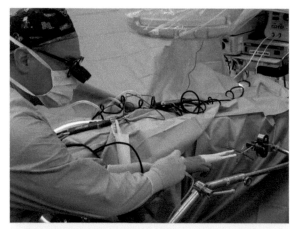

Fig. 12.14 Horizontal position of traction tower to obtain radiographs.

ruling out associated injuries, the scope is transferred to the 6R portal and a 14-gauge needle is advanced through the 3–4 portal into the radiocarpal joint. The arthroscopy tower can be laid horizontally to allow real-time fluoroscopy during arthroscopy (▶Fig. 12.14). The 14-gauge needle is then embedded into the cartilage just radial to the scapholunate ligament at the volar aspect of the proximal pole. The guidewire for the cannulated screw is then aimed at the base of the thumb and advanced through the needle and into the scaphoid along its axis. A second derotational pin may be placed across the fracture but outside the trajectory of the central screw. Reduction of the fracture is confirmed by transferring the arthroscope to the radial and ulnar midcarpal portals. Position of the guidewire and fracture alignment is confirmed on fluoroscopy. The near cortex is predrilled and an appropriately sized screw is advanced as previously described.[26]

Post-op Protocol

Return to play after cannulated headless compression screw varies by location of fracture and type of athlete. For example, scaphoid waist fractures may be started on immediate active ROM protocols, whereas proximal poles should be immobilized for 1 month postoperatively. Athletes such as weightlifters and gymnasts should be restricted until CT scans confirm 50% bridging bone. Rigidly fixed proximal pole fractures will benefit from an accelerated rehabilitation schedule but require 4 additional weeks of immobilization compared to scaphoid waste fractures.[27]

12.2.2 Hamate Fractures

Hamate fractures account for 2 to 4% of all carpal fractures.[28] Hook of the hamate fractures are overly represented in the athletic population, primarily among stick handling athletes. The hook of the hamate protrudes into the palm and is in direct contact with a tightly gripped handle. Injuries sustained in two-handed stick sports, such as lacrosse or hockey, tend to fracture the hamate of the nondominant hand. Inversely, single-handed stick sports, such as racketball or tennis, tend to injure the dominate hand.

Evaluation

The athlete typically presents with a subacute or chronic injury. The patient typically complains of pain in the hypothenar area aggravated by gripping. Occasionally, patients may complain of ulnar nerve paresthesia involving the ring and small fingers and weak grip strength.[29] On physical examination, patients will demonstrate tenderness directly over the hook of the hamate. Patient may also demonstrate pain on resisted ring finger and small finger flexion. Radiographic evaluation requires a carpal tunnel view, as the standard projections of the hand wrist rarely identify the fracture.[30] A CT scan can help characterize the fracture fragments and may identify associated injuries such as a trapezial ridge fracture which occurs via the same mechanism but is rarely identified on X-rays.

Hook of the Hamate

Nondisplaced hook of hamate fractures have demonstrated good outcomes when cast immobilization is initiated in the acute phase.[31] Like the scaphoid, the hook of the hamate has been shown to have tenuous blood supply and time to union typically ranges from 8 to 12 weeks. Furthermore, the hook of the hamate serves as an attachment site for several anatomical structures and is prone to displacement. Position of the wrist is critical in neutralizing deforming forces. It is typically recommended to place the wrist in slight flexion with metacarpals in 90 degrees of flexion. Any displacement warrants surgical intervention.

While both ORIF and excision have been described as a treatment of this troublesome fracture, fixation is difficult owing to the small size of the fracture fragments and time to union remains an obstacle for the athlete's ability to return to play. Previous studies have shown no loss of function with excision and earlier return to sport.[32,33]

Surgical Technique

A longitudinal incision is made in the palm centered over the hook of the hamate. Guyon's canal is released. Careful spreading dissection is carried through the subcutaneous tissue, the ulnar neurovascular bundle is identified, and carefully retracted radially. The motor branch should specifically identified and protected as it runs along the base of the hook of the hamate. The bony fragment is identified and subperiosteal dissection is performed circumferentially around the fragment. The fragment is excised. Any sharp bony edges are smoothed out and the periosteum is closed. The patient may return to sports as tolerated. Any residual hypothenar discomfort may be somewhat mitigated with a well-padded glove.

Body of the Hamate

Body of the hamate fractures are high-energy injuries typically associated with perilunate fracture dislocations. Mechanism of injury commonly involves an axial load of the ulnar metacarpals. Fractures may occur in the coronal or sagittal plane. CT scan is valuable in characterizing the fracture pattern as well as identifying associated injuries. The body of the hamate may be exposed via a dorsal approach. The skin is sharply incised between the ring and small fingers near the base and extended proximally toward the distal radioulnar joint (DRUJ). Dorsal cutaneous branches of the ulnar nerve are identified and protected. Extensor tendons to the small finger are identified and retracted radially. T-shaped capsulotomy is made with the transverse limb along the CMC joint and the longitudinal limb in line with the incision. K-wires can be used for provisional fixation. A cannulated headless compression screw can be used for definitive fixation.[34] Hardware may be directed into the base of the hook of the hamate when fractures are in the coronal plane. Surgeon should take special care to ensure unicortical placement of hardware as prominent hardware may cause injury to the ulnar neurovascular bundle on the palmar aspect of the bone.

12.2.3 Triquetral Fracture

Fractures of the triquetrum are common and account for 3 to 4% of all carpal fractures. Injury to the triquetrum is thought to occur via two mechanisms. The first mechanism involves falling onto an outstretched hand with the wrist hyperextended and ulnarly deviated. A dorsal chip fracture may occur due to impingement of the ulnar styloid on the triquetrum.[35] Alternatively, a fall onto a hyperflexed wrist places excessive tension on the dorsal intercarpal and dorsal radiocarpal ligaments. Avulsion of their insertion of the triquetrum results in a dorsal chip fracture.

Evaluation

The athlete may present to the clinic with dorsal wrist pain and tenderness to palpation directly over the triquetrum. A lateral view of the wrist with slight pronation best projects the dorsal contour of the triquetrum. Treatment of triquetral fractures is typically conservative with immobilization for 4 to 6 weeks. Contact athletes may return to play immediately with a splint or a club cast. Rarely, these fractures may progress to a symptomatic nonunion in which case the offending fragment may be excised and the athlete can return to sports as tolerated.

12.2.4 Pisiform Fractures

The pisiform is not a true carpal bone, instead it is a sesamoid contained within the tendon of the flexor carpi ulnaris (FCU) which articulates with the triquetrum. The typical mechanism of injury involves a direct blow either with an object such as a ball or a fall onto an outstretched hand. Fractures of the pisiform are uncommon, representing 1 to 3% of all carpal fractures. Pisiform fractures are associated with fractures of the distal radius or an adjacent carpal 50% of the time.[36]

On physical examination, the athlete may be noted to have pain with resisted wrist flexion/ulnar deviation. There is often tenderness to palpation directly over the pisiform. There may be crepitus with axial loading of the pisotriquetral joint. Radiographically, the pisiform is best evaluated with a 45-degree, semisupinated lateral wrist view. Nondisplaced fractures of the pisiform can be managed in a short arm cast for 3 to 6 weeks. Articular step-off may progress to pisotriquetral posttraumatic arthritis and chronic ulnar-sided wrist pain. Both comminuted pisiform and pisiotriquetral arthritis may be treated with pisiform excision.[37]

Exposure of the pisiform is gained via volar approach, a stand Bruner's Z-incision made with the horizontal limb in line with the volar wrist crease centered over the pisiform. Full-thickness skin flaps are elevated and the ulnar nerve vascular bundles are identified and protected. The pisiform fragments are then shelled out of the FCU taking care to preserve its fibers. Hemostasis is confirmed and the skin is closed in a typical fashion. Athlete may return to sports as tolerated with a padded glove to mitigate hypothenar discomfort.

12.2.5 Trapezium Fractures

Trapezium fractures account for 1 to 5% of all carpal fractures. These injuries have been classified into two main types, trapezial body and trapezial ridge fractures. The mechanism of injury for trapezial body fractures involves axial loading of the thumb metacarpal, which results in a shear fragment on the radial aspect to the trapezium. The metacarpal then dislocates or subluxates with the shear fragment. The trapezial ridge is bony prominence that extends into the palm of the hand and is vulnerable to direct injury. Body fractures are readily identified on standard projections of the wrist, but ridge fractures are much more difficult to detect. A carpal tunnel view may be helpful but superimposition of the scaphoid tubercle can conceal the fracture. Often a CT scan will be required to identify the fracture. Displaced body fractures are inherently unstable and typically require ORIF for stabilization.[38]

Trapezial body fractures are exposed via a standard Wagner approach. An incision is made at the junction of the glabrous and the hair-bearing skin of the hand over the CMC joint. Incision is extended proximally and palmarly along the wrist flexion crease. Spreading dissection with blunt-tipped scissors is carried down through the subcutaneous tissue to avoid injury to the volar branches of the superficial radial sensory nerve. The thenar musculature is identified and elevated radially. A capsulotomy is performed and the fracture is exposed. The articular surface is scrutinized for articular depression. If present, it is temped up and supported with cancellous autograft obtained from the distal radius or tip of the olecranon. Fracture is then provisionally reduced, then fixed with cannulated headless compression screws.

Trapezial ridge fractures have been subdivided into two types. Type 1 are base fractures and type 2 are tip avulsion fractures.[39] If identified early, nondisplaced type 1 may be amenable to simple short arm cast immobilization for 6 weeks. Delayed presentation and displaced fractures are risk factors for progression to painful nonunion. In the athlete, immediate fragment excision allows for immediate return to play and avoids the need to wait for union.[40] The trapezial ridge may be exposed through the same approach used to gain volar exposure of the scaphoid. After fragment excision, the athlete may return to sport in a well-padded glove to help mitigate palmar discomfort.

12.2.6 Trapezoid Fractures

Trapezoid fractures are rare and represent less than 1% of all carpal fractures. Injury to the trapezoid results from an axial load to the metacarpal of the index finger. Fracture patterns vary from a dorsal chip fracture to a comminuted body fracture with index finger metacarpal dislocation. Although index finger CMC dislocations are readily identified of standard projections, CT scan is often required to identify these fractures. The presence of articular incongruity or CMC instability are indications for surgical intervention. Goals of treatment are to restore articular congruity and CMC stability. Chip fractures with CMC dislocations may be treated with closed reduction and temporary K-wire fixation across the CMC. Two 0.062 K-wires are used. One is driven from the index into trapezoid, the second is driven from the base of the index finger into the base of the long finger. Pins are cut beneath the skin. Wrist is immobilized in a cast for 3 months. Pins are removed at 8 weeks. Contact athletes may return to play in club cast when pins are removed.[41]

12.2.7 Capitate Fractures

Capitate fractures are rare and account for 1 to 2% of all carpal fractures. The capitate may be fractured in isolation or as part of a greater arc perilunate injury. Mechanism of injury involves a fall onto an outstretched radially deviated hand. The capitate typically fractures through its neck.[42] The capitate head is not unlike the proximal pole of the scaphoid, in that it is mostly covered in cartilage and has a tenuous blood supply. Consequently, displaced capitate neck fractures pose treatment challenges similar to scaphoid waist fractures. Capitate neck fractures are prone to delayed union, nonunion, and AVN of the head.[28] The diagnosis can usually be made on standard projections of the wrist. Management and surgical decision making associated with capitate neck fractures mirror that of scaphoid waist fractures. Nondisplaced fractures

are amenable to long arm cast immobilization for 6 to 8 weeks with close radiographic follow-up. Any amount of displacement, delay in presentation, or need for early return to play warrants surgical consideration.

Authors' Favored Surgical Technique

Capitate neck fractures are exposed through a dorsal approach. Incision is made in line with the radial aspect of the long finger and centered over the capitate neck. Full-thickness adipocutaneous skin flaps are elevated and the interval between the third and fourth compartment is identified. A capsulotomy is made in line with the incision and the wrist is hyperflexed to expose the head of the capitate. Depending on the severity of the injury, the capitate head may be hyperextended to 180 degrees.[42] Fracture is reduced, then provisionally fixed with axial guidewires in an antegrade fashion. The capitate can generally accommodate two cannulated headless compression screws. Capsule and skin are closed in a standard fashion. Postoperatively, isolated capitate injuries placed in a volar resting splint for 4 to 6 weeks. Immobilization is extended to 12 weeks if capitate fracture is part of a perilunate fracture dislocation. ROM exercises are started when immobilization is discontinued. Return to play should be delayed until CT demonstrates 50% bony bridging.

12.2.8 Lunate Fractures

Fractures of the lunate are relatively rare and make up 0.5 to 1% of all carpal fractures (Watson 2001). The five patterns of fracture as described by Teisen et al[43] are volar lip, dorsal lip, transverse body, osteochondral and transarticular frontal fractures. Body fractures are thought to occur due to an axial load driving the capitate into the lunate. Dorsal lip fractures occur with hyperextension of the wrist in ulnar deviation. In this position, the dorsal lunate is crushed between the capitate and dorsal rim of the radius. Volar lip fragments are difficult to recognize on plain radiographs. Often the only clue to their presence is subtle volar subluxation of the capitate. A CT scan can further characterize the fracture pattern and aid in preoperative planning. Treatment goals are obtaining anatomical reduction, restoring lunocapitate alignment, and preventing lunate AVN. A missed fracture is thought to be at risk for progression to Kienböck's disease. Nondisplaced body fractures may be treated with cast immobilization with MPs held in flexion to help off load the lunate. Due to the rare nature of these injuries, there is insufficient evidence to guide duration of immobilization or appropriate radiographic follow-up. Clinical resolution of pain and bridging bone on CT should guide the clinical decision making. In the athlete, early ORIF may decrease the time of immobilization and expedite return to play. Chip fractures without evidence of carpal instability have healed well with brief splint immobilization and return to sports when pain resolved. Lip fractures with capitate subluxation require open versus closed reduction and temporary pin fixation. Return to play should follow perilunate dislocation protocols. The athlete should be closely monitored for the development of Kienböck's disease. MRI is helpful in making the diagnosis before lunate collapse or sclerosis occurs.[44,45]

12.3 Scapholunate Injuries

Scapholunate interosseous ligament (SLIL) injuries are postulated to occur due to a fall with the wrist in extension, ulnar deviation, and carpal supination.[46] Mayfield's original description of perilunate instability separated these injuries into four stages, starting with isolated SLIL injury and progressing to lunate dislocation. Contact athletes commonly sustain this mechanism of injury but tend to remain on the lower end of the spectrum. These injuries can be deceptively mild in symptomatology and difficult to detect on screening radiographs. Consequently, the athlete may incorrectly dismiss the injury as a simple "wrist sprain" and may not present for evaluation acutely. Previous biomechanical studies have shown that characteristic dynamic and static patterns, typically attributed to SLIL injuries, require concurrent injury or attenuation of extrinsic carpal ligaments as well.[47] Isolated SLIL injuries demonstrate a predictable clinical pattern of progressive deformity. Delayed treatment has been shown to result worse outcomes.[48] Consequently, treatment of these injuries requires consideration of chronicity and severity of the injury.

12.3.1 Management of Acute Injuries (< 4–6 weeks from injury)

The athlete that presents to the office after recently sustaining a hyperextension injury and point tenderness over the SLIL receives standard three views of the wrist, clenched fist view and radial and ulnar deviation PA of the wrist. If no radiographic evidence of instability is identified, the wrist is immobilized in a splint and patient is reevaluated in 3 weeks. Resolution of symptoms confirm simple wrist sprain and athlete is allowed to return to play. Persistent pain at the 3- to 4-week visit is often indicative of a more severe injury. In our practice, we elect to forgo the MRI and perform a diagnostic arthroscopy to avoid any further delay in treatment. Management of the SLIL is determined based on Geissler's arthroscopic classification of carpal instability.[49] If on initial examination, there was evidence of radiographic dynamic instability, we would progress to immediate diagnostic arthroscopy and treatment. In the presence of static SL diastasis, we employ open primary ligament repair with suture anchors and protect it with SLIC screw (Acumed, Hillsboro, Oregon) augmentation (▶Fig. 12.15, ▶Fig. 12.16, ▶Fig. 12.17, ▶Fig. 12.18, ▶Fig. 12.19, ▶Fig. 12.20).

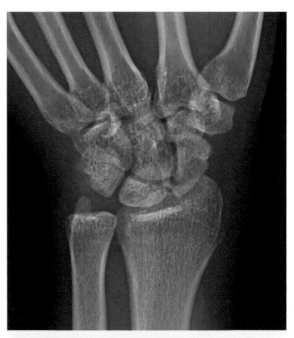

Fig. 12.15 Collegiate running back presented 1 week after wrist injury with Geissler grade IV SLIL.

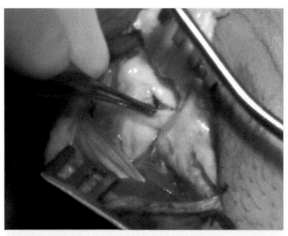

Fig. 12.16 SLIL avulsed off the lunate.

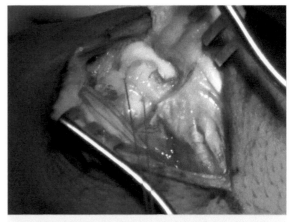

Fig. 12.17 Suture anchor was inserted into the lunate with a horizontal mattress stitch brought up through the substance of the dorsal SLIL.

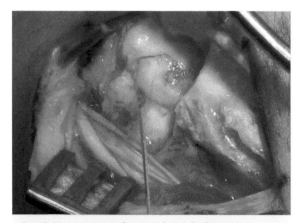

Fig. 12.18 Mattress stitch was tied over the ligament.

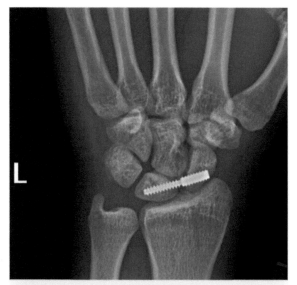

Fig. 12.19 SLIC screw (Acumed, Hillsboro, Oregon) placed instead of K-wires protect repair while allowing early active ROM. Player returned to competitive sports 2 weeks after surgery in a splint.

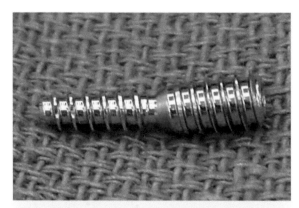

Fig. 12.20 SLIC screw (Acumed, Hillsboro, Oregon) has a ball and socket joint at the junction between the thick and narrow threaded shafts which allows for rotation as well as 15-degree cone of angulation.

12.3.2 Management of Chronic Injuries (> 12 weeks from injury)

The management of chronic injuries is much more controversial. Initial evaluation is aimed at determining whether ligamentous injury is partial or complete. If complete, it is important to determine the presence of SL dissociation and scaphoid subluxation. Lastly, the surgeon must determine if the carpal deformities are fixed or reducible and ensure that there is no cartilage injury. As with acute injuries, work-up starts with the previously mentioned plain radiographs. Unremarkable radiographs prompt diagnostic arthroscopy. In the chronic setting, a dynamic or static deformity on plain film suggests an unrepairable ligament and warrant open ligament reconstruction (reducible SL deformity) or salvage procedure (irreducible or articular damage).[50]

Authors' Favored Surgical Techniques

Arthroscopic SLIL Evaluation and Treatment

The arm is prepared and draped. Sterile tourniquet is applied and the arm is suspended with a wrist arthroscopy tower. The radiocarpal joint is evaluated first. 6U portal is used for inflow. The scope introduced through a standard 3–4 portal. Standard diagnostic arthroscopy is performed to rule out associated lesions. SL ligament and SL interval are evaluated. Attention is then turned to the midcarpal space. Midcarpal radial (MCR) portal is created 1 cm distal to the 3–4 portal in line with the radial aspect of the long finger. Inflow is switched to the scope cannula. A 14-gauge needle is inserted into the midcarpal ulnar (MCU) portal for outflow. SL interval is again evaluated.

Geissler's arthroscopic classification of carpal instability guides intervention. Grade I lesion is characterized by the loss of the normal concave appearance due to stretching of the ligament. Mayfield previously reported that the SL ligament may stretch 225% prior to rupture.[51] When viewed through the midcarpal portals, a grade I lesion maintains a tight congruent SL joint. These injuries are better characterized as a simple sprain in the acute setting and resolved with short-term immobilization and supportive management. In chronic injuries, grade I lesions are likely incidental and probably not related to the patient's symptoms.

In addition to the loss of convexity of the SLIL, grade II lesions are characterized by flexion of the scaphoid which is best identified as an articular step-off from the MCU portal. The ability to pass an arthroscopy probe between the scaphoid and lunate differentiate grade III from grade II lesions. In the nonathlete, these injuries when treated acutely are amenable to percutaneous reduction and pin fixation. However, pin fixation requires 3 months of immobilization which can have significant implications on a high-level athlete. SLIC screw fixation could potentially reduce immobilization time to 6 weeks, but its use in lower-grade injuries is still being studied.

Management of chronic lesions is controversial and have universally demonstrated worse outcomes compared to acute injuries.[48]

Chronic (> 6 weeks) incomplete SLIL tears (grade II or III) have been treated with partial arthroscopic debridement with fair results. All patients underwent splint immobilization postoperatively for 14 days and then began a hand therapy protocol concentrating on ROM and strengthening.[52] Alternatively, Geissler reported on his 19 patient case series on chronic (> 6 months) grades II and III SLIL injuries treated with electrothermal shrinkage. Results demonstrated good or excellent outcomes in 100% grade II injuries and 50% of grade III. Postoperative protocols are still not well established and remain at the discretion of the treating physician.[53] Similarly, Lee et al[54] reported on his retrospective review of 13 grade II SLIL tears treated with thermal shrinkage. Mean duration of symptoms was 11.2 months. Average follow-up was 52.8 months. Modified mayo wrist scores improved from 70 to 94.68. Postoperatively, the splint was used full time for 3 weeks, and a removable cock-up brace was used intermittently for another 2 weeks. Patients began rehabilitation programs, including wrist ROM and strengthening exercises, when the splint was removed.[54]

Grade IV injuries demonstrate complete disruption of the dorsal SLIL and are notable for SL gap large enough to accommodate a 2.7-mm arthroscope. Acutely, complete tears can be treated with open ligament repair. We augment repair with SLIC screw to accelerate the rehab time frame in the athlete. A cast is applied for approximately 4 weeks, and followed by a removable splint for an additional 2 weeks. Digital ROM is started immediately. ROM exercises are started at 6 weeks and a strengthening program initiated at 12 weeks. Chronic reducible lesions have been treated with several different ligament reconstruction techniques such as the Brunelli,[55] 3LT,[56] bone retinaculum bone grafting,[57] scapholunate axis method (SLAM),[58] and reduction association scaphoid and lunate (RASL).[59] To date, no technique has proven superior and none have shown to return patients to their prior level of function. Progression to scapholunate advance collapse (SLAC) is a contraindication for reconstruction. SLAC wrist is typically treated with either proximal row carpectomy or four corner fusion, both of which are rarely performed on the high-level athlete.

References

[1] Emmett JE, Breck LW. A review and analysis of 11,000 fractures seen in a private practice of orthopaedic surgery, 1937–1956. J Bone Joint Surg Am. 1958; 40-A(5):1169–1175

[2] Stark H. Troublesome fractures and dislocations of the hand. Instr Course Lect. 1970; 19:130–149

[3] Weiss AP, Hastings H, II. Distal unicondylar fractures of the proximal phalanx. J Hand Surg Am. 1993; 18(4):594–599

[4] Geissler WB. Cannulated percutaneous fixation of intra-articular hand fractures. Hand Clin. 2006; 22(3):297–305, vi

[5] Kodama N, Takemura Y, Ueba H, Imai S, Matsusue Y. Operative treatment of metacarpal and phalangeal fractures in athletes: early return to play. J Orthop Sci. 2014; 19(5):729–736

[6] Dabezies EJ, Schutte JP. Fixation of metacarpal and phalangeal fractures with miniature plates and screws. J Hand Surg Am. 1986; 11(2):283–288

[7] Low CK, Wong HC, Low YP, Wong HP. A cadaver study of the effects of dorsal angulation and shortening of the metacarpal shaft on the extension and flexion force ratios of the index and little fingers. J Hand Surg [Br]. 1995; 20(5):609–613

[8] Royle SG. Rotational deformity following metacarpal fracture. J Hand Surg [Br]. 1990; 15(1):124–125

[9] Geissler WB, McCraney WO. Operative management of metacarpal fractures. In: Ring DC, ed. Fractures of the Hand and Wrist. New York, NY: Informa Healthcare, Inc. 2007:75–89

[10] Rettig AC, Ryan R, Stone J. Epidemiology of hand injuries. In: Strickland JW, Rettig AC, eds. Hand Injuries in Athletes. Philadelphia, PA: Saunders; 1992:37–48

[11] Borgeskov S, Christiansen B, Kjaer A, Balslev I. Fractures of the carpal bones. Acta Orthop Scand. 1966; 37(3):276–287

[12] Gelberman RH, Menon J. The vascularity of the scaphoid bone. J Hand Surg Am. 1980; 5(5):508–513

[13] Gelberman RH, Wolock BS, Siegel DB. Fractures and nonunions of the carpal scaphoid. J Bone Joint Surg Am. 1989; 71(10):1560–1565

[14] Hanks GA, Kalenak A, Bowman LS, Sebastianelli WJ. Stress fractures of the carpal scaphoid. A report of four cases. J Bone Joint Surg Am. 1989; 71(6):938–941

[15] Olsen N, Schousen P, Dirksen H, Christoffersen JK. Regional scintimetry in scaphoid fractures. Acta Orthop Scand. 1983; 54(3):380–382

[16] Gaebler C, Kukla C, Breitenseher M, Trattnig S, Mittlboeck M, Vécsei V. Magnetic resonance imaging of occult scaphoid fractures. J Trauma. 1996; 41(1):73–76

[17] Sanders WE. Evaluation of the humpback scaphoid by computed tomography in the longitudinal axial plane of the scaphoid. J Hand Surg Am. 1988; 13(2):182–187

[18] Gellman H, Caputo RJ, Carter V, Aboulafia A, McKay M. Comparison of short and long thumb-spica casts for non-displaced fractures of the carpal scaphoid. J Bone Joint Surg Am. 1989; 71(3):354–357

[19] Cooney WP, III. Scaphoid fractures: current treatments and techniques. Instr Course Lect. 2003; 52:197–208

[20] Fernandez DL. Anterior bone grafting and conventional lag screw fixation to treat scaphoid nonunions. J Hand Surg Am. 1990; 15(1):140–147

[21] Eddeland A, Eiken O, Hellgren E, Ohlsson NM. Fractures of the scaphoid. Scand J Plast Reconstr Surg. 1975; 9(3):234–239

[22] Szabo RM, Manske D. Displaced fractures of the scaphoid. Clin Orthop Relat Res. 1988(230):30–38

[23] Lindström G, Nyström A. Natural history of scaphoid non-union, with special reference to "asymptomatic" cases. J Hand Surg [Br]. 1992; 17(6):697–700

[24] Sheetz KK, Bishop AT, Berger RA. The arterial blood supply of the distal radius and ulna and its potential use in vascularized pedicled bone grafts. J Hand Surg Am. 1995; 20(6):902–914

[25] Ford DJ, Khoury G, el-Hadidi S, Lunn PG, Burke FD. The Herbert screw for fractures of the scaphoid. A review of results and technical difficulties. J Bone Joint Surg Br. 1987; 69(1):124–127

[26] Geissler WB. Arthroscopic management of scaphoid fractures in athletes. Hand Clin. 2009; 25(3):359–369

[27] Slade JF, III, Gillon T. Retrospective review of 234 scaphoid fractures and nonunions treated with arthroscopy for union and complications. Scand J Surg. 2008; 97(4):280–289

[28] Rand JA, Linscheid RL, Dobyns JH. Capitate fractures: a long-term follow-up. Clin Orthop Relat Res. 1982(165):209–216

[29] Cameron HU, Hastings DE, Fournasier VL. Fracture of the hook of the hamate. A case report. J Bone Joint Surg Am. 1975; 57(2):276–277

[30] Abbitt PL, Riddervold HO. The carpal tunnel view: helpful adjuvant for unrecognized fractures of the carpus. Skeletal Radiol. 1987; 16(1):45–47

[31] Whalen JL, Bishop AT, Linscheid RL. Nonoperative treatment of acute hamate hook fractures. J Hand Surg Am. 1992; 17(3):507–511

[32] Kadar A, Bishop AT, Suchyta MA, Moran SL. Diagnosis and management of hook of hamate fractures. J Hand Surg Eur Vol. 2017:1753193417729603

[33] Futami T, Aoki H, Tsukamoto Y. Fractures of the hook of the hamate in athletes. 8 cases followed for 6 years. Acta Orthop Scand. 1993; 64(4):469–471

[34] Freeland AE, Finley JS. Displaced dorsal oblique fracture of the hamate treated with a cortical mini lag screw. J Hand Surg Am. 1986; 11(5):656–658

[35] Höcker K, Menschik A. Chip fractures of the triquetrum. Mechanism, classification and results. J Hand Surg [Br]. 1994; 19(5):584–588

[36] Cassidy C, Ruby LK. Fractures and dislocations of the carpus. In: Browner BD, Jupiter JB, Krettek C, Anderson P, eds. Skeletal Trauma: Basic Science, Management, and Reconstruction. Vol. 2, 5th ed. Philadelphia, PA: Elsevier/Saunders; 2015:1343–1403

[37] Arner M, Hagberg L. Wrist flexion strength after excision of the pisiform bone. Scand J Plast Reconstr Surg. 1984; 18(2):241–245

[38] Cordrey LJ, Ferrer-Torells M. Management of fractures of the greater multangular. Report of five cases. J Bone Joint Surg Am. 1960; 42-A:1111–1118

[39] Botte MJ, von Schroeder HP, Gellman H, Cohen MS. Fracture of the trapezial ridge. Clin Orthop Relat Res. 1992(276):202–205

[40] Palmer AK. Trapezial ridge fractures. J Hand Surg Am. 1981; 6(6):561–564

[41] Stein AH, Jr. Dorsal dislocation of the lesser multangular bone. J Bone Joint Surg Am. 1971; 53(2):377–379

[42] Adler JB, Shaftan GW. Fractures of the capitate. J Bone Joint Surg Am. 1962; 44-A:1537–1547

[43] Teisen H, Hjarbaek J. Classification of fresh fractures of the lunate. J Hand Surg [Br]. 1988; 13(4):458–462

[44] Almquist EE. Kienböck's disease. Hand Clin. 1987; 3(1):141–148

[45] Allan CH, Joshi A, Lichtman DM. Kienbock's disease: diagnosis and treatment. J Am Acad Orthop Surg. 2001; 9(2):128–136

[46] Mayfield JK, Johnson RP, Kilcoyne RK. Carpal dislocations: pathomechanics and progressive perilunar instability. J Hand Surg Am. 1980; 5(3):226–241

[47] Meade TD, Schneider LH, Cherry K. Radiographic analysis of selective ligament sectioning at the carpal scaphoid: a cadaver study. J Hand Surg Am. 1990; 15(6):855–862

[48] Rohman EM, Agel J, Putnam MD, Adams JE. Scapholunate interosseous ligament injuries: a retrospective review of treatment and outcomes in 82 wrists. J Hand Surg Am. 2014; 39(10):2020–2026

[49] Geissler WB, Freeland AE, Savoie FH, McIntyre LW, Whipple TL. Intracarpal soft-tissue lesions associated with an intra-articular fracture of the distal end of the radius. J Bone Joint Surg Am. 1996; 78(3):357–365

[50] Paci GM, Yao J. Surgical techniques for the treatment of carpal ligament injury in the athlete. Clin Sports Med. 2015; 34(1):11–35

[51] Mayfield JK. Wrist ligamentous anatomy and pathogenesis of carpal instability. Orthop Clin North Am. 1984; 15(2):209–216

[52] Weiss AP, Sachar K, Glowacki KA. Arthroscopic debridement alone for intercarpal ligament tears. J Hand Surg Am. 1997; 22(2):344–349

[53] Geissler WB, Haley T. Arthroscopic management of scapholunate instability. Atlas Hand Clin. 2001; 6:253–274

[54] Lee JI, Nha KW, Lee GY, Kim BH, Kim JW, Park JW. Long-term outcomes of arthroscopic debridement and thermal shrinkage for isolated partial intercarpal ligament tears. Orthopedics. 2012; 35(8):e1204–e1209

[55] Brunelli GA, Brunelli GR. A new technique to correct carpal instability with scaphoid rotary subluxation: a preliminary report. J Hand Surg Am. 1995; 20(3 pt 2):S82–S85

[56] Garcia-Elias M, Lluch AL, Stanley JK. Three-ligament tenodesis for the treatment of scapholunate dissociation: indications and surgical technique. J Hand Surg Am. 2006; 31(1):125–134

[57] Weiss AP. Scapholunate ligament reconstruction using a bone-retinaculum-bone autograft. J Hand Surg Am. 1998; 23(2):205–215

[58] Yao J, Zlotolow DA, Lee SK. Scapholunate axis method. J Wrist Surg. 2016; 5(1):59–66

[59] Rosenwasser MP, Miyasajsa KC, Strauch RJ. The RASL procedure: reduction and association of the scaphoid and lunate using the Herbert screw. Tech Hand Up Extrem Surg. 1997; 1(4):263–272

13 Special Aspects in Musicians

Philippe Cuénod

Abstract

Carpal and hand fractures in musicians require special consideration, not only to restore the delicate and precise movements needed to play the instrument, but also to take care of the patient as a whole. As any artist, musicians are very sensitive persons and any trauma of their hand or carpus may trigger a fear of not being able to resume their playing and therefore put their career in jeopardy. A surgeon in charge to treat a fracture in a musician's hand should be aware of the artist's needs to play his instruments. The requirements may be very different according to the instrument played. The movements for playing the most common instruments are detailed. The general principles of fracture treatment are the same as for other patients, except that any bone displacement that can interfere with the precise movements, should not be tolerated. Stable fracture fixation to allow early mobilization and rehabilitation is the rule. Stiffness has to be avoided at all costs. Care must be taken to plan the incision in a way to avoid the contact areas of the finger with the instruments. Mini-invasive surgery should be used, as long as it does not increase the risks. In particular, percutaneous screw fixation is useful in selected cases. When the fracture is too bad, joint fusion in a functional position is indicated.

During the whole process of treatment, care must also be taken to discuss with the patient of his or her technical needs with the instrument, to encourage and support him or her psychologically to prevent that a good surgical treatment turns into a catastrophe by emotional complications.

Keywords: musician, hand, carpus, fracture, treatment, special features

13.1 Introduction and Historical Perspective

Being artists, musicians are, by definition, very sensitive persons. Considering the importance of hand representation in the cerebral cortex, it is not surprising that any fracture of the hand, even minor, may have disastrous consequences on the artist's playing ability. Even with a perfect functional result, such an incident can put the musician's career in jeopardy. Musicians are as much concerned by the risk of losing the skills to fulfill a passion as by the risk of losing their job. Historically, there are plenty of examples of musicians who had to stop their career or radically change it, following a hand trauma. It is not clear what caused Schumann's hand problem; was it an attempt to improve the agility of his left fourth finger with a device of his own, then an operation, that resulted in a cripple hand,[1,2] or a focal dystonia[3] that terminated his concert pianist career and obliged him to become a composer?

A missing or handicapped hand may trigger a new career, for example, pianist Paul Wittgenstein, who lost his right arm in world war I, but continued to play piano pieces, specially written for him by famous composers like Ravel, Britten, Korngold, Prokofiev, Strauss, and others.[4,5] Django Rheinhardt, used to play banjo guitar until he sustained a deep second- and third-degree burn of the hand. A retracted scar on the dorsum of the left fourth and fifth rays left him with a cripple hand. He, however, took advantage of his problem to switch to guitar and develop a particular technique to become one of the best ever jazz guitarists[5] (▶Fig. 13.1). In some instances, adjustment of the musical interface can be achieved by tailoring the instrument to the patient's handicap.[6]

The incidence of fractures in musicians has not been reported precisely, but is probably not very different than in the general population. Musicians may be more cautious to avoid accidents and refrain from having dangerous activities, although some admit not taking any special precaution.[7] A survey of the musicians of a symphonic

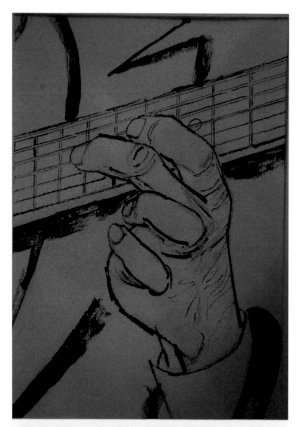

Fig. 13.1 Django Rheinhardt's left hand playing the guitar. Clawing of the fourth and fifth fingers by burn contracture. Drawing © Gani Jakupi. Used with permission.

orchestra is underway to try and determine the incidence and outcome of hand and carpal fractures, but collection of data is a bit tedious. Indeed, as already reported, musicians reluctantly acknowledge any hand trouble fearing to lose their job in the very competitive world of orchestras.[8]

The general technical principles of fracture management, however, apply to the musician's hand. The goal is, of course, to restore the anatomy, but moreover, the function. In this regard, the progress of fracture management, with smaller implants and mini-invasive techniques, may help the surgeon to achieve this goal. It is to be kept in mind that the choice of a technique should be guided by the moto "primum non nocere." It is of vital importance to take the time needed to expose the different treatment options for the patient, the risks, and the expected outcome. This moment is of utmost importance and may be determinant for the result. Unsatisfactory surgical results may not be the end of the musician career. A complete finger function may not be necessary to play an instrument, depending on which one is played. Therefore, the surgeon needs to have some knowledge of the movements required to play the most common instruments to determine the best treatment options or, at least, carefully ask the patient about the technical aspects, if necessary, with the help of his or her instrument.[9–11]

The emotional consequences of a traumatized hand in a musician must not be underestimated. An injury, even minor, may have disastrous consequences in some artists, known to be particularly vulnerable emotionally. Stiffness may prevent the musician to correctly play his or her instrument and interfere with the ability to cope with the handicap through fear, anxious feeling, and depression. On the other end, a crippled hand is not always the end of the skill to play as some musicians can adjust their game in order to continue playing.

13.2 Instruments and Movements Required to Play Them

A quick search on the internet shows that the number of listed music instruments amounts to 888.[12] Most of them are unknown to the author and probably to most of the readers. The hand surgeon should, however, be aware of the interface between the wrist/hand and the most common instruments, in order to understand the needs of the artist and to correctly address his or her lesion.[13]

The standard instruments in western countries compose different types of orchestras or are played as solo. The orchestra of classical music includes four groups of instruments: strings (violin, viola, cello, and double bass), woodwinds (flutes, clarinet, oboe, and bassoon), brass (trumpets, trombones, horns, tuba), and percussion (drums, cymbals, tubular bells, xylophone). Other instruments such as the piano and celesta may sometimes be grouped into a fifth section, such as a keyboard section or may stand alone, as may the concert harp and electric

and electronic instruments. The orchestra, depending on the size, contains almost all of the standard instruments in each group.

The jazz orchestra uses more or less the same instruments but in a different setting. Early ensembles were composed of clarinet, tuba, cornet, baritone, drums, and piano, as were the New Orleans bands. Then the Big Bands were predominantly wind orchestras, containing alto and tenor sax sections, trumpet and trombone sections, along with piano and drums. Later during the Bop period, the alto saxophone and trumpet were played by the major soloists, backed up by piano, string bass, and drums. With the advent of fusion, electric instruments such as the electric guitar and keyboard synthesizer became prominent.

The movements of fingers, hand, and wrist obviously differ from one instrument to another, but also from classical to jazz. It is not rare to see a jazz pianist play with a flexion of the wrist and flat fingers, which is in contradiction with the academic posture of slight wrist extension and midflexion position of the fingers. Thelonius Monk's flat fingers on the keyboard is a well-known feature of a jazz pianist, but classical artists may also have a nonacademic posture, as the Canadian pianist Glenn Gould.[2] The position of the distal interphalangeal (DIP) joint can vary from tight flexion (Count Basie) to hyperextension (Jelly Roll Morton).[9]

13.2.1 String Instruments

String players' right hand holds the bow and the important movements required are extension and flexion of the wrist as well as radial and ulnar deviation. The violinist's left hand is positioned with a hypersupination of the forearm and a wrist flexion and needs a normal flexion of the finger joints to reach to the cords and also an ability to completely stretch the little finger (▶ Fig. 13.2). Viola requires more or less the same movements. As the cello is not held between the jaw and the shoulder, but in

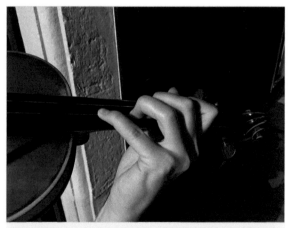

Fig. 13.2 Left hand of a violinist. The three radialmost fingers need an excellent flexion at PIP and DIP joints. The fifth finger requires full extension too.

front of the body, it does not need a hypersupination of the forearm and the hand is therefore in a more direct plane. The left hand mostly plays by flexion of the proximal interphalangeal (PIP) and DIP joints while the metacarpophalangeal (MP) joints are in neutral or slightly flexed (▶ Fig. 13.3). Guitar is played without a bow. The fingers of the right hand play the cords in a movement including flexion at the MP, PIP, and DIP level. Jazz or rock guitarists often play with a plectrum that needs a good pollicidigital pinch. The left hand squeezes the cords in an analogous movement as the violin player, with less extreme position of the wrist (▶ Fig. 13.4). Double bass players' left hand is held in flexion of the MP and PIP joints increase flexion to reach to the cords. The right hand plays with the bow or with the fingers rather straight, especially when playing jazz. The typical movement is a lateral swipe that needs some flexibility, but without too much of a flexion. The skin of the volar and radial aspects of the right fingers is specially exposed when playing that way and any tender

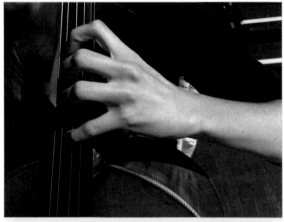

Fig. 13.3 Left hand of a cello player. The MP joints are in neutral or slight flexion and the PIP and DIP need good flexion.

scar resulting from a trauma or operation could interfere with proper playing.

In the contrary to the string players, a pianist does not require an important flexion at the PIP and DIP level, the finger movements taking place mostly in the MP joints, except for the thumb that needs some flexion at the MP and IP joints for the "thumb under" movement (the thumb crossing under the other fingers when playing the scale). Pianists with small joint arthritis of the hand can therefore continue to play on keyboards with some adjustments (▶ Fig. 13.5).

13.2.2 Brass Instruments

Trumpeter's left hand holds the instrument with more or less straight PIP and DIP and about 45 degrees of MP flexion. The thumb just needs opening of the first web space, but can have only little flexion of the MP and IP joints, because its role is mostly static. The hand therefore does not require too much of a movement. The right hand needs little MP flexion, but more PIP flexion to get to the valves with the pulp, although, according to the size of the hand or the style of play, the PIP can be held more in extension. Once again differences of style and techniques exist between musicians, above all jazzmen.

Horn is played with the left hand on the keys, but the right hand is important to modulate the sound by placing the fist in the position of an obstetrician hand into the bell. A good trapezo-metacarpal (TM) flexion is therefore required, but IP needs to extend. The left hand needs MP and PIP motion of second, third, and fourth fingers in order to play the keys. The thumb holds the instrument in a more or less static way, but needs a good IP range of motion to activate a key (▶ Fig. 13.6).

In trombone playing, the right hand holds the instrument, the thumb around the bell brace, the index completely stretched to reach the mouthpiece and the other

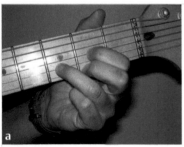
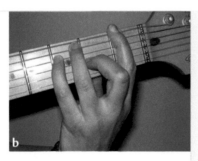
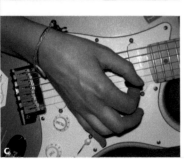
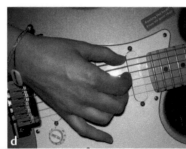

Fig. 13.4 Guitarist's hand. (a) Left hand with MP, PIP, and DIP flexion to pluck the strings. (b) Left hand with straight fingers to bar the strings. (c) Right hand using plectrum. (d) Right hand playing directly with the fingers.

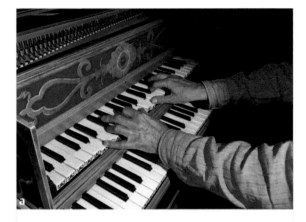

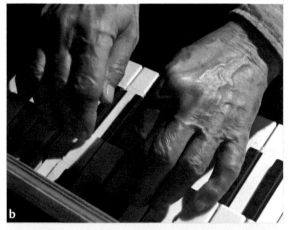

Fig. 13.5 Cembalo player. (a) The fingers are in slight PIP and DIP flexion. (b) Small joints arthritis does not impede playing.

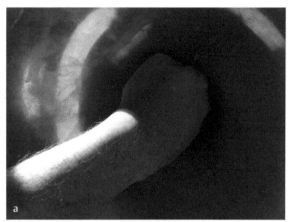

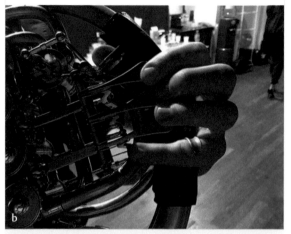

Fig. 13.6 Horn player. (a) The right hand is placed in the bell to modulate the sound. (b) The left hand needs MP and PIP motion of second, third, and fourth fingers in order to play the keys.

fingers flexed at the MP and IP level. The left thumb, index, and third finger hold the slide brace. Index and third finger need MP flexion and IP extension in a more or less intrinsic plus position.

In tuba, the right hand plays the keys and requires more flexion of the MP joint than of the IP. The right thumb is placed in a ring besides the valves to hold the instrument and does not need special movement but extension. The left hand grasps the instrument to hold it and therefore needs to have a good MP and IP flexion for a good grip.

13.2.3 Woodwind Instruments

Flute requires very flexible left index and third finger to allow simultaneous hyperextension of the MP joint and flexion of the PIP to reach the keys, while the ring and little fingers have a much more extended position. The right fingers are gently curved at the level of the MP and PIP without too much range of motion.

The movements to play oboe are less extreme; the index and third finger need some more PIP flexion than the two ulnar fingers that play in a more extended position (▶Fig. 13.7). The gently curved position of the fingers of both hands is the same for clarinet. In saxophone, the fingers are also in a gently curved position, but increased

PIP flexion is required during the play. MP joints have to be capable of some hyperextension in order to release the keys (▶Fig. 13.8).

13.2.4 Percussion

The multiple percussion instruments are divided in three main categories: membranophones, where the sound is produced by the vibrations of a stretched membrane, mainly produced by hitting the membrane, drums for instance; the idiophones, where the instrument as a whole vibrates by hitting (triangle, xylophone, vibraphone, celesta), scraping or shaking (maracas); the chordophones that are kind of string instruments played by percussion, such as berimbau, hammered dulcimer, or cimbalom. Percussion is played either directly by hitting the membrane of a drum with the hand or with sticks. There are different ways of holding the sticks: the traditional grip used to play the tambour with the left hand, the stick resting on the volar aspect of index and long finger, and passing between long and fourth fingers, and held by the thumb making a key pinch with the index. The screwdriver grip is the other way, either with the

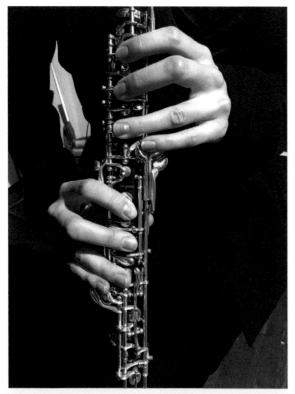

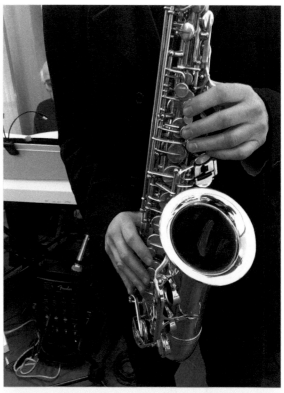

Fig. 13.7 Oboe player. Index and third finger need some more PIP flexion than the two ulnar fingers that play in a more extended position.

Fig. 13.8 Saxophone player. Left fingers are gently curved, but the MP joints have to be capable of some hyperextension.

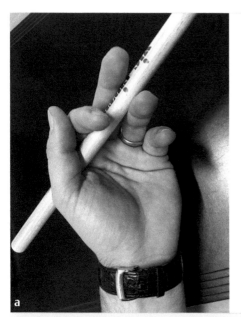
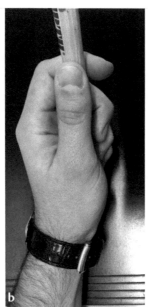
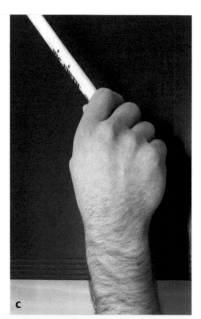

Fig. 13.9 Percussion player. The three ways of holding the sticks. **(a)** Traditional tambour grip. **(b)** Screwdriver grip French style. **(c)** Screwdriver grip German style.

forearm in neutral position (French technique) or in pronation (German technique). The movements with the sticks require an extension of the wrist with rhythmic radial–ulnar reduction for the French technique and an extension–flexion movement for the German technique (▶Fig. 13.9).

The most common instruments in western countries are used for classical music and jazz, but some are more typical for one or the other music. In a constant search for new sounds and harmonies, composers and musicians nowadays include unusual, exotic instruments in their instrumentation. Faced with a musician playing one of these exotic instruments, care must be taken to examine him or her while playing his or her instrument in order to catch his or her needs to be able to play it.

13.3 General Principles and Clinical Examples

The clinical presentation of a hand fracture in a musician does not differ from other persons' traumatized limbs.[2] The condition should be assessed as in any other patient and functional needs analyzed to adjust treatment.[7] The way, however, how the patient presents him-/herself is sometimes more dramatic, due to the emotional involvement in these very sensitive artists. Stress may be an aggravating factor.[2] Preliminary information gathered from professional musicians with traumatized hand show a clear tendency to important psychological impact, ranging from understandable anguish to near-panicking reaction (personal study under way). Patients need to be reassured that the problem has a solution, but it would be nonsensical to underestimate the severity of the lesion and let the patient believe that it is benign, even if it is not so. The surgeon should tactfully explain the nature of the problem, what are the therapeutic options, and what result can be expected. A simple fracture of the phalangeal tuft, although a trivial trauma, can have extraordinary effects on a professional musician, whose swollen and transient hypoesthetic finger pulp may mean for him or her the end of his or her career! A good explanation is sometimes worth weeks of physiotherapy.

Musicians' traumatized hand do not only include fractures, as any traumatic lesion can of course be encountered; in a series of seven musicians with hand trauma, Winspur reported only two fractures,[7] whereas Crabb had no fracture in his six reported cases.[1]

At times, the patient comes secondarily after an operation performed in another hospital with a bad result. In these cases, the challenge is to try and correct the failure without aggravating the situation. A guitarist with a middle phalanx condylar fracture was treated in another clinic with a percutaneous headless compression screw, whose diameter was obviously too large for the small bone, resulting in a necrosis of the condyle. After removal of the screw and physiotherapy without trying to correct the bony deformity, the finger condition improved to such an extent that the patient could resume his guitar playing with some adaptation of his technique (▶Fig. 13.10).

The ultimate goal in treating fractures is to restore the arches, the length, and rotation as close as possible of the normal anatomy, in order for the patient to have the same feeling when he or she plays. Indeed, any angulation or malalignment, in particular at the metacarpal and phalangeal level, that could be tolerated in average persons, may detrimental to the delicate sequence of movements of instrumental play.[7,11] Restoration of stable anatomical normality, even if relative contraindications exist, may be required to achieve a good functional outcome. It should be followed by early mobilization and progressive, careful return to play, avoiding, however, too intense work that might cause a secondary displacement.[7,9] Moreover, too early return to play could trigger compensatory movements with changes in the technique that could be permanently damaging.[9]

The surgical planning is important in order to achieve a good result. According to Winspur, the planning should be focused in three areas: (1) location of the incision to avoid interference with the important tactile areas; (2) surgical exposure, operative technique, and closure designed to facilitate early return to limited playing; (3) adjust any anticipated mechanical compromise to fit the playing position rather than the usual position of function.[9]

Midlateral approach to the PIP and phalanges is favored to decrease the damage to the extensor mechanism. The incision should avoid the critical tactile areas. The areas to be spared have to be precisely determined with the patient prior to the operation. Some usual approaches may not at all be suitable for playing specific instruments. Winspur lists some areas to be avoided.[9] They are summarized in ▶Table 13.1. Obviously, incision on the tip of the pulps of the left fingers in string players, for instance, should be avoided, but one must not overlook personal technique. An analysis of the play with the instrument can be helpful in deciding where to place the incisions.[11]

The value of open reduction and internal fixation followed by early mobilization is illustrated by the case of a 50-year-old professional guitarist who fell on the floor and broke his fourth metacarpal on the left hand. The patient appeared devastated by the deformity and loss of function of his hand, fearing the worst for his playing skills. After a long preoperative talk to explain the possible treatments and outcomes, he decided to undergo a surgical procedure. The fracture was reduced and fixed by lag screw and the patient could resume his play rather quickly (▶Fig. 13.11).

Some fractures, however, can be treated by less invasive methods, as in the case of a 12-year-old pianist who trapped her fourth finger in the door, resulting in a displaced subcapital fracture of the middle phalanx, with scissoring over the neighbor finger. In order to prevent the risk of soft tissue damage, the fracture was reduced and fixed with an intramedullary smooth 0.8-mm K-wire. She could resume playing after 1 week with a good functional result (▶Fig. 13.12). Early return to play is indeed important and even therapeutic; it shows the patient that he/she is able to resume playing and use his or her fingers without losing his/her skills.[9]

The indication of anatomical open reduction with a good fixation must be more liberal than in other cases, even if the risk of operative complications exists.[9,15] The risk is of course increased when facing an open fracture with tendon or nerve laceration. In this situation, the rehabilitation is of utmost importance and must be tailored to the patient needs. A complex regional pain syndrome (CRPS) could develop after an operation with

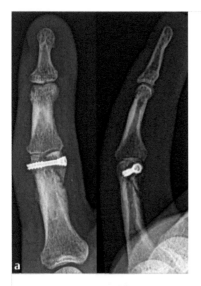
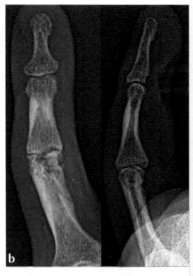

Fig. 13.10 Guitarist with basal phalanx condylar fracture of little finger.
(a) Condylar fracture of P1 D5 treated by too large and too long a compression screw. (b) After removal of implant, partial condylar necrosis with some degenerative changes. (c) Despite PIP and DIP stiffness of fifth finger, play is possible with some adjustments.

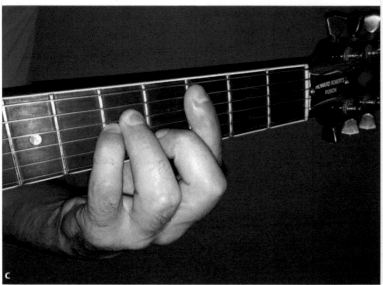

Table 13.1 Areas to be avoided in planning incisions in a musician's hand

Musician	Areas to be avoided
Bagpipe player	Radial border and pulp of the left thumb
Bagpipe player	Pulp of the right little finger
String player	Tips of the pulps of the digits of left hand
String player	Pulp of the thumb, index, long, and little fingers of right hand
Clarinet and oboe player	Ulnar border of the right thumb
Drummer	Radial and ulnar borders of ring and long fingers
Pianist	Pulp of all long fingers and radial border of distal phalanx of thumbs

Beware of nonstandard personal technique involving unusual areas!
Source: Adapted from Winspur.[9]

severe consequences, but this possibility also exists with a conservative treatment.

The open articular fractures could be addressed by a low-invasive technique to minimize the soft tissue damage. For instance, a depressed fracture of a phalangeal base can be realigned by using an owl introduced by a cortical window and fixed by K-wires and/or screws through mini-invasive technique (▶Fig. 13.13). Open fracture of the distal phalanx can be disastrous for the musician, in particular, by the soft tissue lesions. These fractures must be treated with utmost care. The fracture is reduced and fixed with K-wires and the soft tissues repaired. The patient must be warned before the operation that some sensibility troubles are expected. Early occupational therapy is required for the finger to recover as normal a sensibility as possible. In distal phalanx fracture with a dislocated dorsal fragment, reduction and fixation can be achieved with screws using a percutaneous method. A 0.8-mm K-wire is inserted through the skin into the fragment. It is then used as a lever, along with traction and manipulation to reduce the

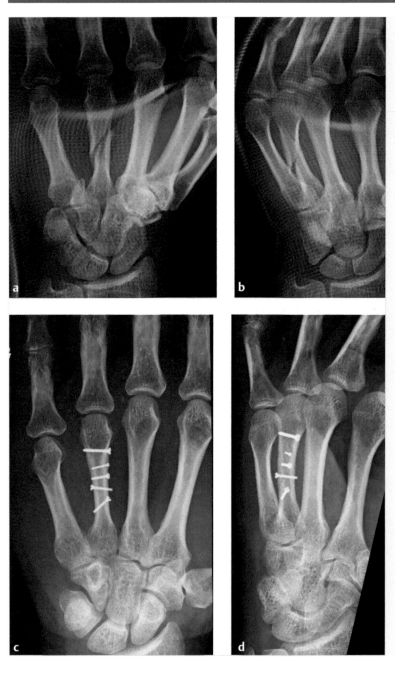

Fig. 13.11 Professional guitar player with a fracture of fourth metacarpal. **(a)** Posteroanterior X-ray view: length of fracture is underestimated. **(b)** Oblique X-ray view better showing the fracture line extending proximally and distally. **(c)** Posteroanterior X-ray view after fixation with multiple lag screws. **(d)** Postoperative oblique X-ray view.

fragment and drilled into the palmar cortex. After radiological control of the reduction, a second K-wire is inserted beside the first and its location radiologically confirmed. It is then withdrawn and replaced by a 1.0 screw inserted through the skin under fluoroscopic guidance. The first wire is then replaced by a second screw and, if the fragment is large enough, the fixation may be completed with a third screw (▶Fig. 13.14). Even if the fracture is fixed, it requires 3 weeks of immobilization in a Stack splint to prevent secondary displacement. Then gentle progressive mobilization out of the splint is authorized up to 6 weeks.

If a loss of motion is anticipated by the severity of the lesion, attempts have to be made to position the finger in a functional position.[9] When the fracture involves a joint and results in arthritis, the situation may or may not be catastrophic. Arthritis is indeed not always painful or motion limiting. The patient may therefore adjust his or her playing according to the handicap. If, however, the joint is stiff and painful, a treatment may be necessary. In distal interphalangeal joint, a fusion is the procedure of choice, although a prosthetic arthroplasty may be used in selected case with good results.[16,17] It will give some painless range of motion that allows to play. If a fusion is indicated, it has to be performed in the best functional position. In a pianist, the joint may be fused with very slight flexion or neutral position, but for the string players' left hand, a more pronounced flexion is required, in order to allow a good contact with the cords.

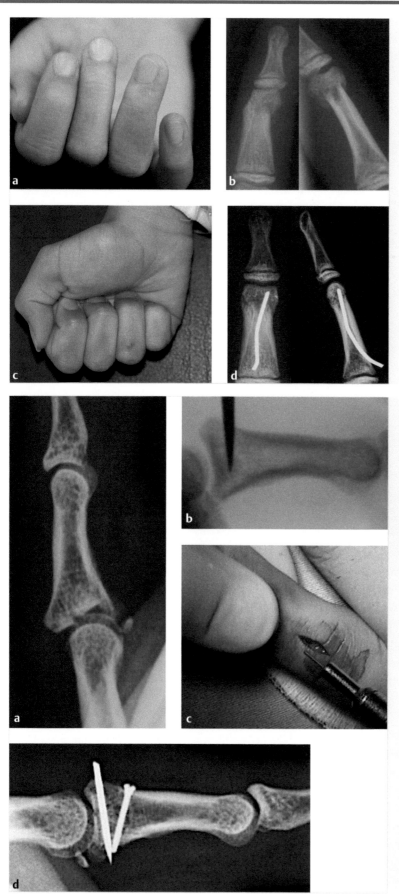

Fig. 13.12 Subcondylar fracture of the middle phalanx in a young pianist. **(a)** Deformity of the fourth finger with scissoring over fifth finger. **(b)** PA and L X-rays: subcondylar fracture with displacement. **(c)** Postoperative view. Full motion. Mini scar on the dorsal base of middle phalanx. **(d)** Postoperative PA and L X-rays: fracture reduced and fixed with intramedullary wire.

Fig. 13.13 Comminuted intra-articular fracture of middle phalanx base ("pilon fracture"). **(a)** Comminution and depressed fragment of the P2 base. **(b)** Minimally invasive approach. Longitudinal traction to align fragments and elevation of the depressed fragments with an owl. **(c)** Percutaneous screw insertion. **(d)** Postoperative lateral X-Ray: screw to fix the main fragment and K-wire buttressing the subchondral bone.

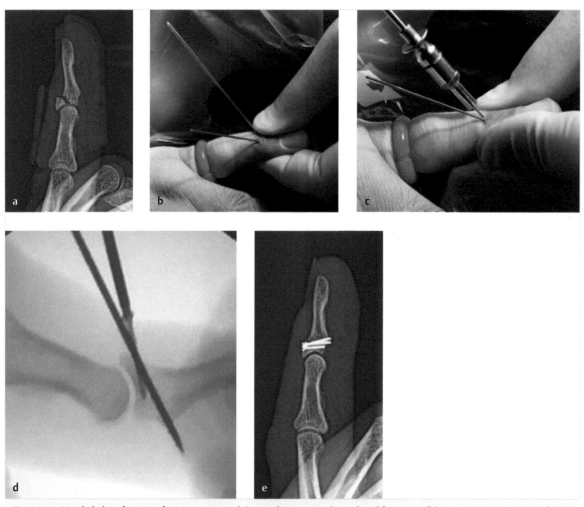

Fig. 13.14 Distal phalanx fracture of D5 in a guitarist. (**a**) Lateral X-ray view: large dorsal fragment. (**b**) Percutaneous K-wire used as lever for fracture reduction and provisional fixation. Second wire insertion. (**c**) Screw insertion after K-wire removal. (**d**) Peroperative X-ray control. (**e**) Postoperative X-ray: fixation with three 1.0 screws.

The angulation must be tailored to the needs of each finger and the DIP of the fifth digit may be fused with a 40-degree flexion.[15] If the PIP joint is involved, again the tactic will depend on the instrument played, the way it is played, and the possibility of adjustment that the musician is capable of. In string players (the left hand), a prosthetic arthroplasty is probably the treatment of choice to give as much range of motion as possible. The keyboard player would also benefit of an arthroplasty, even if a PIP joint fusion could not be incompatible with the performance with some adjustments. For other musicians, the strategy would depend on the movements required. It is important to again stress the importance of some basic knowledge of instruments or to have a thorough interview of the patient with his or her instrument. A stiff PIP joint of the left fourth finger in a bassoonist for instance would not be a problem owing to the fact that this is the functional position of this finger. The angle of fusion can be determined preoperatively with the use of a splint worn by the musician while playing to find the best compromise.[15]

Non- or mal-union requires operative treatment with osteotomy, graft, and fixation to restore the anatomy and function of the hand.[15]

In carpal lesions, there is no doubt that fresh scaphoid fracture should be treated by percutaneous headless screw fixation. This allows an immediate active mobilization and playing the instrument. Another fracture amenable to percutaneous headless compression screw fixation is the fracture of the hook of the hamate. This fracture is, as the scaphoid fracture, prone to nonunion, owing to its poor blood supply. It may also provoke flexor tendon irritation or rupture, which, for a pianist for instance, who performs repetitive finger flexion in ulnar deviation can be painful.

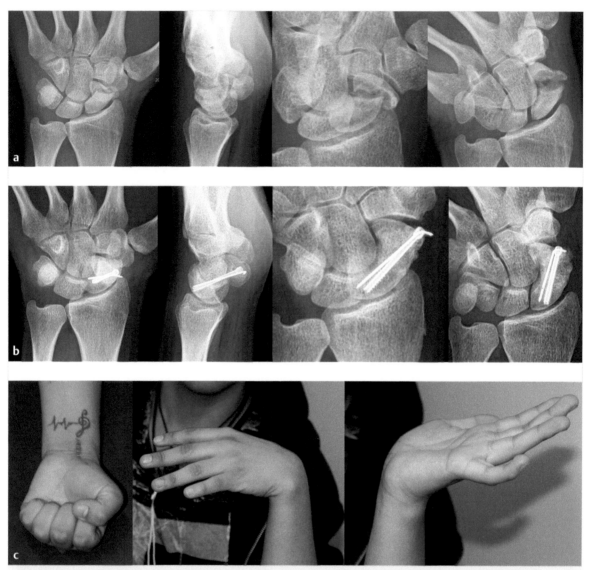

Fig. 13.15 Guitarist with scaphoid nonunion. **(a)** Preoperative X-rays showing a nonunion with bone loss and short distal pole fragment. **(b)** Postoperative X-rays after iliac crest bone graft and fixation with screw and K-wire. **(c)** Functional result.

A percutaneous screw fixation contributes to prevent non-union and alleviates the pain due to the pressure of the flexor tendons on the broken apophysis. It is also possible to treat a hamate hook nonunion without any bone graft. The stability achieved by the screw permits early mobilization. A scaphoid nonunion may impair the instrument playing because of pain and stiffness. The limited wrist flexion is particularly limiting for the string and guitar players' left hand. In young, no smoking patients, a simple scaphoid fixation without bone graft is possible, if there is no bone resorption. In case of bone resorption and carpal instability, reconstruction by bone graft and internal fixation by screw and/or K-wires is indicated. Arthroscopic techniques may be advantageous (see Chapter 8). A young amateur guitar player suffered a left scaphoid nonunion with bony resorption that interfered with his play. The bone was reconstructed with an iliac crest bone graft, headless compression screw, and K-wire. After healing, the patient could resume his playing the guitar like before (▶Fig. 13.15).

13.4 Conclusions

The fractured hand of a musician does not differ very much from other persons' traumatized hand. It, however, requires a slight different approach in the sense that the emotional impact should not be underestimated and the treatment tailored to the musician's need. It is of tremendous importance to talk with the patient, explain him or her the possibilities and the probable outcome, and understand his or her functional needs, at the best with his or her instrument. He or she must be encouraged and reassured in order to be confident that the treatment will be successful. Restoration of anatomy as normal as possible is indicated, even if this requires a surgical procedure. Anatomical reposition and fixation stable enough to allow early mobilization are performed to permit the musician to resume playing as soon as possible.

Acknowledgments: The author wishes to thank all the musicians who allowed him to take pictures of their hands while playing.

References

[1] Crabb DJM. Hand injuries in professional musicians. A report of six cases. Hand. 1980; 12(2):200–208

[2] Amadio PC. Surgical assessment of musicians. Hand Clin. 2003; 19(2):241–245, vi

[3] Ochsner F. La crampe du musicien. A propos de la maladie de Robert Schumann. Rev Med Suisse. 2012; 8(323):66–69

[4] Brofeldt H. Piano music for the left hand alone. http://www.left-hand-brofeldt.dk/index.htm. Accessed on December 27, 2017

[5] Pillet J. Main mutilée et musique. In Tubiana R ed. Traité de chirurgie de la main. Paris: Masson; 1998:664–668

[6] Markinson RE. Adjustment of the musical interface. In: Winspur I, Wynn Parry CB, eds. The Musician's Hand. A Clinical Guide. London: Martin Dunitz; 1998:149–159

[7] Winspur I. Surgical management of trauma in musicians: going the extra mile. In: Winspur I, Wynn Parry CB, eds. The Musician's Hand. A Clinical Guide. London: Martin Dunitz; 1998:101–122

[8] Parry CB. The musician's hand. Hand Clin. 2003; 19(2):211–213

[9] Winspur I. Surgical indications, planning and technique. In: Winspur I, Wynn Parry CB, eds. The musician's hand. A clinical guide. London: Martin Dunitz; 1998:41–52

[10] Amadio PC, Russotti GM. Evaluation and treatment of hand and wrist disorders in musicians. Hand Clin. 1990; 6(3):405–416

[11] Rosenbaum AJ, Vanderzanden J, Morse AS, Uhl RL. Injuries complicating musical practice and performance: the hand surgeon's approach to the musician-patient. J Hand Surg Am. 2012; 37(6):1269–1272, quiz 1272

[12] Wikipedia. List of musical instruments. https://en.wikipedia.org/wiki/List_of_musical_instruments. Accessed on December 27, 2017

[13] Blum J. Examination and interface with the musician. Hand Clin. 2003; 19(2):223–230

[14] Winspur I. Special operative considerations in musicians. Hand Clin. 2003; 19(2):247–258, vi

[15] Schwartz DA, Peimer CA. Distal interphalangeal joint implant arthroplasty in a musician. J Hand Ther. 1998; 11(1):49–52

[16] Sierakowski A, Zweifel C, Sirotakova M, Sauerland S, Elliot D. Joint replacement in 131 painful osteoarthritic and post-traumatic distal interphalangeal joints. J Hand Surg Eur Vol. 2012; 37(4):304–309

14 Fractures of the Hand and Carpus: Complications and Their Treatment

Adnan Prsic, Jing Chen, Jin Bo Tang

Abstract

Complications arising from fractures of the hand and carpus are unavoidable in a hand surgery practice. Metacarpal and phalangeal fractures account for a large percentage of all hand fractures, while fractures of the carpal bones excluding the scaphoid are exceedingly rare and account for a low number of all fractures. The treatment for such fractures are either operative or nonoperative and both carry the risk of complications directly related to the nature of the injury and subsequent treatment. Commonly seen complications are infection and osteomyelitis, malunion, nonunion, bone necrosis, stiffness, posttraumatic arthritis, and hardware-related complications. Knowledge of the causes, indications for treatment, and major surgical techniques of such complications should be a part of every hand surgeon's armory.

Keywords: hand fractures, metacarpal, phalangeal, carpus, complications, nonunion, malunion, surgical correction

14.1 Infection/Osteomyelitis

14.1.1 Causes

Infection in closed fractures of the hand are uncommon, but the risk is increased in open fractures given the reported incidence of open injuries to the finger from 34 to 68% among large studies.[1] In addition, the extent of soft tissue damage, regional ischemia, contamination, and delay to treatment as well as inadequate debridement has been correlated with poorer outcomes and increase in infection in hand fractures.[2,3] Compared to soft tissue infections in open fractures of the metacarpals and phalanges, osteomyelitis—a pyogenic infection caused by direct inoculation of the bone or untreated soft tissue infections—typically has morbid outcomes.

14.1.2 Clinical Judgment and Indication for Surgery

In our experience, nonpurulent open soft tissue infections (cellulitis) should be treated with washout and systemic antibiotics. For purulent infections of open phalangeal and metacarpal fractures with adequate washout, early administration of antibiotics has yielded low rates of soft tissue infection and osteomyelitis.[4]

Compared to purulent soft tissue infections in open fractures of the hand, osteomyelitis has increased morbidity. Diagnosis is established through clinical examination, radiographic imaging and obligatory bone biopsy. X-ray findings suggestive of osteomyelitis are regional osteopenia, periosteal reaction/thickening, bony lysis or cortical loss, and loss of bony trabecular architecture. Computed tomography (CT) and nuclear medicine studies can be useful, but magnetic resonance imaging (MRI) has the highest sensitivity and specificity in diagnosis. We resort to MRI in questionable cases. Positive cultures from a bone biopsy are diagnostic for osteomyelitis.

Systemic antibiotics of 4 to 6 weeks are required in the treatment of osteomyelitis and the patient must be counseled on the duration of treatment. It is very common for infection to lead to delayed union or nonunion (▶Fig. 14.1). The presence of necrotic bone is a true indication for surgical removal of affected bone. Otherwise, surgeons should not aggressively remove bones, because a bony defect is a more serious problem. Poor judgment

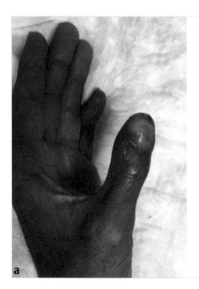
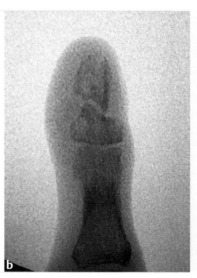

Fig. 14.1 A 32-year-old man with left thumb tip open injury with fracture. He developed infection of the fracture site 8 weeks after incident, resulting in delayed union and local soft tissue infection. The patient was treated with oral antibiotic and local incision and drainage. The infection subsided and the fracture healed 5 weeks later. **(a)** The infected thumb tip. **(b)** The delayed union 8 weeks after incident because of infection, but no bone necrosis was noted in X-ray films.

and improper surgical removal of bone can cause bony defects.

Severe infections refractory to antibiotic use for 1 or 2 months and repeated debridement, resulting in stiffness of multiple joints of a finger, may benefit from amputation. It was reported that although mild forms of osteomyelitis can be treated successfully with antibiotics, it should be noted that overall amputation rates hover around 40%.[5] The percentage of amputations increases to 86% with a delay of more than 6 months from onset of symptoms to diagnosis and definitive treatment, highlighting the urgency with which the suspicion of osteomyelitis should be managed.[5]

14.1.3 Surgical Methods

A combined management plan of antibiotics and surgical debridement is required for treatment of osteomyelitis.[5] Our treatment of osteomyelitis includes monitoring of inflammatory markers such as white blood cell count, C-reactive protein (CRP) and erythrocyte sedimentation rate (ESR), irrigation and debridement of affected bone, and early antibiotic administration. Adequate soft tissue coverage is necessary. If there is a large soft tissue defect, local or regional flaps are indicated. Debridement of bone may result in bony gap which can be filled with antibiotic-impregnated polymethylmethacrylate to serve as a spacer for length and alignment for later reconstruction. Once secondary healing has concluded and infection treated adequately, the void can be filled with cancellous or corticocancellous bone graft and the fracture treated with appropriate internal fixation. We prefer fixation with plates and screws and the distal radius for donor site for cancellous bone. The olecranon, the tibial plateau, and the anterior iliac crest are also valid alternatives for bone graft donor sites.

For any fracture with internal fixation, antibiotic use and local washout should be the primary and essential treatment. Whether the internal fixation should be removed should be judged intraoperatively. If the internal fixation is firm and bony healing is not achieved, the internal fixation should not be removed. If the internal fixation is loose or bony healing is near complete, the surgeons can remove the internal fixation. After surgery, external fixation should be used. If the area of infection is extensive and open wounds left open for egress, an external fixator should be considered.

Infection may cause bony defects. Based on our clinical experience, if a bony defect is less than 1 cm, there is great likelihood of bony regeneration without a bone graft. If the defect is lengthy—1 cm or longer in the finger and carpus—a bone graft is indicated. Cancellous or cortical bone graft or allograft can be used, but the timing of surgery should be carefully planned. Usually, the local tissue should be free from infection following weeks of drainage and dressing changes after debridement or drainage of the abscess. The local bone should be further debrided up to confirmation of healthy bleeding bone before measuring the size of defect and deciding on the size of the bone graft. An iliac bone with cortical bone element is the best site for metacarpal bone defect. Alternatively, bone from dorsal aspect of the distal radius can be used, but the bone quality is usually inferior to good as that from the iliac crest. Therefore, for any larger defect, iliac bone graft should be considered, while the bone taken from dorsal distal radius is reserved for a relatively smaller defect.

14.2 Malunion

14.2.1 Causes

The bony union of a fracture in a nonanatomical position can range from minor nondisabling aesthetic concerns to severe disability for the patient. Malunion of phalangeal and metacarpal fractures can lead to remarkable angulation, longitudinal shortening, joint surface step-offs, and rotation of the bones because of failure in maintaining reduction by splinting, casting, or internal fixation. Sometimes, the malunion is the result of not having applied the proper treatment such as adequate reduction of the fracture, or timely treatment.

14.2.2 Clinical Judgment and Indications for Surgery

Phalangeal malunion varies by the location, complexity, and the nature of the deformity.[6] The location can vary by digit and include proximal, middle, or distal phalanges and be articular versus extra-articular. The complexity of injury can be grouped into isolated malunion, malunion from open fracture, malunion with prior soft tissue injury, or malunion with prior extensor or flexor tendon injury. Different approaches depend on the above factors but more so on apex volar angulation, lateral angulation, rotation, and shortening caused by the malunion.

Angulation in the phalanges is usually hard to be tolerated. Usually less than 10 to 15 degrees of angulation in the coronal plane lead to no functional loss, but sagittal angulation of 10 to 15 degrees is more problematic, and should be corrected at initial reduction. However, if malunion occurs, we must examine the patient carefully to see whether such angulation causes functional impairment. Usually, angular malunion in the coronal plane should be greater than 20 to 30 degrees to indicate corrective osteotomy.

Volar angulated malunions cause shortening of the digit greater than 30 degrees and can cause relative extensor tendon lengthening and a subsequent extension lag at the proximal interphalangeal (PIP) joint. This in turn can cause a fixed flexion contracture at the PIP joint.[6,7]

Patients with tolerable malunion of the metacarpals do not require operative intervention (▶Table 14.1). However, symptomatic patients with disabling shortening secondary to comminution, oblique fractures, angulation, or rotational deformity should be offered surgical correction as we outlined earlier.

Table 14.1 Limits of acceptable deformities in metacarpal fractures

Deformity	Tolerable limit of deformity	Exam findings	Possible complications
Apex dorsal angulation	Neck: IF and MF 10–15° RF 30° SF 50–70° Shaft: IF and MF 10° RF and SF 20–30°	Dorsal prominence	Pseudo-clawing, grip weakness, malunion
Shortening	Up to 6 mm	Loss of prominence of the MCP joint in closed fist Extension lag	Extension lag, grip weakness
Rotation	No tolerable limit	Malaligned nail beds Finger overlap/scissoring in closed fist	Scissoring, grip weakness

Abbreviations: IF, index finger; MCP, metacarpophalangeal; MF, middle finger; RF, ring finger; SF, small finger.
Source: Adapted from Kollitz et al. 2014.[4]

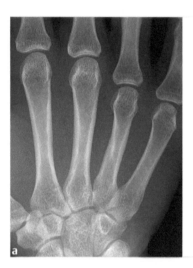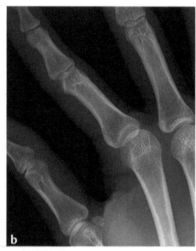

Fig. 14.2 (a) AP and (b) oblique radiographs of malunion and shortening of the fourth metacarpal. Patient has clinical symptoms of extensor lag.

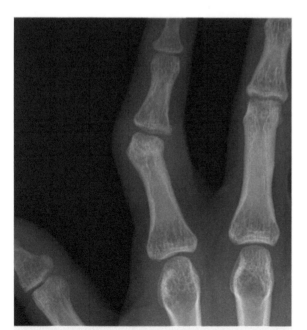

Fig. 14.3 AP radiographs of malunion and ulnar angulation deformity of the index finger proximal phalanx.

In all of the metacarpal bones, rotational angulation is less tolerable than sagittal angulation (▶Table 14.1). The tolerable degrees of sagittal angulation decrease by 5 to 10 degrees moving from the little to index finger. About 1 to 1.5 cm of shortening deformity can be tolerated in all metacarpal fractures.

There is no consensus regarding the permissible step-off in intra-articular fractures in the hand. However, except for the carpometacarpal (CMC) joints in which malunion usually does not require treatment, any step-off of 2 mm would need to be corrected. Patients with articular step-offs, especially when not at the middle portion of the articular surface of the joint, can function well and allow patients to avoid surgical intervention. Development of arthritis is a slow process and if step-offs exist, the surgeon needs to carefully weigh in patients' desire, location of the step-offs, activity levels, and age of the patient (▶Fig. 14.2, ▶Fig. 14.3, and ▶Fig. 14.4).

Mechanical Data and Clinical Outcomes

A study by Strauch et al was performed on fresh frozen cadavers demonstrated a 35-degree extensor lag for a

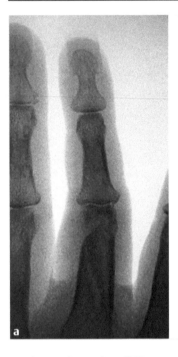
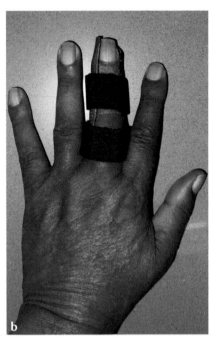

Fig. 14.4 **(a)** X-ray of a proximal phalangeal fracture of the middle finger 5 weeks after applying external fixation using a finger-based splint ulnar deviation at the PIP joint was noted. **(b)** A lateral splinting was used to correct ulnar deviation from week 5. The callus at week 5 is still soft and correctable, because the fracture healing is not yet matured. The callus matures after 6 to 8 weeks, after which correction of deformity is more difficult or impossible.

maximum shortening of 10 mm or 7-degree extensor lag for every 2 mm of shortening for fractures of the second and fifth metacarpal.[8] Based on their findings it is important to consider that metacarpal shortening of 6 mm will still provide for an acceptable range of motion given that the metacarpophalangeal (MCP) joint is able to hyperextend up to approximately 20 degrees and allow motion to full extension despite an extensor lag. Severe angulation of the second and third metacarpals can contribute to weakened and painful grip as a result of the metacarpal head position in the palm.[6,9] However, it is also widely believed that angular deformity and the associated shortening of the fourth and fifth metacarpal caused weakened hand grip.[9,10,11] Westbrook et al studied metacarpal neck and shaft fractures of the fifth finger treated closed versus operatively.[12] They established that the severity of malunion reported as palmar angular deformity did not affect the outcome of those treated nonoperatively. The disabilities of the arm, shoulder, and hand (DASH) survey, sports DASH, and cosmesis scores were significantly better in the nonoperative group compared to the operative group. The literature reports acceptable angular deformities of the second and third metacarpal from 0 up to 10 degrees while the fourth and fifth metacarpal can tolerate angular deformities of 20 and 30, degrees, respectively, without significant adverse functional outcome.[6,13]

Trumble and Gilbert[14] corrected uniplanar and multiplanar deformities with in situ closing wedge osteotomies and dorsal plates fixation without any complications. Del Pinal et al treated malunion of phalangeal base fractures with opening wedge osteotomy, distal radius bone graft, and fixation with titanium lag screws, cerclage wires, or both.[15] He reported decreased distal interphalangeal (DIP) joint motion but achieved functional range of motion in the PIP joint for all patients. Chronic injures of the PIP joint with intra-articular volar lip fracture can benefit from resection of the middle phalangeal base and reconstruction with a hemi-hamate arthroplasty.[16]

14.2.3 Surgical Methods

Correction of angular malunions at the shaft of the phalanges or metacarpals with significant deformity is attempted through either an opening or a closing wedge osteotomy. When possible, closing wedge osteotomies are preferred given the relative technical simplicity compared to opening wedge osteotomy. Closing wedge osteotomies result in minimal shortening given the gain in length from the angular correction. With significantly shortened metacarpals and bone loss, we recommend bone grafting and opening wedge osteotomy. In both cases, fixation with dorsal plate is recommended (▶Fig. 14.5).

Intra-articular malunion is more difficult to correct. For example, condylar fractures with step-off that extend into the joint may produce pain, rotational and angular deformity, stiffness, and degenerative arthritis. Correction with the above-described methods of metacarpal osteotomy, juxta-articular osteotomy, and wedge osteotomies are insufficient to correct step-offs in articular surfaces but are adequate to correct alignment. Instead, an osteotomy should be performed through the articular surface and the fracture line and fixed with a congruent articular surface.

Rotational deformities of the phalanges should be corrected. Our preferred method is to perform transverse phalangeal osteotomies with a power saw at the site of origin as this allows for multiplanar correction. Fixation is performed with Kirschner's wires but can also be done with mini plates. If indicated, tenolysis and capsulotomy can also be performed at the time of osteotomy. The alternative to this is correction through a metacarpal base

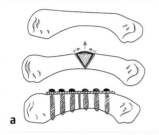
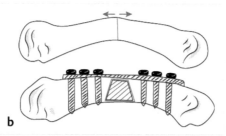

Fig. 14.5 **(a)** Normal metacarpal, malunited metacarpal with closing wedge osteotomy, and metacarpal with rigid fixation and good alignment. **(b)** An opening wedge osteotomy with bone graft and rigid fixation.

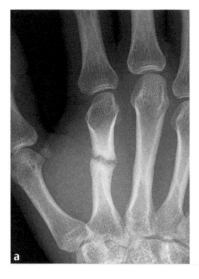
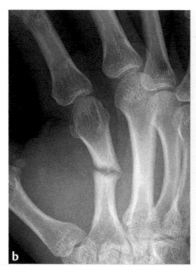

Fig. 14.6 **(a)** AP and **(b)** oblique radiographs of nonunion and shortening of the second metacarpal. Patient has clinical symptoms of tenderness and instability.

osteotomy. The disadvantage of this technique is that it does not allow for multiplanar correction and requires a separate incision if tenolysis and capsulotomy are required to mobilize the digit.

14.3 Nonunion

14.3.1 Causes

Open fractures, severe trauma, infection of the wound, and loss of bone substance all lead to nonunion. This is a severe complication of the fracture. However, its occurrence is rare. The reported prevalence is around 1.5% nonunion of metacarpal fractures and under 1% for phalangeal fractures.[17,18] Nonunions are typically described as atrophic and hypertrophic.

14.3.2 Clinical Judgment and Indications for Surgery

Clinical signs of union are typically seen in 3 to 6 weeks and delayed union and nonunions are mostly associated with open fractures with bone loss, soft tissue injury, and devascularizing injuries. Inadequate fixation and inadequate immobilization, whether from short duration or insufficient stabilization by splint/cast can result in hypertrophic nonunions. Diagnosis should be based on X-rays and clinical examination together,

as radiographical fracture lines can persist for up to a year (▶Fig. 14.6). Although more advanced modalities like CT scan and MRI have been used as adjunct measures, there is still a lack of high-quality studies to encourage routine use of such studies. Clinical signs of nonunion such as hardware failure, tenderness, and instability should strongly be considered as part of diagnosis. Jupiter and colleagues[17] defined nonunion based on radiographical evidence of healing at 4 months after the initial injury. In their study, most nonunions reviewed had inadequate or improper Kirschner's wire fixation. Treatment should consist of stable fixation with plates or lag screws as the treatment of choice. Atrophic nonunions can occur with bone loss as a result of open fractures and soft tissue injury.

14.3.3 Surgical Treatment

Nonunions with good joint range of motion and no associated stiffness, no soft tissue loss or chronic infections, and adequate sensory innervation are amenable to bone grafting and bone lengthening. In the case of stiff fingers, especially with immobile joints, that do not respond to mobilizing treatment (operative or nonoperative) amputation should be strongly considered as an option.

Nonunion sites call for extensive and thorough debridement of fibrous tissue up to fresh and bleeding fracture ends. Some nonunions, caused by osteomyelitis, for example, may require extensive debridement and may result in large bone gaps. If the gaps produce unacceptable shortening, corticocancellous bone grafting is indicated. Autologous bone has remained the standard for bone grafting in the hand. Several options are available for donor sites and most frequently include the distal radius, the tibial plateau, and the iliac crest among others. Despite its frequent use, the iliac crest graft has been found to have high morbidity with 10 to 39% of patients experiencing minor complications like superficial hematomas and 1.8 to 14.3% experiencing major complications such as persistent pain, vascular injury, neurological injury, etc.[19]

For intra-articular and periarticular fractures with severe joint stiffness, arthrodesis of the joint can serve as an alternative. Both the joint surface and adjacent nonunions should be thoroughly debrided to healthy bone. If a large gap remains, it should be bone grafted with corticocancellous bone. Internal fixation should be performed across the joint and the nonunion site to facilitate healing and a stable bony construct. Nonunions in the phalanges and metacarpals are frequently associated with tendon adhesions and therefore concomitant tenolysis and capsulotomy are recommended. Our preferred method of fixation is with a plate fixated either laterally or dorsally.

14.4 Bone Necrosis

14.4.1 Causes

Necrosis of the phalangeal bones and metacarpal bones is a rare occurrence, however, bones of the carpus such as scaphoid and hook of hamate are more prone to necrosis given their vascular anatomy. The blood supply to the scaphoid comes from branches of the radial artery that enter distally through the dorsal ridge and supply the scaphoid distal to proximal. Therefore, the proximal pole is at highest risk for nonunion after fracture and subsequent avascular necrosis (AVN) (see also Chapter 27). Although less frequently, scaphoid waist fracture nonunion can similarly be responsible for scaphoid waist AVN. Similarly, the hook of the hamate is prone to necrosis. There are three vascular pedicles that perfused the hamate and one group of small nutrient arteries arising from the ulnar artery supplies the hook of the hamate. This anatomy is variable and in 79% of people, this nutrient vessel enters at the tip and the rest are at risk for avascular necrosis if the fracture is distal to the insertion of the nutrient vessel. Unlike the scaphoid, the hook of the hamate is amenable to excision with favorable functional outcomes.[20,21]

14.4.2 Clinical Judgment and Indications for Surgery

Patients with scaphoid injuries present with radial-sided wrist pain. It is important to examine the proximal, distal, and waist of the scaphoid. Imaging assistance is used in the form of plain radiographs, CT, and MRI. Plain radiographs will suggest AVN with sclerosis of the proximal

pole. CT scan will display resorptive findings such as sclerosis and collapse in chronic injuries. The use of MRI has been advocated by many to be the ultimate diagnostic modality. However, standard MRI has been shown to have an accuracy of 68% with gadolinium-enhanced MRI increasing it to 83% still leaving room for error.[22] In addition to radiographical modalities, intraoperative examination and debridement to bleeding punctate bone has been held as a standard for evaluating vascularity of the proximal pole of the scaphoid.

14.4.3 Surgical Treatment

Avascular necrosis of the scaphoid is best treated with vascularized bone grafts. Interventions with nonvascularized bone graft such as the Matti–Russe approach have been associated with higher failure rates in cases of absence of punctate bleeding of the proximal pole at the time of surgery.[23] Reports show that vascularized bone grafting can successfully achieve an 88% union rate compared with a 47% union rate with screw and intercalated bone graft fixation in scaphoid nonunions with AVN.[24] Free or pedicled vascularized bone grafts (VBG) have been utilized for treatment of AVN of proximal pole of scaphoid. 1,2-Intercompartmental supraretinacular artery (ICSRA) is a pedicled VBG from the distal radius which has been successfully used in scaphoid nonunions and specifically in AVN of the proximal pole. Another option is the medial femoral condyle (MFC) free VBG which is based off the articular branch of descending geniculate artery. Both have shown to have a good track record in treating AVN of the scaphoid. In both instances, appropriate debridement of the necrotic scaphoid bone is necessary. Fixation with a headless screw after graft harvest is used to achieve rigid fixation of the graft. Scaphoid nonunion advanced collapse resulting from scaphoid AVN can be treated with historically well-tolerated salvage operations such as proximal row carpectomy, four-corner fusion, and wrist arthrodesis. It is our opinion and of others that the use of vascularized bone grafting to the small bones, particularly those with cartilaginous surfaces, is essential for subchondral vascular supply and in preventing degeneration of the joint surface.[25]

14.4.4 Clinical Outcomes

Pedicled VBGs like 1, 2-ICSRA have shown union rates between 93 and 100% in patients with scaphoid nonunion and proximal pole AVN.[26,27] Using the free vascularized MFC bone graft, Jones and colleagues reported on a series of scaphoid nonunions with AVN and achieved 100% union at a mean of 13 weeks.[28] A comparative study examining the free vascularized graft from the MFC to the 1, 2-ICSRA in the treatment of scaphoid nonunions with associated proximal pole AVN and carpal collapse or humpback deformity showed that treatment with MFC achieved union in 100% of subjects compared to 40% of patients treated with the 1, 2-ICSRA.[29] Although there is a paucity of long-term follow-up, both procedures have shown a promise in treating AVN of the scaphoid.

14.5 Complications of Intra-articular Fracture: Osteoarthritis and Stiffness of Ligaments

14.5.1 Causes

Intra-articular fractures of the metacarpals and phalanges can be devastating injuries that can have long-lasting effects on motion of the finger. Specifically comminuted intra-articular fractures are the most difficult to treat. These injuries are typically accompanied by soft tissue injury, extensor tendon injury, collateral ligament injuries, and devascularization of small articular fragments. Early complications are stiffness which results from immobilization for fracture healing, extensor tendon adhesions during the period of immobilization, and infrequently articular incongruity with difficult repairs. Collateral ligament contracture and dorsal capsular contracture are also significant problems caused by immobilization and soft tissue trauma.

14.5.2 Phalangeal Intra-articular Fractures

Intra-articular fractures frequently affect the condyles and are one of the most frequent causes of stiffness of the PIP joint. Posttraumatic and degenerative arthritis of the joint is commonly encountered despite best efforts at reduction, fixation, and restoration of joint congruency.

Appropriate diagnosis of the fracture pattern, displacement, and geometry is of utmost importance. Unicondylar fractures are inherently unstable and nonoperative management is not recommended given poor outcomes and the associated long immobilization period which lead to stiffness. Fixation with lag screws is preferred since it allows for early mobilization and reduction in stiffness. Alternatively, Kirschner's wire fixation can be used. Fixation of bicondylar fractures with minicondylar dorsal plates can also be performed, but some do not see this as a valid option. Studies have shown that plating in fractures with significant soft tissue injury and open fractures should only be used in select instances given the high risk of complications (Wolfe et al., 2017, pp. 231–277).[6] The risk of plates causing extensor tendon adhesions and interference of tendon function should always be a concern. We have not used plating for years for phalangeal fractures. Dynamic traction is another option for restoration of articular surface congruency, which we recommend strongly. This approach is useful, easy, and efficient. No matter the approach, the risk of stiffness in PIP joint injuries is always present; subsequent rehabilitation should always be planned to correct the stiffness. Intra-articular fractures

have great risk of osteoarthritic changes of the joints, even after healing of well-reduced fracture.

DIP joint stiffness or contracture is less of a concern from a functional standpoint as long as the joint is well aligned and not painful. Using rehabilitation to regain adequate function may be difficult, therefore we prefer arthrodesis in the desired position as this may be helpful with function and pain relief. Once painful severe DIP joint arthritis develops, fusion of the DIP joint is indicated.

14.5.3 CMC Joint Arthritis

Injuries to the first CMC joint are often encountered as a Bennett fracture. Reduction of a smooth articular surface is the goal of treatment. Often percutaneous pinning is necessary, with one pin through trapezium lateral to the base of the first metacarpal base and another from the shaft of the first metacarpal to the second metacarpal bone with the thumb pulled and pronated to achieve articular reduction under X-ray images. A displaced first metacarpal bone can rarely be reduced stably without pinning. Reduction of smooth joint surface is important; otherwise, arthritis of the first CMC joint occurs resulting in impairment of thumb function.

Different from the first CMC joint fracture, fracture or fracture dislocations of the fifth CMC joint do not result in remarkably great displacement, and notably, restoration of smooth articular surface is not an important consideration. Closed reduction and cast or plaster splint fixation are most often used for stably reduced CMC dislocation or fracture dislocation. If the reduction is not stable, percutaneous pinning fixation has been used to help keep reduction. There is no risk of symptomatic fifth CMC joint arthritis. The articular surface does not need complete reduction. The intra-articular fractures of the fifth metacarpal base are very different from Bennett's fracture (the first CMC joint intra-articular fracture). The treatment goal is not to restore complete smooth articular surface, rather to reduce to a stable status of the joint. Once the reduction is achieved, almost all of these fractures can be treated with plaster fixation or at most percutaneous pinning, followed by 4 to 5 or 6 weeks of immobilization. Fractures involving the second, third, and fourth CMC joint are also seen, but it is not required to restore smooth articular surface. Usually cast or splint fixation should be sufficient to treat these fractures. Development of osteoarthritis is not a concern of treatment.

14.6 Summary of Clinical Points to Aid in Prevention of Complications

- Complications of the fractures of the hand and carpus are unavoidable; however, they are the direct result of the injury leading to the fracture, the treatment of the fracture, delay in treatment, and lack of treatment.

- Attempts at avoiding infections can be aided with early and thorough washouts of open fractures, debridement of necrotic tissue and bone, as well as meticulous tissue handling.
- Attempts to decrease rates of nonunion can also be aided by meticulous tissue handling to avoid further devascularization of fracture fragments.
- Early follow-up of patients can help detect inadequate immobilization and adherence to splinting or casting.
- Interval to long-term follow-up can help detect early signs of nonunion such as pain and instability. It can also help recognize stiffness.

14.7 Special Clinical Points in Judgment and Surgical Treatment

- In pediatric patients, bony healing may not be accompanied by dense callus at the fracture site and visible on X-ray, which can lead to a false impression of delayed union of the fracture. Delayed unions and nonunions of closed pediatric fractures are very rare. The surgeon should not rush to a surgical intervention with the intention to treat delayed union or nonunion of the pediatric fracture.[30] If any concern, slightly prolonged external fixation should allow calcification, and it is not necessary to wait to see "remarkable" callus prior to the removal of the cast or splint.
- In question of infected wound at a fracture site, do not rush to remove the internal fixation during surgical washout. Without internal fixation, a deformity of finger or hand will usually occur. It is essential to perform a thorough irrigation and drainage but less so to remove the internal fixation, such as a K-wire.
- Great attention should be paid to local use of antibiotics (antibiograms) and locally applied antiseptic solution. The use of iodine solution (5–10 minutes of immersing the fingertip into iodine) along with daily dressing changes is a very useful technique for reduction of bacterial burden in fingertip infections.
- When complications cannot be treated with conservative measures and surgical treatment is necessary, plan the surgery carefully. Staged surgical interventions are necessary for infected cases, but for patients with malunion, one-stage surgery should be planned based on evaluation of multidirectional deformities.
- Intra-articular fracture of the PIP joint is the most difficult to treat and has the highest complication rate. Dynamic traction can be very effective in reducing early complications and restoring a relatively smooth articular surface. Later surgical option such as joint replacement may need to be considered if joint stiffness develops. Both treatment of articular fracture and joint replacement are not discussed in this chapter,

which can be found in other related chapters of the book (Chapter 18).

References

[1] Chow SP, Pun WK, So YC, et al. A prospective study of 245 open digital fractures of the hand. J Hand Surg [Br]. 1991; 16(2):137–140

[2] McLain RF, Steyers C, Stoddard M. Infections in open fractures of the hand. J Hand Surg Am. 1991; 16(1):108–112

[3] Swanson TV, Szabo RM, Anderson DD. Open hand fractures: prognosis and classification. J Hand Surg Am. 1991; 16(1):101–107

[4] Kollitz KM, Hammert WC, Vedder NB, Huang JI. Metacarpal fractures: treatment and complications. Hand (NY). 2014; 9(1):16–23

[5] Reilly KE, Linz JC, Stern PJ, Giza E, Wyrick JD. Osteomyelitis of the tubular bones of the hand. J Hand Surg Am. 1997; 22(4):644–649

[6] Wolfe SW, Hotchkiss RN, Pederson WC, Kozin SH, Cohen MS. Green's Operative Hand Surgery. 7th ed. Philadelphia, PA: Elsevier; 2017

[7] Vahey JW, Wegner DA, Hastings H, III. Effect of proximal phalangeal fracture deformity on extensor tendon function. J Hand Surg Am. 1998; 23(4):673–681

[8] Strauch RJ, Rosenwasser MP, Lunt JG. Metacarpal shaft fractures: the effect of shortening on the extensor tendon mechanism. J Hand Surg Am. 1998; 23(3):519–523

[9] van der Lei B, de Jonge J, Robinson PH, Klasen HJ. Correction osteotomies of phalanges and metacarpals for rotational and angular malunion: a long-term follow-up and a review of the literature. J Trauma. 1993; 35(6):902–908

[10] Ali A, Hamman J, Mass DP. The biomechanical effects of angulated boxer's fractures. J Hand Surg Am. 1999; 24(4):835–844

[11] Freeland AE, Jabaley ME, Hughes JL. Stable Fixation of the Hand and Wrist. New York, NY: Springer-Verlag; 1986

[12] Westbrook AP, Davis TR, Armstrong D, Burke FD. The clinical significance of malunion of fractures of the neck and shaft of the little finger metacarpal. J Hand Surg Eur Vol. 2008; 33(6):732–739

[13] Balaram AK, Bednar MS. Complications after the fractures of metacarpal and phalanges. Hand Clin. 2010; 26(2):169–177

[14] Trumble T, Gilbert M. In situ osteotomy for extra-articular malunion of the proximal phalanx. J Hand Surg Am. 1998; 23(5):821–826

[15] Del Piñal F, García-Bernal FJ, Delgado J, Sanmartín M, Regalado J. Results of osteotomy, open reduction, and internal fixation for late-presenting malunited intra-articular fractures of the base of the middle phalanx. J Hand Surg Am. 2005; 30(5):1039. e1–1039.e14

[16] Calfee RP, Kiefhaber TR, Sommerkamp TG, Stern PJ. Hemi-hamate arthroplasty provides functional reconstruction of acute and chronic proximal interphalangeal fracture-dislocations. J Hand Surg Am. 2009; 34(7):1232–1241

[17] Jupiter JB, Koniuch MP, Smith RJ. The management of delayed union and nonunion of the metacarpals and phalanges. J Hand Surg Am. 1985; 10(4):457–466

[18] Zura R, Xiong Z, Einhorn T, et al. Epidemiology of fracture nonunion in 18 human bones. JAMA Surg. 2016; 151(11):e162775

[19] Myeroff C, Archdeacon M. Autogenous bone graft: donor sites and techniques. J Bone Joint Surg Am. 2011; 93(23):2227–2236

[20] Devers BN, Douglas KC, Naik RD, Lee DH, Watson JT, Weikert DR. Outcomes of hook of hamate fracture excision in high-level amateur athletes. J Hand Surg Am. 2013; 38(1):72–76

[21] Smith P, III, Wright TW, Wallace PF, Dell PC. Excision of the hook of the hamate: a retrospective survey and review of the literature. J Hand Surg Am. 1988; 13(4):612–615

[22] Cerezal L, Abascal F, Canga A, García-Valtuille R, Bustamante M, del Piñal F. Usefulness of gadolinium-enhanced MR imaging in the evaluation of the vascularity of scaphoid nonunions. AJR Am J Roentgenol. 2000; 174(1):141–149

[23] Green DP. The effect of avascular necrosis on Russe bone grafting for scaphoid nonunion. J Hand Surg Am. 1985; 10(5):597–605

[24] Merrell GA, Wolfe SW, Slade JF, III. Treatment of scaphoid nonunions: quantitative meta-analysis of the literature. J Hand Surg Am. 2002; 27(4):685–691

[25] Deng AD, Innocenti M, Arora R, Gabl M, Tang JB. Vascularized small-bone transfers for fracture nonunion and bony defects. Clin Plast Surg. 2017; 44(2):267–285

[26] Henry M. Collapsed scaphoid non-union with dorsal intercalated segment instability and avascular necrosis treated by vascularised wedge-shaped bone graft and fixation. J Hand Surg Eur Vol. 2007; 32(2):148–154

[27] Waitayawinyu T, McCallister WV, Katolik LI, Schlenker JD, Trumble TE. Outcome after vascularized bone grafting of scaphoid nonunions with avascular necrosis. J Hand Surg Am. 2009; 34(3):387–394

[28] Jones DB, Jr, Moran SL, Bishop AT, Shin AY. Free-vascularized medial femoral condyle bone transfer in the treatment of scaphoid nonunions. Plast Reconstr Surg. 2010; 125(4):1176–1184

[29] Jones DB, Jr, Bürger H, Bishop AT, Shin AY. Treatment of scaphoid waist nonunions with an avascular proximal pole and carpal collapse. A comparison of two vascularized bone grafts. J Bone Joint Surg Am. 2008; 90(12):2616–2625

[30] Xing SG, Tang JB. Surgical treatment, hardware removal, and the wide-awake approach for metacarpal fractures. Clin Plast Surg. 2014; 41(3):463–480

15 Rehabilitation of Hand and Finger Fractures

Jürgen Mack

Abstract

Hand therapy, like hand surgery, has developed into a separate discipline in physical therapy. For successful treatment, the problems that can occur must be taken into consideration in order to be able to react with the appropriate measures. This is only possible if we specialize in hand therapy and have experience in this area of expertise. In rehabilitation of fractures of the wrist, metacarpals and the fingers, a detailed assessment is very important. This is the basis for the treatment in order to proceed to an appropriate therapy method. For a good result, treatment should start as soon as the surgeon allows the therapy to begin. The next step for the therapist is to use the right techniques, which will vary depending on the location and classification of the fracture. There are different techniques that may be used for the wrist, metacarpals and the fingers. Moreover, it depends on what the patient can cope with. There should be regular assessments to get feedback on the progression. A valuable key point for a successful treatment is for the patient to be always informed regarding the therapy and to be provided with homework. The exercises must be thoroughly explained to the patient and the progress should be monitored regularly. If all these steps are strictly followed, a good result can be accomplished.

Keywords: assessment, techniques, treatment for fractures in the wrist/metacarpals/fingers, home exercises, problem solving

15.1 Challenges in Rehabilitation of Hand and Wrist Fractures

There are several specific problems in hand rehabilitation, some of which are the following:
- Beginning too late with the therapy causes stiffness of the fingers and the wrist.
- Being in a resting position for too long also causes stiffness of the fingers and the wrist.
- Immobilization in a wrong position leads to stiffness as well. Usually, patient tends to hold their fingers in flexion so they have less pain. But only intrinsic plus position avoids contractures.
- Improper healing of the bones (nonunion or malunion).

- Avoiding rotational deformity with scissoring of the fingers when making a fist.
- Persistent swelling.
- Inadequate exercises of the patient (bad compliance).
- Beginning of complex regional pain syndrome (CRPS).

15.2 Patient Evaluation before Therapy

An extensive assessment of the patient is required before therapy. It should include the following information from the patient and the doctor:
- The date of assessment.
- The date of the trauma or operation.
- Taking pictures of the hand, to locate where the problems are: wrist/metacarpals/finger and left or right hand.
- Description of trauma mechanism: how and where it happened (at work, during sports, at home).
- Type of fracture: straight/oblique/debris/, affected joint.
- Age of the patient.
- If it is the dominant hand, the therapy is significant to decide when the patient can go back to work or carry on with sport.
- Profession, to be able to decide accordingly when work can be resumed.
- Hobbies, so the patient is able to use his fingers during his favorite activities.
- Smoker or nonsmoker.
- Pain classification, quality and exact location so we can decide if it is a regional pain syndrome or a peripheral pain.
- Instruction from the surgeon, guidelines for the treatment.
- Is the patient wearing a splint and has he been properly instructed how to wear it?
- X-rays, especially if the patient had surgery. We have to see where the wires and screws are (finger and metacarpal, close to a joint) or a plate at wrist fractures.

15.2.1 Tools for Measurement

For measurement of the angle, we use the neutral zero method with the finger goniometer (▶Fig. 15.1). An alternative is the documentation on pictures that are taken at regular intervals (▶Fig. 15.2).

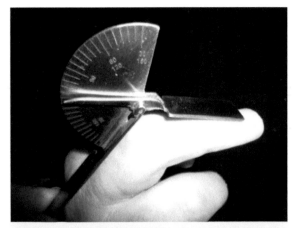

Fig. 15.1 The neutral zero method.

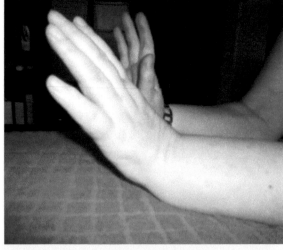

Fig. 15.2 Taking pictures for comparing both sides.

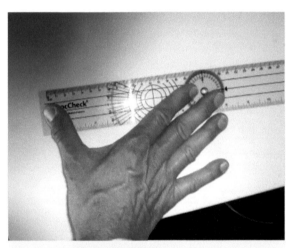

Fig. 15.3 Thumb to index distance.

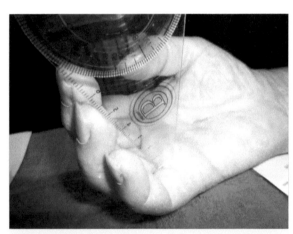

Fig. 15.4 Finger-hollow of the hand distance.

15.2.2 Measuring the Hand Span Distance and Incomplete Closure of the Fist

At the thumb, the distance between the thumb tip and the fingertip of the second finger is measured (▶Fig. 15.3) for measuring the first webs pace. For handspan evaluation, the distance between the tips of the thumb and the fifth finger is measured while spreading the fingers as far as possible.

The distance from the fingertip to the distal flexion crease of the palm can be measured with the fingers (▶Fig. 15.4).

15.2.3 Neurological Evaluation

In the case of neurological signs, the 2-point discriminator can be used to measure the nerve innervation density (▶Fig. 15.5); monofilaments with different pressure intensities can be used to measure the sensitivity (▶Fig. 15.6) and we use the Tinel sign to test the renervation process (▶Fig. 15.7).

15.2.4 Circumference and Volume

In the acute phase, the circumference is measured with the tape measure (▶Fig. 15.8). When the wound healing is complete, the hydrometer can be used (▶Fig. 15.9).

15.2.5 Measuring Force with the Jamar Dynamometer

To measure the hand force, the Jamar dynamometer is used (▶Fig. 15.10).

15.3 Techniques Used in Rehabilitation

15.3.1 Manual Therapy

An essential part of hand therapy is mobilization with manual therapy. With this therapy, we improve the rolling

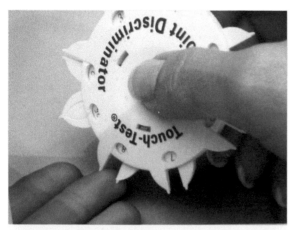

Fig. 15.5 Two-point discriminator, static or dynamic.

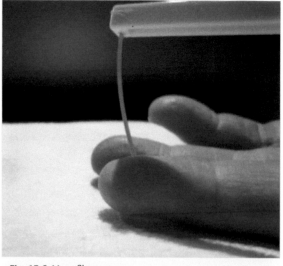

Fig. 15.6 Monofilaments.

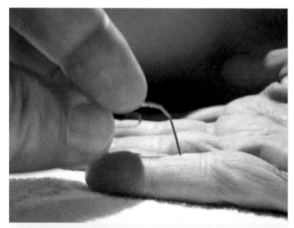

Fig. 15.7 Tinel's sign.

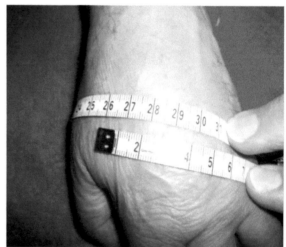

Fig. 15.8 Hydrometer.

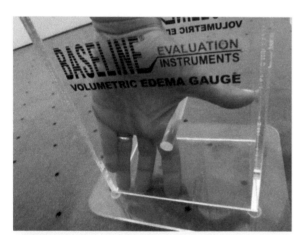

Fig. 15.9 Using a measuring tape.

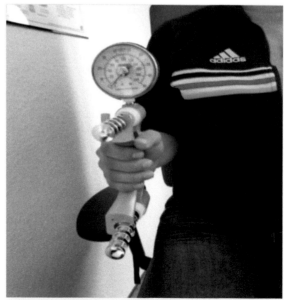

Fig. 15.10 Using a dynamometer.

and gliding of the partners involved in the movement. This is shown in ▶Fig. 15.13: fixation of the forearm and the distal carpal row is moved dorsally. ▶Fig. 15.14 shows the fixation of the head of the second metacarpal and the proximal phalanx which is displaced dorsally and ventrally.

To be able to work with manual therapy, we have to know the exact location and classification of the fracture. The X-ray images are very important (▶Fig. 15.11).

The fixation for mobilization of the finger or the wrist depends on where the fracture is (▶Fig. 15.12).

For the right position, we need a wedge and good positioning of the patient.

For the therapy, we need a stable storage and exact grip techniques (▶Fig. 15.13 and ▶Fig. 15.14).

15.3.2 Flossing

For this method, we use broad elastic rubber bands. We wrap the finger from distal to proximal. It has to be wrapped very tightly. Once it is wrapped, we start moving the joints (▶Fig. 15.15), which creates pressure on the tissue and helps solve the problems of adhesions and nonphysiological crosslinks.

The finger will be wrapped for 2 minutes (▶Fig. 15.16). During this time, the finger is moved in flexion and extension.

Another effect is increased lymph flow and softened scar tissue.

A good example for using flossing is when the movement does not improve. There is no scientific evidence yet, but practical experience has shown this method to be effective.

15.3.3 Lymphatic Drainage

This technique is used to reduce the edema, which indirectly improves range of motion. So it is mandatory to reduce swelling in the hand and fingers. For controlling the effect, we can measure with a hydrometer or measure the circumference. It is important to always measure at the same point of time, especially during the first days and up to 2 to 3 weeks after the fracture. Therefore, lymphatic drainage is very important for this purpose. To make the treatment successful, we have to note that the lymph nodes are on the back of the hand (▶Fig. 15.17). So we start at the palm of the hand and go to the dorsum of the hand.

For self-treatment, the patient has to be explained very accurately what is to be done.

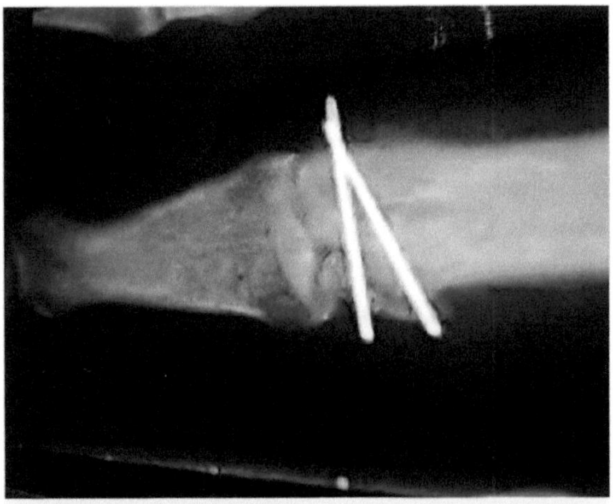

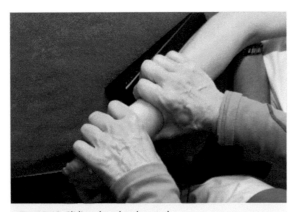

Fig. 15.11 X-ray of the finger.

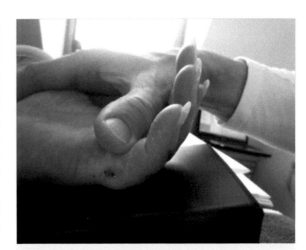

Fig. 15.12 Manual therapy hand fixation for mobilization.

Fig. 15.13 Sliding dorsal and ventral.

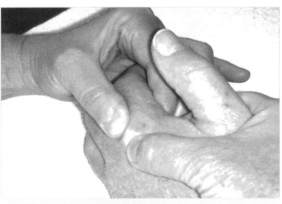

Fig. 15.14 Mobilization in flexion.

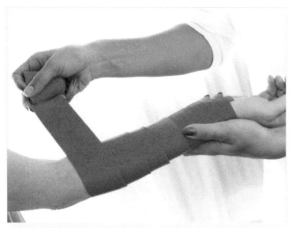

Fig. 15.15 Flossing the forearm.

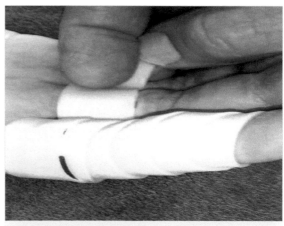

Fig. 15.16 Flossing of the finger.

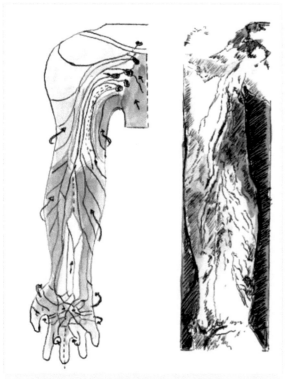

Fig. 15.17 Direction of the drainage.

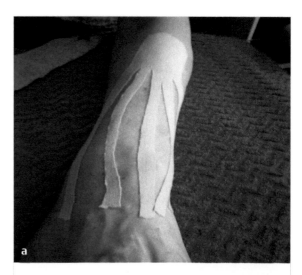

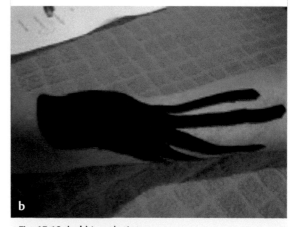

Fig. 15.18 (a, b) Lymphatic tapes.

Another option is to apply a lymphatic tape with kinesiology tape. This holds for several days and reduces the swelling significantly (▶Fig. 15.18). Finger compression sleeves with silicone lining are a good option to reduce finger edema. Care must be taken not to wear it 24 hours due to potential macerati---on of the skin (▶Fig. 15.19).

15.3.4 Mirror Therapy

Mirror therapy has to begin as soon as possible so the patient keeps his mind on movement.

The injured hand is behind the mirror. With their unaffected hand, the patient exercises and watches the exercises in the mirror. This gives the illusion of the injured hand moving.

In the beginning, the injured hand does not make any movement. After several treatments, the patient starts working with the injured hand, training to do the same movements the unaffected hand does (▶Fig. 15.20 and ▶Fig. 15.21).

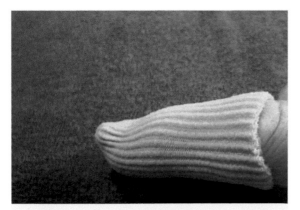

Fig. 15.19 Finger sleeves made out of silicon.

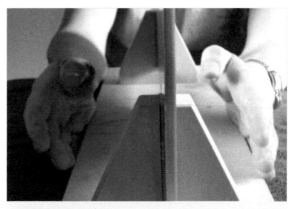

Fig. 15.20 Mirror therapy.

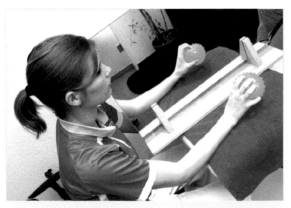

Fig. 15.21 An example of working with mirror therapy.

It is very important that the patient has his/her eyes on the mirror all the time while moving the unaffected hand.

15.4 Extension and Traction

15.4.1 Extension Therapies with Extension Sleeve

For improvement of the movement, we take this extension trainer. We can do it intermittently or with a constant traction. The traction stretches the ligaments and makes the joints more supple.

The patient can do it by themselves or it could be done by the therapist (▶ Fig. 15.22a, b).

15.4.2 Training of Sensibility

Training for sensibility is required when you have hypersensitive scars. It is done with several training materials (▶ Fig. 15.23).

The patient starts by touching the sensitive area with a texture that is perceived as comfortable. With decreasing threshold, the patient uses materials that are more and more coarse.

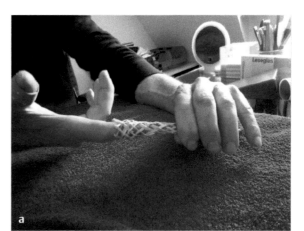

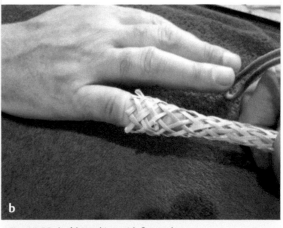

Fig. 15.22 (a, b) Working with finger sleeves.

▶ Fig. 15.24 is a depiction of a hypersensitive scar and what it can look like.

15.4.3 Scar Treatment

Fascia rings for the wrist and fingers are shown in ▶ Fig. 15.25 and ▶ Fig. 15.26. The rings are pushed back and forth over the scar area. This leads to a significantly better circulation and the layers of the skin dissolve through the manual stimulus. It has to be done several times a day.

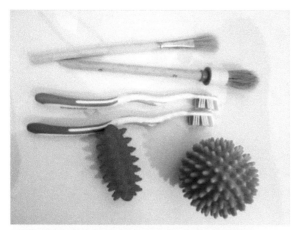

Fig. 15.23 Examples of tools that can be used to train sensitivity.

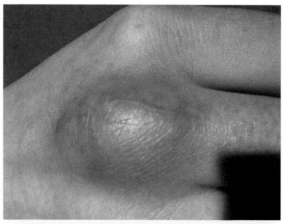

Fig. 15.24 Hypersensitive scar.

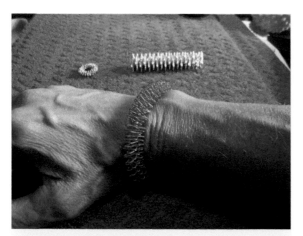

Fig. 15.25 Fascia rings for the wrist.

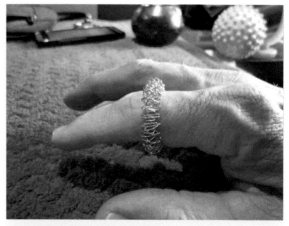

Fig. 15.26 Fascia rings for the finger.

In this area, the patient will face a lot of problems if there is a scar. This will cut movement enormously. In such cases, cupping glasses can be used. Cupping for scar treatment is depicted in ▶ Fig. 15.27.

Therapeutical massage can also be used for this. For this scar, we need silicon plaster (▶ Fig. 15.28). The patient has to wear it as often as possible.

15.4.4 Splints

There are different kinds of splints. Static splints used to improve mobility are shown in ▶ Fig. 15.29, ▶ Fig. 15.30, ▶ Fig. 15.31.

It is very important to explain to the patient accurately how to wear the splint. This must include the following:
- How to carry.
- Presence and absence of pressure points.
- Watching if the hand or fingers are swelling.
- If it is advisable or not advisable to move the splint to clean the hand.
- Ideally, a splint is the passport where everything is written.

Another individual way to improve movement is shown in ▶ Fig. 15.32.

15.4.5 Home Exercises

Home exercises are very important for the fingers and the wrist. They have to be given to the patient and explained and shown precisely. This must include how often (per day and per week) the patient should repeat the exercises and what is to be done exactly. Moreover, the therapist has to monitor the exercises on a regular basis.

Here's an example:

The patient is instructed precisely and can control the exercises (▶ Fig. 15.33). This could be given in pictures or with an exact plan.

Exercise 3: Coin counter.

Frequency: The patient has to perform this exercise 3 times daily. Each session should consist 3 passes with 10 repetitions in each pass and 30 seconds of rest between the passes.

2. Intensification: Thumb opposition back and forth.

Frequency: The patient has to perform this exercise 3 times daily. Each session should consist 3 passes with 10

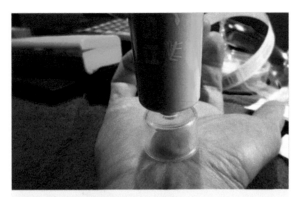

Fig. 15.27 Cupping for scar treatment.

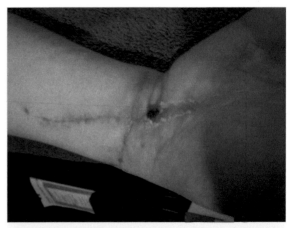

Fig. 15.28 Scarred wrist.

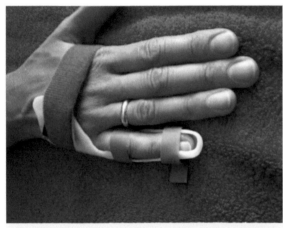

Fig. 15.29 Static extension splint.

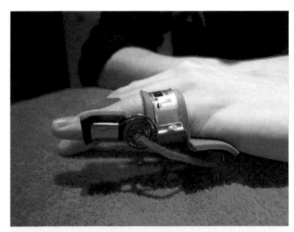

Fig. 15.30 Dynamic extension splint.

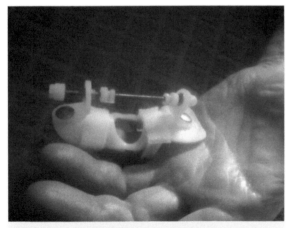

Fig. 15.31 Splint for gradually increasing flexion.

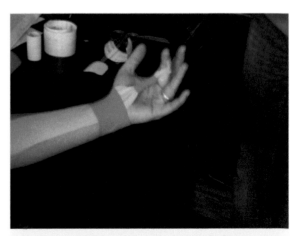

Fig. 15.32 Correction with tape for improve the flexion.

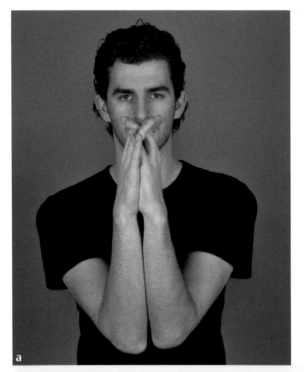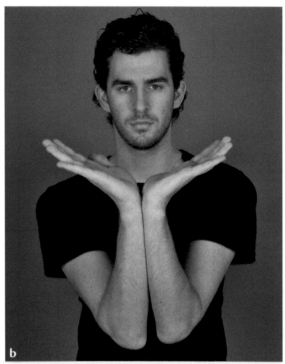

Fig. 15.33 **(a)** Flexion. **(b)** Extension. (Reproduced with permission of the Department of Hand Surgery, University of Ulm.)

repetitions in each pass and 30 seconds of rest between the passes.

This is an exercise day.

17

Documentation for week 5:

Exercises 3 times per day accomplished (the following times are just a guideline):

Day 1	morning ☐	noon ☐	evening ☐
Day 2	morning ☐	noon ☐	evening ☐
Day 3	morning ☐	noon ☐	evening ☐
Day 4	morning ☐	noon ☐	evening ☐
Day 5	morning ☐	noon ☐	evening ☐
Day 6	morning ☐	noon ☐	evening ☐
Day 7	morning ☐	noon ☐	evening ☐

15.4.6 Rehabilitation of the Wrist

We have to distinguish whether we are dealing with conservative treatment or treatment after surgery. This concerns usually the distal radius fracture and the fracture of the scaphoids, which is the most common location of carpal bone fractures.

In conservative treatment, if the patient is wearing a cast, it is important to ensure:

- Positioning of the arm and the hand in the cast is correct.
- Patient is well instructed in performing finger motion exercises.
- Cast fits well and is not too tight.

In therapy, we can start with lymphatic drainage and finger mobilization. Later on, we have to control the home exercises and the cast. From the fifth to the sixth week, with the agreement of the surgeon, we can start with active motion and adapted manual therapy.

From the seventh/eighth week, we start with manual therapy for the joints that are close to the operated bones to improve the range of motion.

Additionally, the patient is encouraged to use his hand for activities of daily living, which is always the best therapy (e.g., playing an instrument, do the dishes).

In the 12th week, we reach full movement and start weight training.

15.4.7 Operation

In an operation with stable angle plate osteosynthesis, the improvement in mobility can be started as soon as possible after the operation. For this purpose, the patient is instructed with a home program. It is also taken care that the finger agility is maintained. By the 12th week, the patient can be fully charged again.

15.4.8 Problems

Some of the problems that may arise include the following: swelling, CRPS, hypersensitive scar, too tight splints (►Fig. 15.34, ►Fig. 15.35, ►Fig. 15.36, and ►Fig. 15.37).

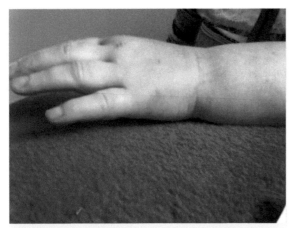

Fig. 15.34 Persistent swelling and suspicion of CRPS.

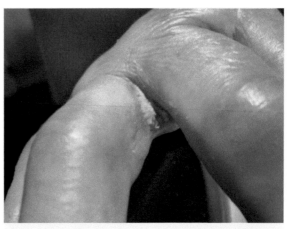

Fig. 15.35 Sensitive scar.

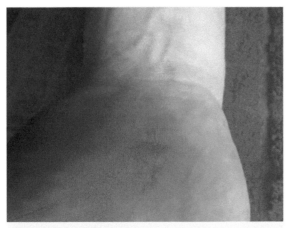

Fig. 15.36 Hypersensitive scar.

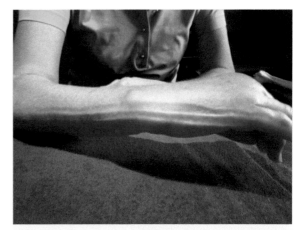

Fig. 15.37 Marks after too tight cast.

15.4.9 Rehabilitation of Metacarpal Fractures

We need to know where the fracture is located. In metacarpal neck fractures, the mobilization must be done cautiously to avoid secondary displacement.

Until the fourth to sixth week, lymphatic drainage is necessary to diminish the swelling of the hand and to treat the scar to reduce adhesions. Functional training for the fingers leads to better range of motion.

Starting at week 6, we can continue with stronger training of finger motion (kneading ball, working with corn; ▸Fig. 15.38 and ▸Fig. 15.39).

At the same time, manual therapy should be started to improve range of motion of the metatarsophalangeal and interphalangeal joints.

The patient has to be instructed for exercises and how to use his hand till the 6th week.

As shown in ▸Fig. 15.40 and ▸Fig. 15.41, it is not always possible to get a good result. This young patient could not reach total extension and flexion in MCP4 after 1 year. Another surgery and the metal removal did not improve the movement.

15.4.10 Rehabilitation of Phalange Fractures

In most cases, treatment is surgically with plates, Kirchner's wires or Herbert's screw.

Concerning hand therapy, we have to know where the fracture is located (▸Fig. 15.42). For this issue, it is helpful to have access to the X-rays (▸Fig. 15.43). X-rays show us where we can do our fixation and where the joints can be moved. This has to be done very precisely.

Active motion is needed to prevent adhesion of the tendons to prevent loss of function. Caution is advised if the fracture is close to the joint.

All joints (as well as the wrist and metacarpals) that are not injured have to be moved to avoid contractures.

The patient has to be instructed what training is mandatory for him. Active and passive exercises are possible.

Another important point is scar treatment, especially scars on the dorsal side. It is essential to treat them as soon as possible to avoid adhesions and contractures (▸Fig. 15.44). Often the patient needs hand therapy sessions at least three times a week (▸Fig. 15.45).

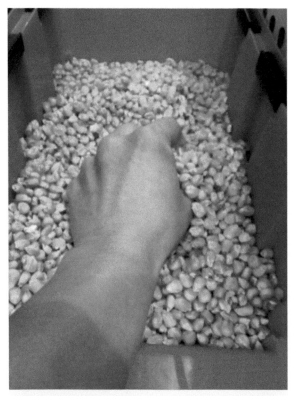

Fig. 15.38 Working with corn.

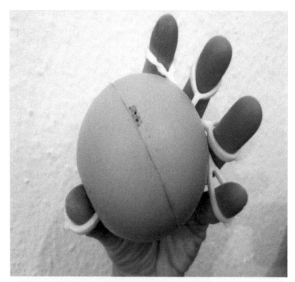

Fig. 15.39 Kneading ball.

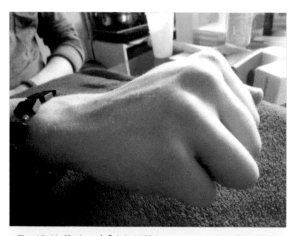

Fig. 15.41 Flexion deficit in MCP4, same case as in ▶Fig. 15.40.

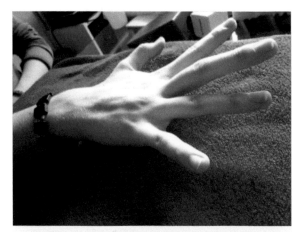

Fig. 15.40 Extension deficit in MCP4 after fracture of the 4th metacarpal.

Frequently we are faced with problems after fractures of the first phalanx of the fifth finger. Very often, it is not possible to reach total extension due to extensor tendon adhesions, as can be seen in ▶Fig. 15.46 and ▶Fig. 15.47.

15.5 Summary

Hand therapy has to start as soon as possible. However, a detailed assessment is necessary before the beginning of therapy. X-rays and a medical report from the surgeon are required.

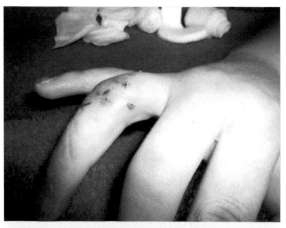

Fig. 15.42 Fracture involving the PIP-joint, fixed with K-wires.

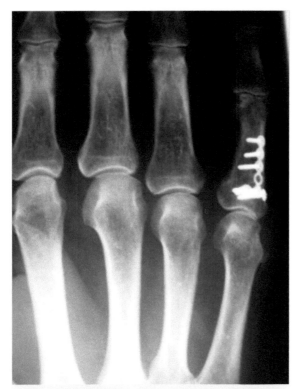

Fig. 15.43 X-ray demonstrating a fracture of the 5th proximal phalanx after ORIF.

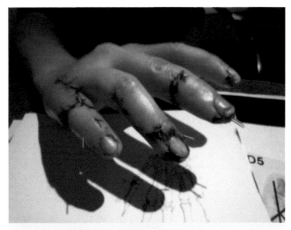

Fig. 15.45 Multiple fractures necessitating intensive hand therapy.

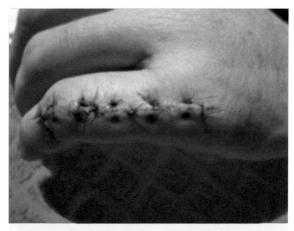

Fig. 15.44 Dorsal surgical approach to a fracture of the proximal phalanx. Scar therapy is essential to avoid adhesions.

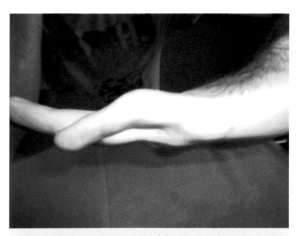

Fig. 15.46 Flexion contracture of the PIP joint due to adhesions.

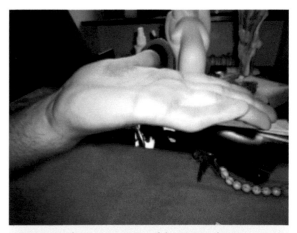

Fig. 15.47 Flexion contracture of the PIP joint due to adhesions.

We start with lymphatic drainage. All joints that need no immobilization must treated be actively and passively to prevent contractures.

The therapist needs to know the treatment frequency required for optimal results. The patient has to perform home exercises, which must be explained in detail and controlled constantly. The therapy must be adapted to the healing process as well as the techniques used. If the patient wears a splint, correct fitting of the splint has to be controlled.

These treatment processes should be followed strictly to achieve the goal of hand therapy, which is to assist the patient in regaining full use of their hand in everyday life.

Section II

Phalangeal Fractures

16 Fractures at the Base of the
   Proximal Phalanx   *159*

17 Extra-articular Fractures of
   the Phalanges   *163*

18 Intra-articular Fractures of the
   Proximal Interphalangeal Joint   *175*

19 Avulsion Fractures of the
   Flexor and Extensor Tendons   *185*

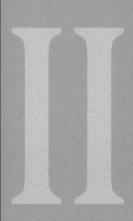

16 Fractures at the Base of the Proximal Phalanx

Lars S. Vadstrup

Abstract

Treatment of base fractures in the proximal phalanx depends on the fracture type, the degree of displacement, and whether fracture reduction is stable or not. In this chapter, intervention options are reviewed focusing on restoration of finger function and to a lesser extent on exact reposition of the fractured digit. Conservative treatment and immediate mobilization are first choice for undisplaced fractures. If osteosynthesis are required to maintain an acceptable position of the fracture after closed reduction, K-wire fixation should be considered, with respect for the anatomy of the extensor apparatus. Open reposition and internal plate fixation is a specialist procedure, where absolute stability is needed, so that immediate mobilization of the finger can be initiated soon after surgery.

Keywords: conservative treatment, Buddy Loops, early mobilization

16.1 Trauma Mechanism

Hyperextension and abduction of one of the fingers tend to cause a base fracture of the proximal phalanges, most frequently to the fourth or fifth finger. An extra-articular transverse or oblique fracture is often the outcome of the described trauma, whereas torsion injuries might cause an oblique or spiral fracture of the shaft. A direct blow creating an axial load to the finger may result in a comminuted, intra-articular base fracture. If coronal forces are applied to a finger, intra-articular avulsion fractures of the base of the proximal phalanx are a consequence of ligament strength superior to bone strength. This type of fracture results in evident joint instability (►Fig. 16.1).

A phalangeal fracture is the most common injury to the skeletal system and accounts for approximately 10% of all fractures. The trauma is most likely related to sports activities in the 10-to 30-year-olds, work related in the 30- to 70-year-olds, and due to fall from a standing position in people above 70 years of age.[1–3] The fracture often results in a dorsal angulation at the fracture site in the base of the proximal phalanx. This deformity tends to be maintained by the intrinsic muscle insertion on the base of the proximal phalanx (dorsal interossei) and the extension force of the central slip across the proximal interphalangeal (PIP) joint (palmar interossei and lumbricals insertion into lateral bands of the extensor hood). Unlike diaphyseal fractures, these do not tend to cause appreciable rotational deformity.

16.2 Classification

The AO Foundation divides the base fractures of the proximal phalanx into proximal metaphyseal and proximal articular. The proximal metaphyseal fractures are extra-articular and segmented into transverse and oblique types. The proximal articular fractures are subdivided into avulsion, shearing, and multifragmentary fractures. Upon consideration of the subsequent treatment of the fractured phalanx, stability, angulation, and possible rotation of the fracture should be observed.

16.3 Clinical Signs and Tests

When evaluating a proximal phalanx fracture, it is important to pay attention to the tendon function of

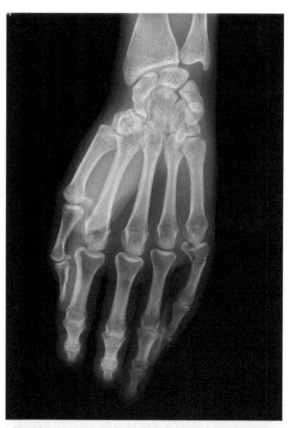

Fig. 16.1 An intra-articular avulsion fracture of the base of the proximal phalanx is a consequent of ligament stability superior to bone strength.

the involved digit, as the bottom of the flexor tendon sheath is constituted of the palmar aspect of the phalangeal bone. Test of ligament stability is performed on the metacarpophalangeal (MP), PIP, and distal interphalangeal (DIP) joints taking a possible intra-articular base fracture of the proximal phalanx into account. If any doubt about the function of the flexor tendons or ligament stability of the finger, the finger should be examined under local anesthesia (finger block anesthesia). With the finger anesthetized, the examiner also gets the best possible evaluation of a possible rotation deformity of the finger, comparing the plane of the digits nails, as the patient actively flexes and extends the affected finger. Rotational deformity is a clinical diagnosis, not assessed on radiographs, and no rotational deformity can be accepted.

16.4 Investigatory Examinations

Plain radiographs (posteroanterior [PA] and lateral views) of the injured finger should always be performed when a fracture is suspected. Proper assessment of the injured hand should also include radiographs of the entire hand, to rule out associated fractures.

In adults a dorsal fracture angulation, up to 25 degrees is acceptable in an extra-articular fracture, but no more than 10 degrees of lateral of volar angulation should be accepted. Malunion causes impairment of digital function, and causes loss of equilibrium between flexor and extensor tendons. Clinically, the shortening of the proximal phalanx leads to loss of full extension at the PIP joint due to laxity of the extensor mechanism, and the dorsal angulation to hyperextension at the fracture site and MP joint. Sonography of the flexor tendons can be used in case of doubt concerning tendon lesions. Computed tomography (CT) scan is rarely needed.

16.5 Possible Concurrent Lesions of Bone and Soft Tissue

Evaluation of the soft tissues, nerves, and tendons of the injured finger is mandatory when the treatment method is to be determined. Reduced motion of the injured finger(s) may be the result of tendon adhesions (either flexor or extensor) or capsular contracture. Associated joint injury and soft tissue injury are contributing factors to reduced mobility of the fractured finger.[4] When treating a combined fracture and tendon lesion, it is necessary to achieve absolute stability in the fixation of the fracture, to enable early active mobilization of the tendon injury. Nerve lesions are usually associated to open injuries.

16.6 Evidence

Fractures of the metaphysis of the proximal phalanx can be transverse, oblique, or comminuted. Reduction is achieved by traction and digital manipulation. When the fracture is undisplaced and stable or displaced, and stable after closed reduction, it can be treated nonoperatively with "buddy taping" and immediate active mobilization for 5 weeks.[5] Reduced fractures are prone to displace and radiographical monitoring after 1 and 2 weeks treatment is advised.

Displaced fractures, that are unstable after closed reduction, require stable pin or percutaneous screw fixation. Pins or screws should be placed in the plane that crosses the fracture plane and at least two pin/screw diameters from the fracture line. When using lag screws, maximal fracture compression is obtained. Nerve and tendon anatomy should be taken into consideration when planning pin or screw placement. Postoperatively, a plaster of Paris in intrinsic-plus position is applied for 1 to 2 weeks followed by "buddy taping" and active mobilization for 5 weeks. Pin removal is done after 3 to 4 weeks.

Comminuted fractures are treated with either closed reduction and external fixation, or open reduction and internal fixation (ORIF). When addressing a comminuted fracture, one must consider whether the soft tissues tolerate further mobilizing or not. Closed reduction and external fixation provides stabilization with minimal risk of worsening the soft tissue lesion caused by the trauma. The use of plates and screws requires that a rigid osteosynthesis is obtained during surgery, as immediate mobilization is needed after open surgery to secure an acceptable function by avoiding adhesion of the soft tissues to the bone.[6-8]

16.7 Author's Favored Treatment Option

Treatment of base fractures at the proximal phalanx is a compromise between fixation and mobilization in retrieval of full range of motion (ROM) of the finger.[3,9-12] Surgical fixation tends to cause a substantial loss of motion when percutaneous K-wire fixation or open reduction and internal fixation is performed.[13-15] Standard treatment strategy for base fractures of the proximal phalanx should focus on function and to a lesser extent exact reposition of the fractured digit. In my practice "buddy taping" is always used if the fracture is nondisplaced and stable, or displaced and stable after closed reduction allowing immediate mobilization (▶ Fig. 16.2).

Displaced (> 2 mm) radial/ulnar avulsion or shearing fractures of the proximal metaphysis needs closed or open reduction and internal fixation, as joint stability may be compromised. The fracture can be addressed with K-wires (1–1.25 mm) with a percutaneous technique. If

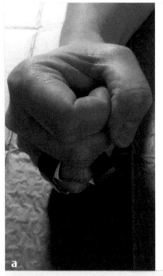
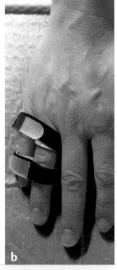

Fig. 16.2 (a, b) Buddy taping of the fourth and fifth finger allowing for full flexion and extension of both fingers.

open surgery is required for fracture reposition, a volar approach is recommended.[16] Brunner incisions are used at the level of the MP joint. The digital nerves and arteries are identified and the A1 and proximal part of A2 pulley are divided to expose the fracture as the flexor tendons are kept aside. A rigid osteosynthesis should be obtained, as early mobilization after 1 to 2 weeks is necessary to secure a satisfactory functional outcome (▶Fig. 16.3).

16.8 Alternative Treatment Options

Numerous nonoperative and operative methods are described in treating base fractures of the fingers. Fok et al's study[17] reports on 10-year results of managing proximal phalangeal fractures with dynamic splinting. A dynamic splint that kept the MP joint maximally flexed while allowing free movement of the PIP and DIP joints of the injured finger was applied for at least 4 weeks. About 75% of patients attained excellent or good results. Figl et al[12] describes the use of a similar dorsopalmar plaster splint keeping the extensor aponeurosis taut covering two-thirds of the proximal phalanx. About 86% showed full ROM at follow-up.

The use of percutaneous K-wires is useful in extra-articular base fractures of the proximal phalanx[18,19] minimizing further injury of the soft tissue and the extensor apparatus. Oblique fractures are reduced with reduction forceps and fixated with two or more parallel K-wires. Cross pinning technique is ideal for transverse fractures, keeping in mind that K-wires should never cross at the fracture site, but either proximal or distal to the fracture with firm anchorage in the proximal

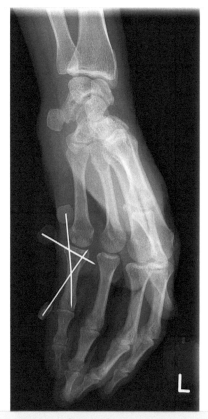

Fig. 16.3 ORIF K-wire fixation of an intra-articular avulsion fracture (same patient as ▶Fig. 16.1).

and distal metaphysis. Attention to safe corridors using percutaneous pinning is mandatory.[20] The central part of the extensor tendon is identified dorsally at the MP joint, and on either side of this, there is a triangular safe zone at the base of the proximal phalanx. Care should be taken to avoid penetrating the lateral bands of the extensor apparatus when introducing K-wires at the diaphysis of the proximal phalanx (▶Fig. 16.4). External fixation is indicated for open fractures with concomitant soft tissue injury.

16.9 Prognosis

Patients with fractures at the base of the proximal phalanx treated conservatively with immediate mobilization report excellent or good results (ROM, absence of pain) in the majority of cases, when examined at a minimum of 1 year after the trauma.[5,12,17] If internal fixation is indicated, closed reduction and K-wire stabilization[6–8] has a better prognosis than open reduction and internal fixation with plates and screws, as the latter in general has been reported to carry a rather high risk of complications, such as reduced mobility, infection, and sympathetic dystrophy and to require reoperation to remove hardware or perform tenolysis.[13–15]

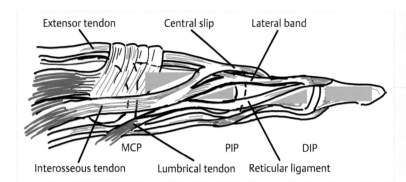

Fig. 16.4 Safe zones for K-wiring are marked with green color.

Extensor tendon · Central slip · Lateral band

MCP · PIP · DIP

Interosseous tendon · Lumbrical tendon · Reticular ligament

References

[1] van Onselen EB, Karim RB, Hage JJ, Ritt MJ. Prevalence and distribution of hand fractures. J Hand Surg [Br]. 2003; 28(5):491–495

[2] Hove LM. Fractures of the hand. Distribution and relative incidence. Scand J Plast Reconstr Surg Hand Surg. 1993; 27(4):317–319

[3] Henry MH. Fractures of the proximal phalanx and metacarpals in the hand: preferred methods of stabilization. J Am Acad Orthop Surg. 2008; 16(10):586–595

[4] Strickland JW, Steichen JB, Kleinman WB, et al. Phalangeal fractures: factors influencing digital performance. Orthop Rev. 1982; 11:39–50

[5] Vadstrup LS, Jørring S, Bernt P, Boeckstyns ME. Base fractures of the fifth proximal phalanx can be treated conservatively with buddy taping and immediate mobilisation. Dan Med J. 2014; 61(8):A4882

[6] Belsky MR, Eaton RG, Lane LB. Closed reduction and internal fixation of proximal phalangeal fractures. J Hand Surg Am. 1984; 9(5):725–729

[7] Brei-Thoma P, Vögelin E, Franz T. Plate fixation of extra-articular fractures of the proximal phalanx: do new implants cause less problems? Arch Orthop Trauma Surg. 2015; 135(3):439–445

[8] Kurzen P, Fusetti C, Bonaccio M, Nagy L. Complications after plate fixation of phalangeal fractures. J Trauma. 2006; 60(4):841–843

[9] Collins AL, Timlin M, Thornes B, O'Sullivan T. Old principles revisited—traction splinting for closed proximal phalangeal fractures. Injury. 2002; 33(3):235–237

[10] Fess EE. A history of splinting: to understand the present, view the past. J Hand Ther. 2002; 15(2):97–132

[11] Hornbach EE, Cohen MS. Closed reduction and percutaneous pinning of fractures of the proximal phalanx. J Hand Surg [Br]. 2001; 26(1):45–49

[12] Figl M, Weninger P, Hofbauer M, Pezzei C, Schauer J, Leixnering M. Results of dynamic treatment of fractures of the proximal phalanx of the hand. J Trauma. 2011; 70(4):852–856

[13] Faruqui S, Stern PJ, Kiefhaber TR. Percutaneous pinning of fractures in the proximal third of the proximal phalanx: complications and outcomes. J Hand Surg Am. 2012; 37(7):1342–1348

[14] Ouellette EA, Freeland AE. Use of the minicondylar plate in metacarpal and phalangeal fractures. Clin Orthop Relat Res. 1996;(327):38–46

[15] Stern PJ. Management of fractures of the hand over the last 25 years. J Hand Surg Am. 2000; 25(5):817–823

[16] Kuhn KM, Dao KD, Shin AY. Volar A1 pulley approach for fixation of avulsion fractures of the base of the proximal phalanx. J Hand Surg Am. 2001; 26(4):762–771

[17] Fok MW, Ip WY, Fung BK, Chan RK, Chow SP. Ten-year results using a dynamic treatment for proximal phalangeal fractures of the hands. Orthopedics. 2013; 36(3):e348–e352

[18] Ip WY, Ng KH, Chow SP. A prospective study of 924 digital fractures of the hand. Injury. 1996; 27(4):279–285

[19] Eberlin KR, Babushkina A, Neira JR, Mudgal CS. Outcomes of closed reduction and periarticular pinning of base and shaft fractures of the proximal phalanx. J Hand Surg Am. 2014; 39(8):1524–1528

[20] Rex C, Vignesh R, Javed M, Balaji SC, Premanand C, Zakki SA. Safe corridors for K-wiring in phalangeal fractures. Indian J Orthop. 2015; 49(4):388–392

17 Extra-articular Fractures of the Phalanges

David J. Shewring

Abstract

Diaphyseal fractures of the phalanges are common and the vast majority of these should be treated nonoperatively. Judicious fixation, when appropriate, has several advantages, but these fractures are unforgiving. The best chance of obtaining a good result is at the first surgical intervention and so the planning and execution of treatment should be undertaken by an experienced surgeon. Various methods of fixation can be employed including wires, screws, and plates and each of these methods has particular indications, advantages, and disadvantages. These are discussed within this chapter along with the treatment of specific configurations of fracture pattern affecting the phalangeal diaphysis. The aim in all cases should be to restore comfort, stability, and timely return to function, with a hand that is pain free, but sensate and with joints that are mobile but stable. For both operative and nonoperative treatment, the services of a team of skilled hand therapists are essential to achieve those goals. This chapter also discusses the management of particularly difficult situations such as delayed presentation of complicated fractures, severely comminuted fractures, and the management of malunion.

Keywords: fracture, phalanges, diaphyseal, internal fixation, nonoperative, hand therapy, lag screws, k-wires, malunion, comminution, osteotomy

17.1 Trauma Mechanism

The mechanism of the injury will dictate the configuration of the fracture and will often have a bearing on how the fracture is treated. A crush injury (▶Fig. 17.1) may result in a comminuted but undisplaced phalangeal fracture. The periosteum is likely to be intact and therefore, despite the comminution, the fracture may be relatively stable. This will allow early mobilization after initial symptomatic treatment. Crush injuries may, however, be associated with more severe soft tissue damage and a higher incidence of complex regional pain syndrome (CRPS), and this will also influence management. A direct blow to the finger may result in a transverse fracture (▶Fig. 17.2). The degree of displacement and comminution will reflect the energy of the injury. Such fractures tend to be unstable and may be open. An axial injury to a digit may result in an intra-articular fracture such as a die punch or pilon fracture with crushing and deformation of the cancellous bone (see Chapter 18). In the case of a spiral fracture, the trauma will have been indirect. The shape of the fracture and any deformity of the digit reflects the rotational nature of the force involved. These fractures often occur as the result of a fall, assaults, injury during contact sport, or as the result of the finger having become entangled in the reign of a horse, or dog lead. Displaced spiral fractures tend to be unstable,

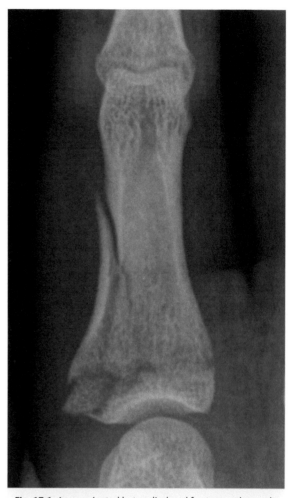

Fig. 17.1 A comminuted but undisplaced fracture as the result of a crush injury.

due to tearing of the periosteum and the configuration of the fracture.

Injuries caused by motorized tools such as mechanical saws or lawnmowers result in complex lesions including comminuted fractures and extensive soft tissue lacerations.

17.2 Classification

- Fractures of the proximal and middle phalanx
  - Metaphyseal
  - Diaphyseal
- Spiral and oblique fractures
- Transverse fractures
- Comminuted fractures
- Fractures of the distal phalanx
  - Shaft fractures
  - Tuft fractures

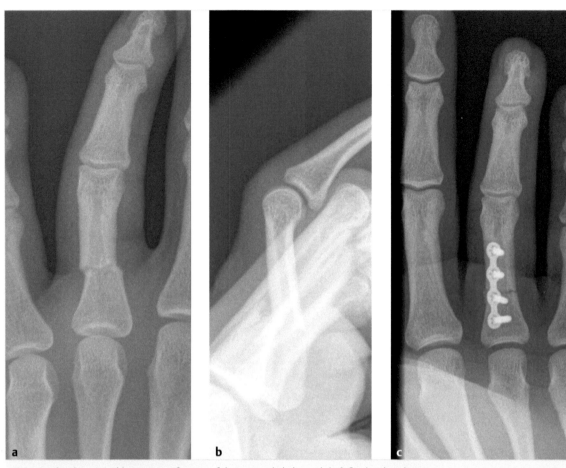

Fig. 17.2 (a–c) An unstable transverse fracture of the proximal phalangeal shaft fixed with a plate.

Fractures can be undisplaced, laterally displaced, angulated, rotated, or displaced in a combination of these.

17.3 Clinical Signs and Tests

Although a spiral fracture may appear undisplaced, this is relative, as the very fact that the fracture is visible on a radiograph will indicate some displacement.

The finger will need to be inspected carefully for signs of malrotation. This can be done by either gently flexing the digits, which will make any malrotation more obvious or by inspecting the relative orientation of the fingernails (▶Fig. 17.3). If malrotation is present, it must be corrected or significant morbidity will result, as well as potential litigation. It is essential that all strapping be removed **before** the finger is examined or radiographs obtained. Failure to do so will not permit adequate examination and radiographs taken with strapping in place will also be inadequate.

17.4 Investigatory Examinations

Initial radiographs taken in the accident unit are often inappropriate. All too often a request for "X-ray hand" has

been made and the resulting images include the whole hand rather than specific views of the relevant digit or joint. It is important that a specific request is made and that posteroanterior (PA) and true lateral views of the relevant digit or joint are obtained.

The advent of computerized radiology with the ability to rotate, expand, and change the contrast of images as well as accurate measurement of angles has made planning the treatment of small bone fractures significantly easier.

17.5 Concurrent Soft Tissue Lesions

Crush injuries may be associated with severe soft tissue damage and a higher incidence of CRPS, and this will influence management. Crush injuries to the fingertip are frequently open fractures, associated with a laceration to the nail matrix.

Severe fingertip injuries may be sustained when the fingers are inadvertently inserted into the path of the rotating blades of a lawnmower resulting in severely comminuted fractures of the phalanges, associated with significant soft tissue injuries, often with tissue loss.

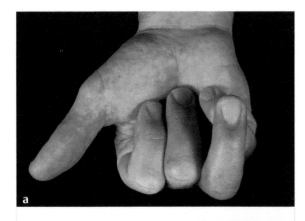

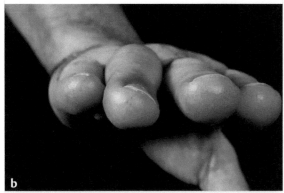

Fig. 17.3 (a, b) Malrotation following fracture of a proximal phalanx. The orientation of the fingernails has been lost and the malrotation is enhanced by flexing the fingers.

17.6 Evidence

Fractures of the phalanges and metacarpals are the most common fractures of the skeletal system[1] and account for 10% of all fractures. Along with fractures of the carpal bones, they represent 55% of upper extremity fractures. Proximal phalangeal fractures are among the most common affecting the hand, accounting for 17% of hand fractures.

Although over the last few decades there has been an increased tendency to treat many of these fractures with internal fixation, the vast majority of hand fractures are stable and can (and should) be treated nonoperatively.[2] If surgical fixation is considered, then it must be appreciated that some hand fractures, particularly those affecting the proximal phalangeal shaft and intra-articular fractures, can be unforgiving.[3,4]

The background to the injury is important and how the patient is treated will be influenced by numerous factors. The age, comorbidities, priorities, demands, occupation, and potential compliance of the patient must be established. What may be correct treatment for a phalangeal fracture in a 60-year-old professional violinist may not be appropriate for the same fracture in a 23-year-old player of contact sport.

It is imperative that the clinician does not fall into the trap of treating the *radiograph* rather than the *patient* that it relates to a sadly all too common scenario.

Many patients with hand fractures have a tendency toward irresponsibility, which must be taken into account. It is also worth considering that in most people, the hand, like the face, is the only part of the anatomy which is on display at all times and so cosmetic defects as the result of fractures (and their treatment) may be poorly tolerated.

At the cornerstone of treatment should be the services of skilled specialized hand therapists. During nonoperative treatment, they can, if necessary, splint injured digits leaving noninjured ones free. They can give patients advice on mobilization and correct care of the injured hand and their involvement will free up time for clinicians in busy clinics. Ideally, the therapists should be present in the trauma clinic so that plans can be formulated jointly and treatment plans discussed with surgeon, therapist, and patient present. If complex fixations are being attempted, then postoperative supervision by a specialized hand therapist is absolutely essential. If the therapists are encouraged to check matters at crucial junctures and bring patients back if they are concerned, then this will allow early discharge to their care.

Above all, it is essential to ensure that the patient is not made worse by the treatment, which is surprisingly commonplace. It is extremely depressing to encounter patients who would have had a far better outcome had they simply not come to a hospital.

"Do no harm."

17.7 Author's Favored Treatment Options

The vast majority of phalangeal fractures should be treated nonoperatively. Treated poorly, with a lack of respect and if the wrong tools are used in the wrong way and in the wrong hands, then the results may be catastrophic and irretrievable (▶Fig. 17.4). Good or perfect results can be obtained, but these may be hard won, demanding careful planning with consideration of all the various methods in the surgical armamentarium. As the best and often only chance of obtaining a good result is at the first surgical intervention, these fractures should not be delegated to unsupervised more junior members of the surgical team. There is also no place for the surgical treatment of difficult hand fractures by the occasional hand surgeon. It is better to delay fixation by a few days until the best expertise is available. However, it is important to establish the exact amount of time that has elapsed between the date of the injury and the first consultation with the clinician who is going to provide the definitive treatment. There may have been delays, due to late presentation by the patient or tardy referral by the accident service.

When making a decision on what will be the most appropriate mode of treatment for a patient with a hand fracture, it is important to be aware of all the available options and to select that which is most likely to result in a good outcome. This may depend on many factors: the

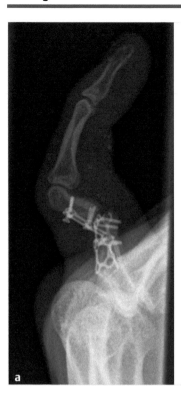
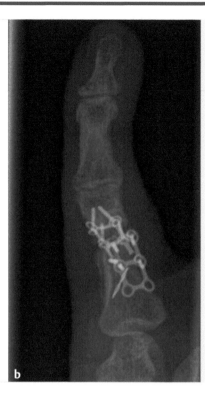

Fig. 17.4 (a, b) A poorly fixed proximal phalangeal fracture, which has failed.

intrinsic qualities of the patient, the skillset of the surgeon, and the availability of facilities, equipment, and specialized hand therapy. Surgeons treating hand fractures should favor the method with which they are most familiar and competent. Consideration should also be given as to which technique utilizes the least health care resources.

There are, of course, several advantages to judicious internal fixation. The anatomy can be restored and stability established. The fracture may be effectively "neutralized" so that efforts can be concentrated on the rehabilitation of the soft tissues, with mobilization of associated joints. It should also be remembered, however, that surgical fixation represents a further insult to an already injured hand and that this is cumulative. The aim in all cases should be to restore comfort, stability, and timely return to function with a hand that is pain free, but sensate and with joints that are mobile but stable.

If fixation is indicated, then there is a spectrum of available techniques, which can be tailored to each fracture. At one extreme would be a robust fixation, such as a plate (▶Fig. 17.2). Although this would have the advantage of more stability and reliability, the increased trauma to the finger involved in its application could potentially compromise the result. At the other end of the spectrum would be a minimal fixation such as a single wire, inserted closed (▶Fig. 17.5). Although this would have the advantage of having inflicted minimal added trauma to the hand, the fixation may not be robust enough to allow vigorous mobilization.

17.7.1 K-wires

K-wires do not provide a high degree of stability of fixation, but they can be used as what are effectively

bone sutures. They provide augmentation of conservative treatment, making it more reliable. They can be used to maintain length and rotation to enable effective splintage and allow some movement.[5–7] K-wires have some disadvantages. They may protrude, causing soft tissue interference to skin and adjacent joints.[8] The pin site is vulnerable to infection and will need regular cleaning. They do not provide a stable enough fixation for vigorous mobilization and they usually need to be removed, although if they are left protruding through the skin, this can be done in clinic. When inserting more than one wire, it is important to avoid them crossing at the fracture site. If this occurs, then the fracture may be held in distraction resulting in a nonunion of the fracture. It is also important to avoid inserting them near the proximal interphalangeal (PIP) joint. This joint is particularly unforgiving (see Chapter 18) and stiffness will often ensue if this joint is compromised in any way (▶Fig. 17.6). It is preferable and easier to insert the wires from the base of the phalanx. The wire can be guided between the metacarpal heads. The rim of the base of the phalanx can be felt with the wire and the wire inserted up the medullary canal, either up to the subchondral bone or to engage the lateral cortex (▶Fig. 17.5).

They are, however, cheap and can be inserted quickly. When inserted closed, the integrity of the soft tissue envelope is preserved. Furthermore, if the fracture is highly comminuted and associated with significant soft tissue damage, as in the case of a crush injury (▶Fig. 17.7), then K-wires provide an invaluable option of stability without the further soft tissue injury consequent to dissection.[9]

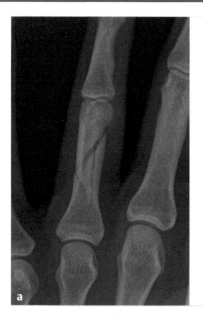
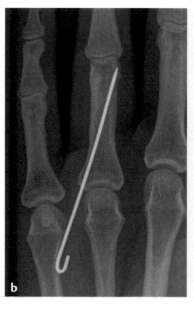

Fig. 17.5 (a, b) A comminuted diaphyseal fracture of the proximal phalanx stabilized with a single K-wire inserted from the base.

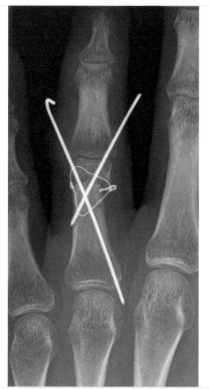

Fig. 17.6 An example of a phalangeal diaphyseal fracture treated with K-wires using poor technique. The wires have been inserted adjacent to the proximal interphalangeal joint, compromising that joint. The wires also cross near the fracture site. A nonunion with marked stiffness of the PIP joint ensued.

17.7.2 Lag Screws

Over the last 20 years, there has been a considerable improvement in the technology of implants used for internal fixation in the hand. Screws are now smaller and self-tapping. The screw heads are lower profile and

the instrumentation for insertion has become more refined.[10,11] As the result of this, as well as there being more widespread expertise in the operative management of hand fractures, the scope for internal fixation has increased. Metalwork should ideally be kept to a minimum, so that there is minimal interference with the soft tissues. This applies particularly to phalangeal shaft fractures. For a displaced spiral fracture with no or minimal comminution, fixation with one or two lag screws is ideal (▶Fig. 17.8). The reduction, however, must be absolutely perfect and accurate. If not, then the stability will not be enough for mobilization and the patient may be left with the worst of all options.

17.8 Alternative Treatment Options

17.8.1 Plates

The use of plates is indicated only occasionally for proximal phalangeal fractures. Although the implants have become lower profile in recent years, they are still relatively bulky and it may be difficult to close the soft tissues over the implant. Application of a plate necessitates significant soft tissue stripping, which is tolerated less over the phalanges than in the metacarpal region. As the phalanx has an elliptical shape in cross-section, they are more easily applied to the dorsal aspect of the bone through a dorsal approach. The "mini condylar plate" is a particularly unforgiving implant.

17.8.2 Cerclage Wire

As with a plate, a cerclage wire or "Lister loop" provides a robust fixation (▶Fig. 17.9). The Lister loop technique[12] is likely to involve more extensive dissection and soft tissue stripping and is technically more exacting. For either

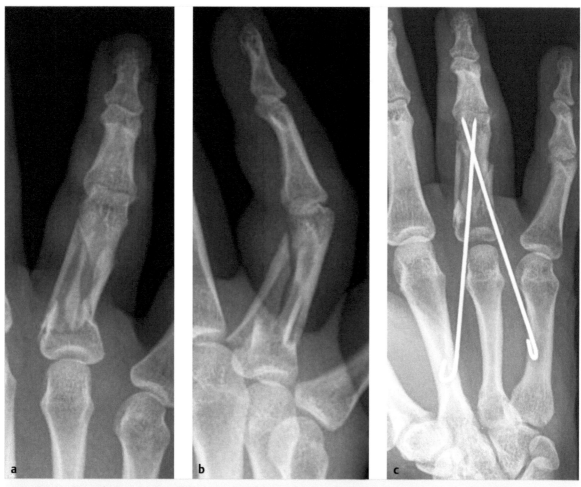

Fig. 17.7 (a–c) Use of two K-wires to stabilize a comminuted open fracture with preservation of the soft tissue envelope.

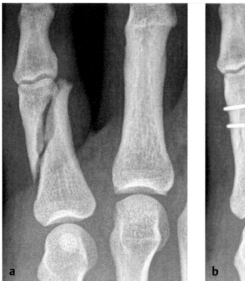
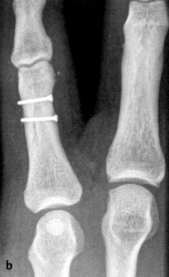

Fig. 17.8 (a, b) Displaced spiral phalangeal fracture fixed with lag screws.

technique the surgeon, therapist, and patient should be prepared for a period of stiffness, with extension lag of the PIP joint, which although usually temporary, may be protracted.

Other alternative options are *external fixation* (see Chapter 7) and *intramedullary screw fixation* (see Chapter 5).

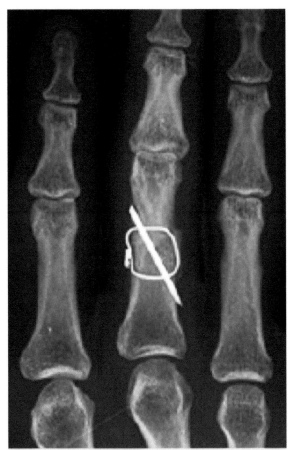

Fig. 17.9 Midshaft phalangeal fracture treated with a "Lister Loop" and oblique K-wire.

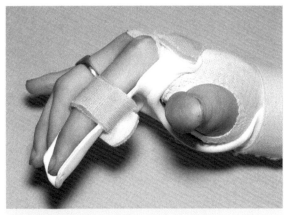

Fig. 17.10 A custom-made thermoplastic splint.

17.9 Treatment of Specific Fracture Configurations

17.9.1 Proximal Phalangeal Fractures

Proximal phalangeal fractures are among the most common affecting the hand, accounting for 17% of hand fractures. Although many of these fractures can be treated nonoperatively, they can be unforgiving, particularly phalangeal shaft fractures.

Undisplaced Fractures

For many undisplaced extra-articular fractures, simple "buddy taping" to the adjacent digit may be enough. However, if the fracture has an unstable configuration, then it may have a tendency to displace, particularly if the patient has an irresponsible nature. It may be wise to augment this with a protective splint, at least for the initial 1 to 2 weeks. The digit should be splinted in the "intrinsic-plus" position with the MP joint flexed and the IP joints in extension. A thermoplastic, custom-made splint can be fabricated by the hand therapists (▶Fig. 17.10).

The splint should be removed and the finger allowed to mobilize when the patient is in a safe environment and at night. Care must be taken not to "over-splint," as stiffness may readily occur.

Spiral Fractures

Spiral fractures are the most common configuration affecting the diaphysis. For unstable fractures that reduce easily, a single K-wire may suffice. Ideally, protrusion of the wires through the distal end of the phalanx should be avoided as the PIP joint is intolerant of injury and any interference with the collateral ligaments of that joint invites trouble. It is preferable and easier to insert the wire from the base of the phalanx and guide it up the medullary canal either up to the subchondral bone or to engage the lateral cortex (▶Fig. 17.5). It is not necessary to use a wire bigger than 1.2 mm for phalangeal fractures. Wires usually remain in place for approximately 3½ weeks, although further protection with "buddy taping" may be necessary for several weeks more. Although initial gentle mobilization will be possible, this will need to be augmented by splintage.

Alternatively, the combination of a precise reduction of the interdigitations of a fresh fracture and compression with lag screws will provide a very stable fixation and will permit immediate mobilization.

A lateral approach for this type of fracture (▶Fig. 17.11a–c) is more difficult than a dorsal approach, but this avoids violation of the plane between the extensor mechanism and the periosteum, which is a potent cause of adherence and stiffness. For uncomplicated spiral factures, this is therefore recommended.

Careful consideration is given to which side to approach the fracture. If an ulnar approach is made, an extra assistant may be required to keep the arm rotated. If the distal fracture line involves the attachment of the collateral ligament, then there may be soft tissue interposition. Any branches of the digital nerve are protected and the extensor tendon edge is identified. The periosteum is incised beneath this and elevated with a small periosteal elevator.

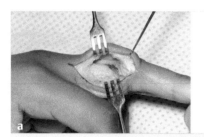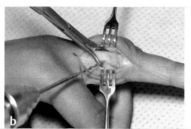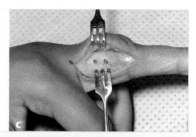

Fig. 17.11 **(a)** Lateral approach to expose a fracture of the phalangeal diaphysis. **(b)** Fracture reduced. **(c)** Lag screws inserted.

The fracture is then opened up and cleared of any fibrinous material, which may prevent accurate reduction. The fracture is reduced and held. It is worth taking extra time to make sure that it is as perfect as possible. Two lag screws are usually adequate. The drill reamings can be collected to use as graft, which can be smeared into the fracture site. This is particularly useful if there has been some slight comminution of the fracture edges. The finger can then be mobilized early. It is adequate to dress the finger and bandage it to an adjacent finger, without plaster.

Transverse Fractures

Transverse fractures of the midshaft are relatively uncommon but pose particular challenges. These fractures are often caused by a direct blow to the finger and so may be comminuted and open. The position of the wound, usually dorsal, will determine the surgical approach, if necessary.

It is possible to treat these with an intramedullary K-wire as described above, but these fractures take longer to unite than spiral fractures, and so the wires may need to be in place for longer.

Either an intraosseous "Lister" wire loop[12,13] or a plate may be necessary. Both provide a robust fixation. The Lister loop technique is technically more exacting and is likely to involve more extensive dissection and soft tissue stripping. A plate will require a dorsal approach and acts as a "tension band" type device (▶Fig. 17.2). A dorsal approach will allow better access, which is valuable if the fracture is comminuted. For either technique, the surgeon, therapist, and patient should be prepared for a period of stiffness with extension lag of the PIP joint, which although usually temporary, may be protracted.

Metaphyseal Fractures

Fractures at the base of the proximal phalanx, through metaphyseal bone, usually result from a simple fall and are common, particularly in the middle aged and elderly. They present their own specific problems due to their configuration (see also Chapter 16).

These fractures tend to angulate, with the distal segment being pulled into dorsiflexion. The angulation can be easily corrected, but the pull of the intrinsics will tend to cause reangulation of the fracture and so conservative treatment is generally unsuccessful.

If the fracture is allowed to heal in such a position, then the normal action of the intrinsics will be reversed.

The pull of the lumbrical tendons normally passes palmer to the axis of rotation of the MP joint (▶Fig. 17.12a), and they therefore have a flexor influence on that joint.

If a metaphyseal fracture heals with dorsal angulation, then the line of pull of the intrinsics is shifted dorsal to the axis of rotation of the MP joint and they then have an extensor influence on the MP joint, their action being reversed (▶Fig. 17.12b).

This will result in significant loss of flexion at the MP joint and of power grip, which no amount of therapy will overcome. An osteotomy may then be necessary.

These fractures can be effectively treated with a single intramedullary K-wire inserted between the metacarpal heads and then through the rim of the proximal phalangeal base, avoiding transfixion of the collateral ligaments. It is driven up through the base of the phalanx, either to subchondral bone, or to engage the opposite cortex (▶Fig. 17.12c). This can be done under local anesthetic.

MP joints are immobilized in flexion with a thermoplastic splint to prevent irritation of the skin by the wire. The interphalangeal joints are mobilized under supervision by the hand therapists and the pin site is cleaned regularly. The wire is removed in clinic at 3½ weeks and the hand is then fully mobilized.

Comminuted Fractures

Occasionally, very difficult phalangeal fractures will be encountered. There may be significant comminution and delay in presentation. Although nonoperative means may not achieve a good position, surgical fixation may have the significant potential for making the situation worse, with the combination of an extensive dissection of an already compromised digit and a poorly fixed fracture that cannot be mobilized. It may be preferable to accept the less perfect position and deal with problems which occur as the result of this at a later stage.

An example of this would be a six-week-old fracture with a bony spike blocking flexion of the base of the middle phalanx and thus limiting PIP joint flexion (▶Fig. 17.13). When the fracture has consolidated, flexion can be restored by excising the palmar spike of

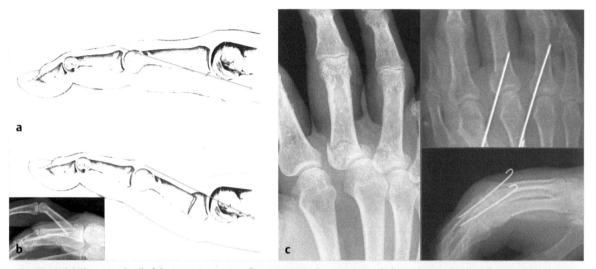

Fig. 17.12 **(a)** The normal pull of the intrinsics exerts a flexor action at the metacarpophalangeal joint. **(b)** After fracture through the metaphyseal region of the proximal phalanx, with dorsal angulation of the distal shaft, this action is reversed. **(c)**. Metaphyseal fractures of the proximal phalanx treated with K-wiring from the base.

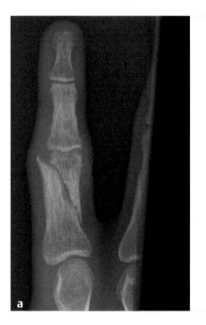

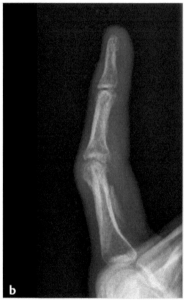

Fig. 17.13 **(a, b)** A 6-week-old fracture of the proximal phalangeal diaphysis with a bony spike blocking flexion of the base of the middle phalanx.

bone through a lateral approach and recreating the retrocondylar fossa using a dental bur; a relatively easy and hazard-free procedure.

Malrotated Fractures

If rotational malunion occurs, then this can be a significant problem. The approach is to obtain consolidated union, remove any preexisting metalwork, and, importantly, to get as full a range of movement as possible of the digit before embarking on corrective surgery to address the malrotation. There is debate about the ideal site for the osteotomy. Metacarpal osteotomy has been advocated as it is thought to be less hazardous, but it makes sense to perform the correction as close to the site of deformity as possible. If the osteotomy is performed

through cancellous bone at the base of the phalanx (▶Fig. 17.14a), then bony healing should not be a problem. The surgery is well away from the PIP joint and the central slip and a good correction can be achieved. The robust fixation means that the digit can be mobilized early and vigorously (▶Fig. 17.14c,d).

17.9.2 Distal Phalangeal Fractures

Tuft and Shaft Fractures

Distal phalangeal fractures often result from crush injuries to the fingertip and are frequently open fractures, associated with a laceration to the nail matrix. These are extremely common injuries in small children as the result of entrapment in the hinge of a door. If an undisplaced

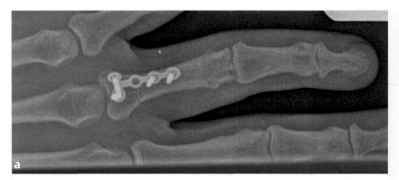

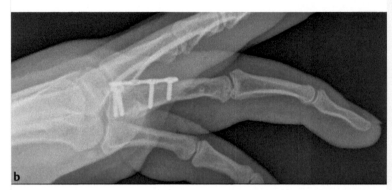

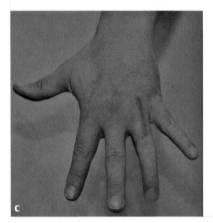

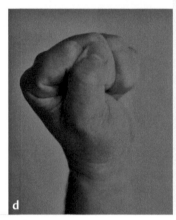

Fig. 17.14 **(a, b)** Osteotomy for malrotation performed through the metaphyseal bone at the base of the phalanx. **(c, d)** The robust fixation allows for vigorous mobilization, seen here at 4 weeks after surgery.

fracture of the phalangeal tuft is associated with a subungual hematoma, but there is no disruption of the nail plate, the hematoma can be evacuated by trephining the nail, but leaving it in place. If the fracture is displaced or if there is dislocation of the proximal nail plate from the eponychium (▶Fig. 17.15), then the nail matrix is likely to require repair. If this is not done, then a poor nail plate may result, with a poor, cosmetic, and functional result, which may be irretrievable. Soft tissue interposition of the matrix into the fracture site may also occur. At best, this may result in a nonunion and a poor nail plate; at worst, infection of the fracture site and loss of the terminal segment of the digit.

To assess these injuries adequately, the nail plate will often have to be removed. Repair of the matrix can then be performed using fine absorbable sutures. Use of microsurgical instruments makes this much easier. If available, the nail can be replaced, as this acts as

an effective splint for the repaired tissues as well as the underlying fracture. It can be held in place with a figure-of-eight suture between the pulp and eponychium (▶Fig. 17.16). In adults, this can be done under a local anesthetic, but small children may necessitate general anesthesia. The majority of these injuries have no tissue loss and if the anatomy is replaced and repaired in an appropriate way, excellent results can be expected.

Severe fingertip injuries may be sustained when the fingers are inadvertently inserted into the path of the rotating blades of a lawnmower. Although mowers are routinely fitted with a handle that interrupts the servomotor to the blades when released, resourceful individuals find ways around this, to "save time" when clearing the grass box. This may result in severely comminuted fractures of the distal phalanges, which are associated with significant soft tissue injuries, often with tissue loss. Such injuries constitute a reconstructive challenge, often requiring

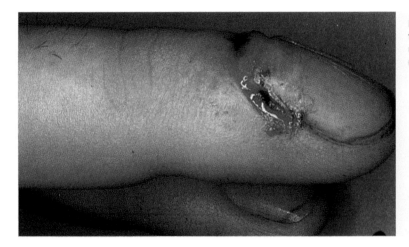

Fig. 17.15 Displacement of the nail plate from the eponychium indicates that the underlying fracture is open and that the nail matrix will require repair.

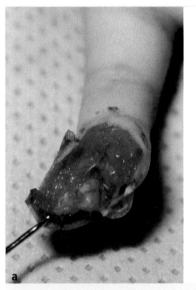
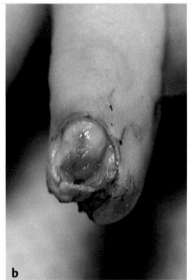
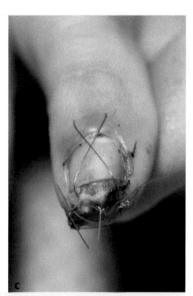

Fig. 17.16 (a–c) Repair of a severe pulp and nail bed injury. The nail plate has been replaced as a dressing/splint and is held in place with a "figure-of-eight" suture.

advancement flaps to preserve the digital tip and nail bed. Ablation of the matrix and terminalization may be necessary.

17.10 Prognosis

Time to union and subsequent consolidation of a hand fracture will depend on numerous factors: age of the patient, concurrent disease and nutrition, type and severity of fracture, and method of treatment. A minimally or undisplaced, uncomplicated phalangeal shaft fracture will usually be stable enough to mobilize without adjuvant support at 3½ weeks. It is not necessary to wait until there is radiological evidence of bony union. K-wires can therefore usually be removed at this stage, although some protection such as buddy taping may still be necessary. The fracture will not be consolidated, however, with complete bony healing, until 5 months.[14] This will have to be taken into account with regard to the level

of protection required for return to work and contact sport.

Malunion, not the least malrotation, and joint stiffness may cause significant functional problems and these complications should be prevented by careful primary treatment. There is no place for the surgical treatment of difficult hand fractures by the occasional hand surgeon. For both operative and nonoperative treatment, the services of a team of skilled surgeons and hand therapists are essential to achieve optimal results.

17.11 Tips and Tricks

- The vast majority of hand fractures are stable and can (and should) be treated nonoperatively.
- Surgical fixation represents a further insult to an already injured hand and this is cumulative.
- There is also no place for the surgical treatment of difficult hand fractures by the occasional hand surgeon.

- Surgeons treating hand fractures should favor the method with which they are most familiar and competent.
- It is important that PA and true lateral views of the relevant digit or joint are obtained.
- Fractured fingers need to be inspected carefully for signs of malrotation.
- The services of a team of skilled hand therapists are essential to achieve good results.

References

[1] Day CS, Stern PJ. Fractures of the metacarpals and phalanges. In: Wolfe SW, Hotchkiss RN, Pederson WC, Kozin SH, eds. Green's Operative Hand Surgery. 6th ed. Philadelphia, PA: Elsevier Churchill Livingstone;2011:239–290

[2] Barton N. Internal fixation of hand fractures. J Hand Surg [Br]. 1989; 14(2):139–142

[3] Horton TC, Hatton M, Davis TRC. A prospective randomized controlled study of fixation of long oblique and spiral shaft fractures of the proximal phalanx: closed reduction and percutaneous Kirschner wiring versus open reduction and lag screw fixation. J Hand Surg [Br]. 2003; 28(1):5–9

[4] Page SM, Stern PJ. Complications and range of motion following plate fixation of metacarpal and phalangeal fractures. J Hand Surg Am. 1998; 23(5):827–832

[5] Hornbach EE, Cohen MS. Closed reduction and percutaneous pinning of fractures of the proximal phalanx. J Hand Surg [Br]. 2001; 26(1):45–49

[6] Belsky MR, Eaton RG, Lane LB. Closed reduction and internal fixation of proximal phalangeal fractures. J Hand Surg Am. 1984; 9(5):725–729

[7] Green DP, Anderson JR. Closed reduction and percutaneous pin fixation of fractured phalanges. J Bone Joint Surg Am. 1973; 55(8):1651–1654

[8] Al-Qattan MM. Displaced unstable transverse fractures of the shaft of the proximal phalanx of the fingers in industrial workers: reduction and K-wire fixation leaving the metacarpophalangeal and proximal interphalangeal joints free. J Hand Surg Eur Vol. 2011; 36(7):577–583

[9] Al-Qattan MM. K-wire fixation for extraarticular transverse/short oblique fractures of the shaft of the middle phalanx associated with extensor tendon injury. J Hand Surg Eur Vol. 2008; 33(5):561–565

[10] Ford DJ, el-Hadidi S, Lunn PG, Burke FD. Fractures of the phalanges: results of internal fixation using 1.5mm and 2mm A. O. screws. J Hand Surg [Br]. 1987; 12(1):28–33

[11] Shewring DJ, Thomas RH. Avulsion fractures from the base of the proximal phalanges of the fingers. J Hand Surg [Br]. 2003; 28(1):10–14

[12] Lister G. Intraosseous wiring of the digital skeleton. J Hand Surg Am. 1978; 3(5):427–435

[13] Al-Qattan MM. Closed reduction and percutaneous K-wires versus open reduction and interosseous loop wires for displaced unstable transverse fractures of the shaft of the proximal phalanx of the fingers in industrial workers. J Hand Surg Eur Vol. 2008; 33(5):552–556

[14] Smith FL, Ryder DL. A study of the healing of one hundred consecutive phalangeal fractures J Bone Joint Surg. 1935; 17A:91–109

18 Intra-articular Fractures of the Proximal Interphalangeal Joint

David J. Shewring

Abstract

Intra-articular fractures of the proximal interphalangeal joints (PIPJs) occur frequently through a variety of mechanisms. The PIPJ is a particularly important joint for the function of the hand and is unforgiving. Condylar fractures are unstable and so are difficult to treat nonoperatively, although success may be more likely in children due to the thicker periosteum. Most will need operative stabilization. This is best achieved with a single lag screw through a lateral approach, after which the finger can be mobilized immediately. These fractures can still be taken down several weeks after injury and although the results are not as good as when treatment is undertaken earlier, this is still better than the prospect of an intercondylar osteotomy. Fractures of the base of the middle phalanx include dorsal and palmar lip fractures, die-punch injuries, and pilon fractures. Dorsal lip fractures can be treated as for a Boutonnière injury if the fragment is very small, or internally fixed if the fragment is larger. Small palmar lip avulsion fractures are very common. They are stable and can be treated with immediate mobilization. Larger fractures may be less stable but can be treated with extension block splintage or a trans-articular wire, depending on patient compliance. A dynamic external fixator can also be used. Die-punch and pilon fractures represent some of the greatest challenges in hand surgery. Selected cases are amenable to internal fixation. A knowledge of the mechanics through which these fractures are created and careful analysis of the fracture pattern will facilitate this. Dynamic external fixation can also be used. Osteochondral hemi-hamate autografting can be used for acute cases and for late reconstruction.

Keywords: fracture, phalanges, internal fixation, nonoperative, condylar, pilon, die-punch, avulsion, hand therapy, lag screws, K-wires, malunion, flexion contracture, comminution

18.1 Trauma Mechanism

Fractures affecting the PIPJ are common.[1] The PIPJ is particularly unforgiving after injury, which is reflective of the complicated bony contours of this joint as well as the complex soft tissue arrangements surrounding it. Stiffness following significant injury, particularly loss of full extension, is common.

The history will give an indication of the configuration of the injury. This will reflect the variety of mechanisms through which injuries to the PIPJ occur. Hyperextension injuries to the joint may damage the palmar plate. A forced flexion injury with simultaneous extension of the joint may disrupt the extensor mechanism, particularly the central slip. Twisting injuries from a dog lead or horse's reigns may damage the collateral ligaments. The patient often gives a history of a dislocation, reduced at the time of injury. This may have been the case, but the same history of "dislocation" is often given when a displaced fracture has been reduced at the time of injury, or immediately after a rupture of the central slip of the extensor when the patient moves the finger from flexion into extension, often with a "clunk."

An axial force through an extended digit, such as when miscatching a ball, or tripping up the stairs is transmitted through the proximal phalangeal head and into the base of the middle phalanx and may result in a condylar or pilon fracture. Various patterns of fracture can be formed. If no central element forms, then a T-shaped fracture pattern may arise resulting in a pilon fracture (►Fig. 18.1a). If a central element is formed, then a die-punch fracture is created (►Fig. 18.1b).

18.2 Classification

- Condylar fractures
- Middle phalangeal base fractures
  - Dorsal lip fractures
  - Palmar lip fractures with or without dislocation
- Pilon fractures
- T-shaped fractures
- Die-punch (i.e., comminuted) fractures

18.3 Clinical Signs and Tests

The finger will be painful and will often have a fusiform swelling and reduced range of movement of the joint. If a displaced fracture is present, there may be deformity.

18.4 Investigatory Examinations

The primary investigation is a plain radiograph with anteroposterior and lateral views of the joint. It is important that specific views of the injured digit are obtained, rather than radiographs of the whole hand which are commonly requested in the emergency department. It is also imperative that a true lateral view of the joint is obtained. If the view is oblique, then a subluxation of the joint may be missed (►Fig. 18.2). If slight incongruency of the joint is present after reduction of a dislocation, this is always significant and may herald soft tissue interposition into the joint requiring exploration. Occasionally, a computed tomography (CT) scan will provide useful information; if the plain radiographs are of good quality, this would be unusual.

175

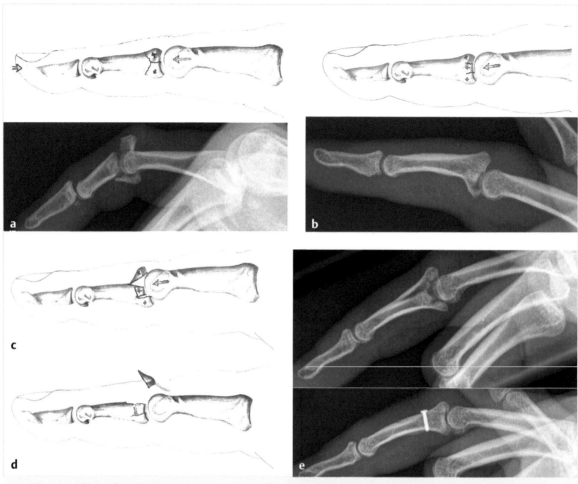

Fig. 18.1 An axial force through the digit may result in a fracture of the base of the middle phalanx. If no central element forms, then a T-shaped pilon fracture is created. **(a)** If a central element forms, then a die-punch fragment is created. **(b)** For this to occur, the two lateral columns have to separate, although one column may remain intact. **(c)** The die-punch fragment can be accessed by an approach via the fractured column, in this case dorsally. **(d)** An example whereby the die-punch has been reduced by hinging the dorsal column fracture on the central slip and then internal fixation using a lag screw **(e)**.

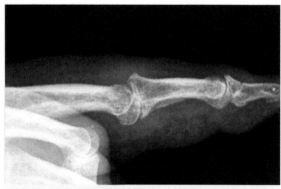

Fig. 18.2 A substandard radiograph of the PIP joint. The obliquity of the view may result in the dislocation being missed.

18.5 Evidence

18.5.1 Condylar Fractures

Condylar fractures of the phalanges are relatively common. They may occur as the result of avulsion through the collateral ligament or as the result of axial loading of the digit resulting in tilting at the joint and a shearing stress. Most of these fractures will require stabilization since the oblique fracture pattern of the typical condylar fracture renders them inherently unstable (▶ Fig. 18.3). Malunion will result in deformity and articular incongruity (▶ Fig. 18.4) with the possibility of late osteoarthrosis. If axial loading is central and high energy, they may be bicondylar (▶ Fig. 18.5). The articular surface may be buckled and the subchondral cancellous bone

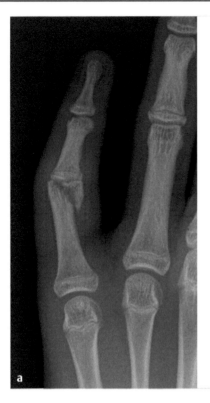
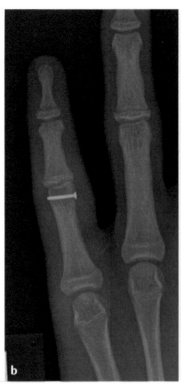

Fig. 18.3 (a, b) A condylar fracture stabilized with a single lag screw. The oblique fracture pattern makes these injuries inherently unstable.

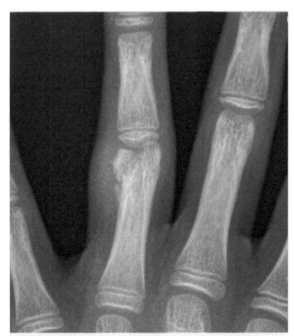

Fig. 18.4 Malunion of a condylar fracture resulting in deformity and articular incongruity.

compressed (▶Fig. 18.6), making accurate reduction difficult. In these cases, it is as well that the surgeon is prepared and the patient warned.

If the fracture presents in an undisplaced position and nonoperative treatment is initially embarked on, close monitoring with weekly radiographs will be required, as these fractures will frequently displace. Undisplaced condylar fractures in children may be more stable, due to the thickness of the periosteum, which may be intact, but vigilance is still necessary.

Displaced condylar fractures will require open reduction and internal fixation. If there is marked displacement (▶Fig. 18.7), then there will be significant soft tissue disruption, with tearing of the periosteum and this will herald instability. It is unlikely that an acceptable result would be obtained by nonoperative means and internal fixation is the method of choice for these fractures.[2]

18.5.2 Middle Phalangeal Base Fractures

Dorsal Lip Fractures

These fractures occur as the result of an avulsion of the insertion of the central slip of the extensor mechanism.

Palmar Lip Fractures

Palmar Lip Fractures without Dislocation

Small avulsion flake fractures of the palmar lip (▶Fig. 18.8) occur as the result of hyperextension injuries,

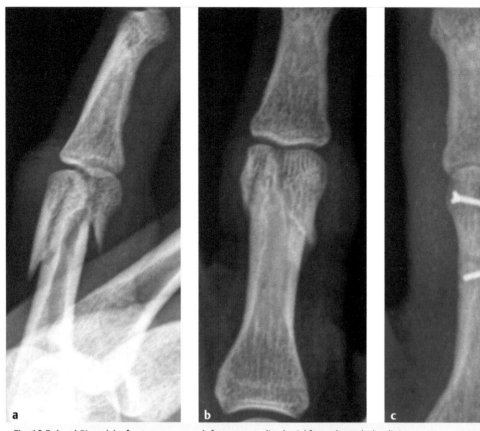

Fig. 18.5 (a–c) Bicondylar fractures may result from a centralized axial force through the digit.

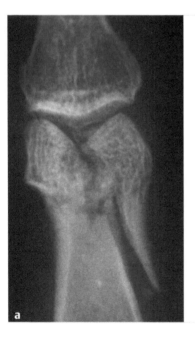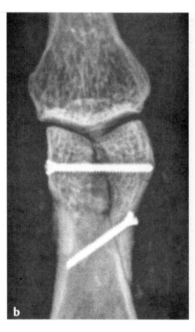

Fig. 18.6 (a, b) High-energy injuries may result in comminution, crushing, and deformation of the fragments precluding an accurate reduction.

often during sports such as netball or basketball and are as the result of traction through the palmar plate. They most commonly affect the long finger and the prognosis is generally good,[3] particularly as they tend to occur in a younger age group. Simple advice and early mobilization is all that is usually needed.[3,4]

Palmar Lip Fractures with Dislocation

Dorsal fracture dislocations of the middle phalangeal base (▶Fig. 18.9) are relatively common and occur as the result of an axial injury to the digit, either during contact sport, miscatching a ball, or when tripping while

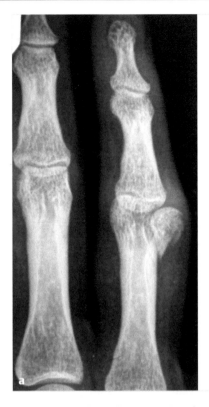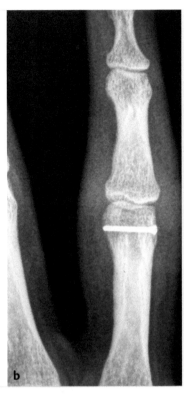

Fig. 18.7 (a, b) Severe displacement of a condylar fracture mandates an open reduction.

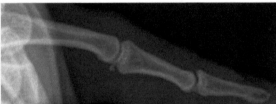

Fig. 18.8 An avulsion fracture of the base of the middle phalanx through the palmar plate (palmar lip fracture).

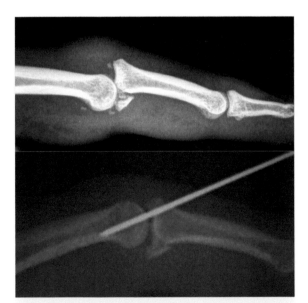

Fig. 18.9 Dorsal fracture dislocation of the PIP joint reduced and stabilized with a transarticular wire.

ascending the stairs. It is imperative that a true lateral of the joint is obtained (▶Fig. 18.2). The stability of the joint is governed by how much of the articular surface of the base of the middle phalanx has been fractured, although this is not exact. If less than 30% of the base has been fractured, then the joint will usually be stable. Between 30 and 40%, the joint may be stable but has a tendency to instability. Over 40% and the joint will be unstable.[5] Assessing the congruency of the joint is important. If, on a true lateral radiograph, the intact dorsal base of the middle phalanx forms a "V" with the dorsal aspect of the proximal phalangeal head, then the joint is incongruent and this should be corrected. If the joint is slightly subluxed, this will herald instability. These injuries are readily reduced closed with traction and flexion of the joint.

Pilon Fractures

These intra-articular fractures can be among the most challenging of all hand fractures. They range from die-punch fractures to the more disastrous T-shaped pilon fractures (▶Fig. 18.10). All represent a considerable management problem. The main problem with these injuries is the resulting articular incongruity and also the intolerance of the PIPJ itself to injury in general. In contrast to condylar fractures, the opportunity for optimum treatment for these fractures is lost fairly quickly. It is important to make clear to the patient at the outset of treatment that these are severe injuries and that poor results are common.

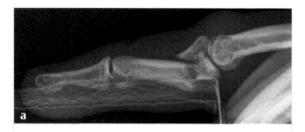

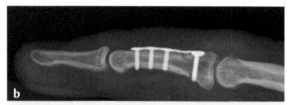

Fig. 18.10 (a, b) A pilon fracture of the middle phalangeal base stabilized with a dorsal plate.

18.6 Author's Favored Treatment Options

It is important to establish exactly how old the injury is. Patients often present late and referral from other centers may result in delays. The window for effective surgical treatment of some (but not all) of these injuries is short. When planning treatment, it is as well to warn the patient that injuries to the PIPJ are poorly tolerated. Even minor injuries may result in discomfort and stiffness that lasts longer than expected and after significant injuries, poor results are common.

18.6.1 Condylar Fractures

A single lag screw is a simple, safe, and effective method to fix these fractures (▶Fig. 18.3, ▶Fig. 18.7). The conical head of the screw will countersink into the softer cancellous bone of the condyle, so that there is minimal interference with the collateral ligament. If the fracture is reduced accurately, the interdigitations of the fracture combined with the compression provided by the screw will provide a strong and stable fixation. This is robust enough to permit vigorous early mobilization, limited only by postoperative discomfort. This, supervised by hand therapy, will help minimize any residual stiffness. Although some authorities have recommended a minimum of two screws, we have found this to be unnecessary. As long as the fracture is relatively fresh, the interdigitations of the fracture surface will provide rotational stability and there is usually no need for a second screw.[2]

Although it is easier to fix these fractures at an earlier stage, a few days delay makes no difference to the outcome and it is preferable to do these semielectively on a designated list. Occasionally, these fractures present after several weeks, either as the result of delayed presentation of the patient or late referral. With a combination of sharp dissection and gentle indirect traction through the collateral ligament, condylar fractures can be taken down and fixed even up to 8 weeks after initial injury. The reduction becomes more difficult and less stable with the passage of time, as the fracture interdigitations become less pronounced and tend to round off. Furthermore, the patients who underwent fixation at a later stage have more residual stiffness of the affected joint, particularly at more than 5 weeks after injury. This, however, may be preferable to the prospect of an intercondylar osteotomy for a healed malunion, which is a significant technical challenge.[6]

Approaches

A *dorsal* approach to the fracture has been advocated, between the central slip and lateral band of the extensor apparatus. In this approach, the screw is inserted dorsal to the collateral ligament.

A *lateral* approach, elevating the periosteum and extensor tendons in one layer (▶Fig. 18.11a–c) gives excellent access to the fragment. Adherence between the periosteum and the extensor mechanism can be a potent cause of postoperative stiffness. With careful technique, using the lateral approach, violation of this plane can be avoided and adherence minimized.

The collateral ligament, attached to the fragment, is identified and carefully preserved. The condyle can be flipped out into the wound and the fracture surfaces cleaned. The fracture is then reduced. The collateral ligament is elevated slightly from the condyle, in order to place the screw beneath it. A little dent can be created in the surface of the condyle to stop the drill bit skiving off, aiding accurate placement of the screw. After 2 to 3 days of rest and elevation, the dressings can be reduced and mobilization commenced under supervision of the hand therapists.

18.6.2 Middle Phalangeal Base Fractures

Dorsal Lip Fractures

If the fragment is small and undisplaced with no subluxation of the joint, they can be treated by immobilization of the PIPJ in extension for 3 to 4 weeks. The adjacent joints can be mobilized during this period.

If the fragment is large enough, then the injury can be treated with internal fixation using a small lag screw (▶Fig. 18.12) through a dorsal approach. The joint can be gently mobilized under supervision after a few days.

Palmar Lip Fractures without Dislocation

The finger can be protected with "neighbor strapping" to the adjacent digit on return to sporting activity.

Palmar Lip Fractures with Dislocation

It should be made abundantly clear to the patient that these are significant injuries and some long-term

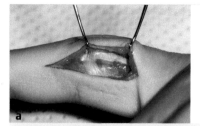
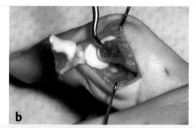
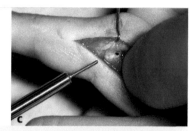

Fig. 18.11 A lateral approach avoids violating the plane between periosteum and extensor mechanism. **(a)** The vertical retinacular fibers, seen here, are incised and later repaired. **(b)** The collateral ligament is carefully preserved. The condyle can be flipped out and the fracture site cleaned. **(c)** The collateral ligament can be elevated slightly from the condyle to allow placement of the screw.

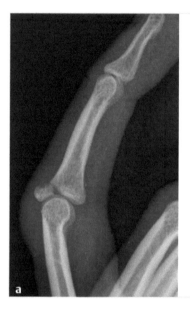
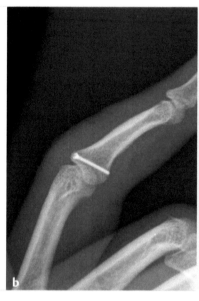

Fig. 18.12 (a, b) An avulsion fracture (dorsal lip fracture) through the central slip of the extensor tendon, fixed with a lag screw.

stiffness of the joint is to be expected, whichever treatment method is used.

Nonoperative Treatment

After reduction, the injury is more stable with the joint in flexion and so if the injury is to be treated nonoperatively, flexion is encouraged and full extension of the joint is prevented through an "extension blocking splint" applied to the dorsal aspect of the digit, continued for 4 to 6 weeks. The joint extension is initially limited by 45 degrees, allowing full flexion for 2 weeks. After this, at weekly intervals, the allowed extension is increased by 10 degrees and the splint can be dispensed with at 4 weeks. The finger can then be mobilized although a fixed flexion deformity of 10 to 20 degrees is usual. Close supervision with serial lateral radiographs, as well as a compliant patient will be required, as redislocation readily occurs.

Operative Treatment

An alternative method of treatment is to insert a percutaneous transarticular K-wire across the PIPJ.[7] A relatively small wire (1 mm) should be used, with the transfixed joint in as much extension as is feasible to minimize

the resulting flexion contracture but enough flexion to maintain reduction (▶ Fig. 18.9). The wire is removed at 4 weeks and the joint mobilized.

18.6.3 Pilon Fractures

These injuries are longitudinally unstable and, as such, are not amenable to K-wiring.

The ideal situation is to restore the anatomy as accurately as possible with correction of the incongruity and a fixation stable enough for immediate mobilization. This, however, may not always be achievable. In such cases, a dynamic external fixator is a useful option.[8,9]

The base of the middle phalanx can be considered in terms of three columns: a central column (the die-punch) and two peripheral columns. For the die-punch fragment to be created, the two peripheral columns have to move apart to allow "access" for the proximal phalangeal head. One of the two peripheral columns may remain intact, but at least one must be fractured to allow the "die-punch" element to occur (▶ Fig. 18.1c).

If surgery is considered for a die-punch injury, the approach can then be made from the side of the broken column giving access to the die-punch fragment. The broken column can be reflected on the central slip or the

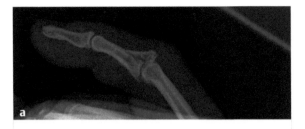

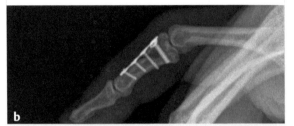

Fig. 18.13 Comminuted pilon fracture of the base of the middle phalanx treated with a plate using a dorsal approach.

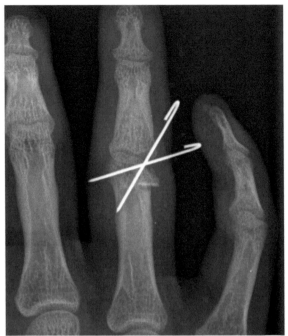

Fig. 18.14 Multiple attempts at K-wiring may result in comminution of the small fragments.

palmar plate, giving access to the die-punch, which can then be reduced (▶Fig. 18.1d).

The die-punch fragment has no soft tissue attachment, and so no amount of indirect traction will realign it. This cannot be achieved by closed means and external fixation traction devices are ineffective in this respect. Bone graft can be added to support the elevated fragment if necessary. The intact column remains as a buttress for fixation. If compression is applied across the two peripheral columns, a sandwich is created with the die-punch fragment as the filler.

If the peripheral column fragment is not comminuted, a lag screw can be used (▶Fig. 18.1e). A crucial factor when planning the approach is to carefully examine the contours of the two peripheral columns and to decide which one is intact. If comminution is present, then a plate may be necessary (▶Fig. 18.13). In such cases, the approach is dictated by surgical ease.

Although patient compliance is important in the rehabilitation after internal fixation, it is not as crucial as when using an external fixation frame, but the surgical techniques are more exacting. There is really no place for the occasional surgeon to treat these injuries and expect a good result.

18.7 Alternative Treatment Options

18.7.1 Condylar Fractures

K-wires tend to interfere with the soft tissues, particularly the collateral ligament and do not really give enough stability for immediate mobilization. Repeated attempts to place the wire may comminute the fragment and when a K-wire is inserted into a small fragment without the benefit of a predrilled hole, there is a risk of explosion of the fragment (▶Fig. 18.14).

Other ways of fixing these fractures are available such as the "bone tie."[10] The device is relatively bulky and may impinge on the collateral ligament. It may be difficult to maintain an accurate reduction during application and application of the device may involve significant soft tissue stripping with a bilateral approach. Use of the "condylar blade plate" has also been advocated for these fractures. This is a bulky device, which is technically difficult to apply and is likely to interfere with the soft tissues such that the movement of the joint will be significantly compromised. Its use is not recommended.

18.7.2 Middle Phalangeal Base Fractures

Extension blocking wires for palmar lip fractures with dislocation have been advocated, on the basis that the joint could be mobilized into flexion. This method is less reliable at maintaining reduction and it is unclear how much the joint could be flexed, as the central slip of the extensor mechanism would be transfixed. However, as the wire is not transarticular, this method avoids further damage to an already injured middle phalangeal base. Dynamic external fixators[8–10] and open reduction and internal fixation[11,12] have also been recommended.

18.7.3 Pilon Fractures

The more comminuted pilon fractures can be treated with indirect traction through an external fixator (▶Fig. 18.15). Various designs are available and these are relatively

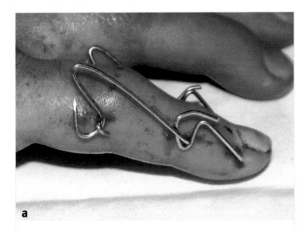

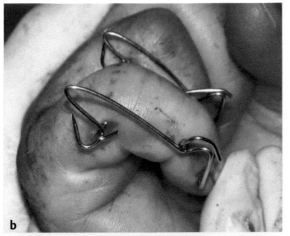

Fig. 18.15 (a, b) Dynamic external fixator used to treat a pilon fracture of the middle phalangeal base as described by Hynes and Giddins.

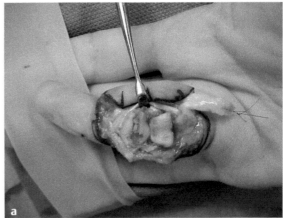

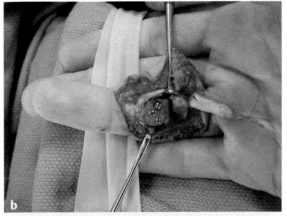

Fig. 18.16 (a, b) Shotgun approach to the PIPJ with insertion of a hemi-hamate osteochondral autograft. (These images are provided courtesy of eatonhand.com.)

straightforward to apply. These devices work through the principle of exerting a longitudinal traction force across the PIPJ. A proximal wire is passed through the axis of rotation of the proximal phalangeal head. The joint can then effectively rotate around that, with the joint and base of middle phalanx distracted. A second wire is passed through the intact distal shaft of the middle phalanx and the wires linked together,[8] by bending them or using a rubber band construct.[9] The joint is actively mobilized under supervision and the wires are removed at the 5-week stage. Thereafter the finger is mobilized freely. These devices allow early mobilization, but a high degree of patient compliance is necessary. As reduction of the joint surface is imperfect, this technique relies on some degree of remodeling, which does occur.

In conclusion, an understanding of the mechanism of injury can aid planning.

The anatomy can be restored or at least improved and the joint mobilized early to facilitate remodeling and avoid stiffness.

Use of osteochondral hemi-hamate autografts have been advocated for both late reconstruction[13] and treatment of acute cases,[14] to replace the damaged base of the middle phalanx. The graft is harvested from the distal dorsal articular ridge of the hamate and secured to the palmar defect of the base of the middle phalanx through a "shotgun" approach (▶Fig. 18.16). A systematic review by Frueh and colleagues[15] examined 13 full text articles with the results of 71 cases. Mean overall PIPJ range of motion was 77 degrees at a mean of 36 months' follow-up with a complication rate of 36%. About 50% of patients showed radiographic signs of osteoarthritis, but few complained of pain or impaired finger motion.

18.8 Prognosis

The PIPJ has a wide range of movement from 0 to 120 degrees of flexion. As it is situated in the center of the finger, these joints put the fingertips through a large arc of movement. For the fingers to function properly, they need this range of movement, as well as stability and comfort. Therefore, injuries to these joints, which frequently result in pain and stiffness, will have a significant impact on the function of the entire upper limb. On the radial side of the hand, the digits interact more with the thumb and so stability is more important. On

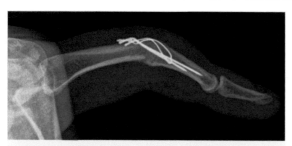

Fig. 18.17 PIPJ fused with a tension band wire technique.

the ulnar side of the hand, the fingers contribute more to the generation of power grip and so range of movement is more important.

The prognosis of small palmar lip flake avulsions is generally good.[3]

Although there may be some remodeling of articular fractures of the base of the middle phalanx and some patients may be naturally more tolerant of the injury with supervised early mobilization, the usual result is a painful joint with stiffness, swelling, and crepitus if articular congruency is not corrected. In any case, patients should be warned that the PIPJ is intolerant of injury and that the digit may be swollen and stiff for several months. There should be a low threshold for referral to hand therapy, to reduce development of a fixed flexion deformity. Patient compliance is important.

Despite all best efforts, the patient may be left with a joint that is stiff and painful and which compromises the function of the rest of the hand. In such cases, it may be necessary to take a pragmatic view. As a stiff but pain free joint is undoubtedly preferable, a fusion may be the best option (▶ Fig. 18.17).

References

[1] Day CS, Stern PJ. Fractures of the metacarpals and phalanges. In: Wolfe SW, Hotchkiss RN, Pederson WC, Kozin SH, eds. Green's Operative Hand Surgery. 6th ed. Philadelphia, PA: Elsevier Churchill Livingstone; 2011;239–290

[2] Shewring DJ, Miller AC, Ghandour A. Condylar fractures of the proximal and middle phalanges. J Hand Surg Eur Vol. 2015; 40(1):51–58

[3] Gaine WJ, Beardsmore J, Fahmy N. Early active mobilisation of volar plate avulsion fractures. Injury. 1998; 29(8):589–591

[4] Phair IC, Quinton DN, Allen MJ. The conservative management of volar avulsion fractures of the PIP joint. J Hand Surg [Br]. 1989; 14(2):168–170

[5] Hastings H, II, Carroll C, IV. Treatment of closed articular fractures of the metacarpophalangeal and proximal interphalangeal joints. Hand Clin. 1988; 4(3):503–527

[6] Teoh LC, Yong FC, Chong KC. Condylar advancement osteotomy for correcting condylar malunion of the finger. J Hand Surg [Br]. 2002; 27(1):31–35

[7] Newington DP, Davis TRC, Barton NJ. The treatment of dorsal fracture-dislocation of the proximal interphalangeal joint by closed reduction and Kirschner wire fixation: a 16-year follow up. J Hand Surg [Br]. 2001; 26(6):537–540

[8] Hynes MC, Giddins GE. Dynamic external fixation for pilon fractures of the proximal interphalangeal joints. J Hand Surg [Br]. 2001; 26(2):122–124

[9] Suzuki Y, Matsunaga T, Sato S, Yokoi T. The pins and rubbers traction system for treatment of comminuted intra-articular fractures and fracture-dislocations in the hand. J Hand Surg [Br]. 1994; 19(1):98–107

[10] Sammut D, Evans D. The bone tie. A new device for interfragmentary fixation. J Hand Surg [Br]. 1999; 24(1):64–69

[11] Aladin A, Davis TRC. Dorsal fracture-dislocation of the proximal interphalangeal joint: a comparative study of percutaneous Kirschner wire fixation versus open reduction and internal fixation. J Hand Surg [Br]. 2005; 30(2):120–128

[12] Deitch MA, Kiefhaber TR, Comisar BR, Stern PJ. Dorsal fracture dislocations of the proximal interphalangeal joint: surgical complications and long-term results. J Hand Surg Am. 1999; 24(5):914–923

[13] Williams RM, Kiefhaber TR, Sommerkamp TG, Stern PJ. Treatment of unstable dorsal proximal interphalangeal fracture/dislocations using a hemi-hamate autograft. J Hand Surg Am. 2003; 28(5):856–865

[14] Burnier M, Awada T, Marin Braun F, Rostoucher P, Ninou M, Erhard L. Treatment of unstable proximal interphalangeal joint fractures with hemi-hamate osteochondral autografts. J Hand Surg Eur Vol. 2017; 42(2):188–193

[15] Frueh FS, Calcagni M, Lindenblatt N. The hemi-hamate autograft arthroplasty in proximal interphalangeal joint reconstruction: a systematic review. J Hand Surg Eur Vol. 2017; 40(1):24–32

19 Avulsion Fractures of the Flexor and Extensor Tendons

Michael Solomons

Abstract

Except for the mallet fractures, avulsion fractures of the tendons are rare injuries. Unlike flexor digitorum profundus (FDP) avulsion injuries where most surgeons agree on the need for intervention, the indications and nature of intervention in mallet fractures can generate lively discussion. Much academic energy has gone into defining the role of fracture size to joint subluxation, but this chapter will remind us that these two issues are related not causal. Even the surgeon who believes strongly that most of these can be treated nonoperatively will eventually encounter a case where the volar subluxation needs to be addressed to correct the normal joint kinematics of rolling and not hingeing.

Keywords: mallet injury, mallet fracture, jersey finger, flexor digitorum profundus avulsion

19.1 Extensor Avulsion Fractures

19.1.1 Mallet Fractures

Trauma Mechanism

The typical mallet injury with a small fragment or no fragment is caused by forced flexion of the fingertip against resisted extension. This can be in domestic accidents or on the sport field.

Axial load in extension causes a larger fragment dorsally and the likelihood of volar subluxation of the joint. This will be described later.

Classification

There is much confusion related to the concept of a fracture of the dorsal aspect of the terminal phalanx. The literature continues to wrestle with the issues of the size of the fragment, the displacement, and whether there is volar subluxation of the joint. Doyle's classification of mallet finger injuries (▶ Table 19.1) separates the 4B from 4C on the size of the fragment as it relates to the articular surface, but does not mention the volar subluxation of the joint.[1]

Recent literature has tried to identify a specific percentage of joint surface involvement that will be a predictable cause of volar subluxation[2,3] and this figure seems to hover around the 43 to 52% mark.

Kim and Kim[3] also suggest that a delay to extension splinting and therefor ongoing unresisted FDP activity is a major cause of volar subluxation.

Table 19.1 Doyle's classification of mallet finger injuries

Type	Description
1	Closed injury with or without small avulsion fracture
2	Open injury (laceration)
3	Open injury (deep abrasion involving skin and tendon substance)
4	Mallet fracture
	A: Distal phalanx physeal injury (pediatric)
	B: Fracture fragment involving 20–50% of articular surface
	C: Fracture fragment involving > 50% of articular surface

An unfortunately forgotten paper going back to 1983 gives us the answer to this issue.[4] A forced flexion against resisted extension force, the classic mallet mechanism, such as catching a ball, will result in a true avulsion fracture that by definition will be small and not result in volar subluxation.

If the force strikes the finger as an axial load in slight extension, the fracture produced is by shear, not avulsion, and will be a large fragment by definition. Langer and Engber called this the hyperextension mallet. This volar shear moment is what causes the volar subluxation. The mechanism of injury dictates the size of the fragment and whether there is volar subluxation or not. These two are associated not causal. The truth is that most patients cannot recall exactly what position the finger was in at the time of force and what direction the force was applied. To reiterate, the size of the fragment is not the cause of whether there is volar subluxation or not (▶ Fig. 19.1 and ▶ Table 19.2).

Indications for surgery have also been much debated over time. Fractures involving more than 30% were considered indications for intervention. Marked displacement of the dorsal fracture, and therefore the potential for delayed or nonunion, is considered by some as an indication for surgery, but this remains a very subjective decision. What is agreed by most surgeons is that this joint does have an incredible ability to remodel over time and that long-term arthrosis is rarely a problem unless there has been volar subluxation. While not universally accepted, many hand surgeons would consider volar subluxation an indication for intervention.

Clinical Signs, Tests, and Investigations

The typical posture of a mallet finger is an extensor lag at the distal interphalangeal joint (DIPJ). It usually takes a few months to develop a fixed flexion deformity.

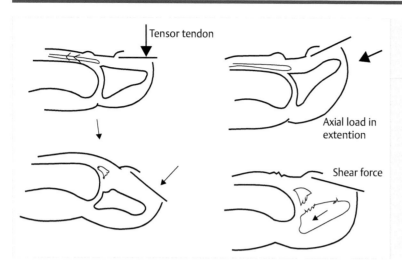

Fig. 19.1 Flexion mallet versus hyperextension mallet.

Table 19.2 Our proposed classification and treatment options

Type	Description	Treatment
1	Closed injury	Extension splint
2	Open injury (laceration)	Repair and K-wire
3	Open injury (deep abrasion involving skin and tendon substance)	Soft tissue reconstruction and K-wire
4	Mallet fracture	
	A: Distal phalanx physeal injury (pediatric)	Might need surgery if nail bed incarcerated In physis (Seymour's lesion)
	B: Typical flexion mallet with fracture and no joint subluxation	Mallet splint unless markedly displaced and risk of nonunion
	C: Extension type mallet with large fracture and joint subluxation	Needs surgery

Any bruising or dorsal tenderness is suspicious of a fracture and an X-ray should be taken. It is important to request a true lateral centered on the DIPJ and the condyles of the head of the middle phalanx should be superimposed and seen as one.

Evidence

A 2004 Cochrane Database review by Handoll and Vaghela[5] suggested there was insufficient evidence to determine when surgery is indicated. Most authors agree that splinting is indicated for all nonbony mallets as well as fracture mallets without joint subluxation. There is no trial looking at only volar subluxed mallet fractures randomized into splintage versus surgery.

Treatment Options

How to correct the volar subluxation and reattach the bone fragment is also a matter of much debate. There have been numerous intervention techniques offered. Widely used is the extension blocking K-wire concept.

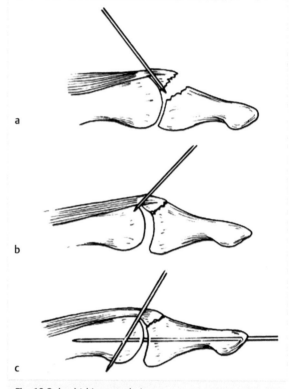

a

b

c

Fig. 19.2 (a-c) Ishiguro technique.

This involves flexing the joint and passing a K-wire proximal to the dorsal fragment to block its dorsal and proximal movement. The joint is then extended to reduce the fracture and a second retrograde wire is passed to immobilize the DIPJ (▶Fig. 19.2).[6]

There are two issues with this technique. The first is that the dorsal wire passes through an exceptionally thin soft tissue envelope and is essentially intra-articular. Any wire sepsis has a real risk of a destructive septic arthritis of the DIPJ. The second issue is that because this is a hyperextension injury, any extension of the joint at the end of the procedure is likely to exacerbate the volar subluxation, which is the indication for surgery in the first place. The surgeon has to take great care not just to extend the terminal phalanx but to translate dorsally as well before placing the retrograde wire.

If the fragment is large enough, then direct open reduction internal fixation (ORIF) can be used, but beware of fracturing the already tiny fragment. Usually, 1- or 1.3-mm screws are used. Tension band suturing or wire has been used by Jupiter and Damron.[7,8]

Pullout sutures tied over a button and gauze on the volar aspect of the pulp, all inside techniques,[9,10] and even external fixation has been attempted. All techniques risk wound breakdown, nail deformity, arthrosis, and stiffness.

Author's Preferred Technique

Indications

- Any fracture with volar joint subluxation.
- Significantly displaced dorsal fragment that does not reduce on extension splinting (irrespective of size). The author acknowledges that deciding on which fracture gaps are at increased risk of delayed or nonunion is a very subjective decision.

Surgical Strategy

- If the size of the fragment is deemed large enough to accept a 1-mm screw without risking fragmentation, then this is preferred (rare).
- For most mallet fractures, we do a transosseous suture technique.

Surgical Technique

The surgical procedure is performed either under general anesthetic or regional anesthetic (Bier's block).

The patient lies supine with the arm placed outstretched on a hand operating table. A bloodless field is created with the use of a tourniquet. A dorsal Y-shaped (Mercedes Benz) incision is utilized (▶Fig. 19.3). Full-thickness skin flaps are elevated with careful protection of the germinal matrix.

At this stage, care needs to be taken to elevate the fracture from distal to proximal. Obviously, it would be a catastrophic surgical error to attempt to create a dissection plane between the fracture and the extensor tendon. The fracture is carefully elevated from the fracture bed and reflected proximally. The fractured terminal phalanx can be seen sitting in a volar subluxed position. Careful curettage of the fracture bed should remove most of the hematoma and/or early soft callus. Usually, the terminal phalanx can be reduced from the volar subluxed position, but in the case of a substantial delay, it might be necessary to perform a limited release of the collateral ligaments.

At this stage, the very small fragment is held with an Adson forceps. A 23-gauge needle is then chosen as a drilling device. The hub needs to be removed and the needle placed into a wire driver. Two holes are drilled parallel starting from the raw fracture surface of the fragment and exiting on the dorsal base at the insertion of the extensor tendon (▶Fig. 19.4).

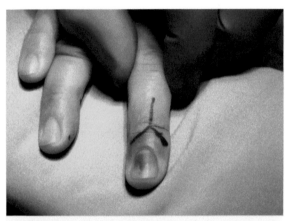

Fig. 19.3 Mercedes Benz incision.

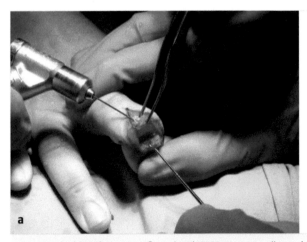

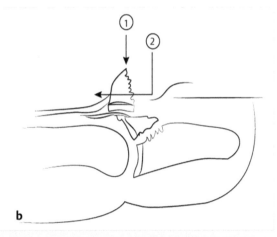

Fig. 19.4 (a, b) '1' fragment reflected and '2' 23-gauge needle used to drill two parallel holes subchondral from fracture surface to exit extensor insertion.

Subsequently, two 23-gauge needles are inserted from dorsal to volar through the small fragment. They are passed through until the very tips of the bevel are visible in the fracture site. It is important now to reduce the dislocation and to reduce the fracture as best as possible. Using a finger drilling technique on the 23-gauge needles, holes are drilled through the volar component of the terminal phalanx. This assures that the sequential holes in the two separate fragments are continuous. If this were not the case, then one would encourage displacement as the suture is tightened (▶Fig. 19.5).

Once the starter holes are made in the fracture bed of the terminal phalanx, then the fracture fragment can be retracted and the rest of the procedure just performed by passing needles freehand through the terminal phalanx using the starter holes as a positioning guide. The two needles are passed through the volar cortex and delivered into a second separate longitudinal volar incision at the base of the terminal pulp. It is important to get the dissection all the way down to the flexor insertion at the level of the periosteum. It is mandatory that no soft tissue gets trapped by the suture material (▶Fig. 19.6).

A prolene suture is pretensioned and the needle is removed. The two ends are passed through the bevels of the 23-gauge needles to exit dorsally through the fracture site. Then the two ends are pulled so that the sutures lie snug against the volar periosteum with no evidence of any soft tissue impingement and most importantly no neurovascular compromise (▶Fig. 19.6). The same is done again for the dorsal fragment using two 23-gauge needles and the 3/0 prolene is passed through from volar (▶Fig. 19.7).

The next stage involves reducing the joint and passing a K-wire in a prograde and then retrograde direction. It is desirable to try and pass the K-wire through the intact volar cartilage. Failing this, one runs the risk of blocking the reduction of the fracture due to the K-wire transgressing the fracture site. If this is not possible, then it is necessary to pass the K-wire through the fracture site and withdraw it so that no part of the K-wire is visible in the fracture site (▶Fig. 19.8).

On reducing the fracture, one can then pass the K-wire carefully across the DIP joint in a retrograde manner. Our choice is for a 0.035-in K-wire (0.9 mm). Using two

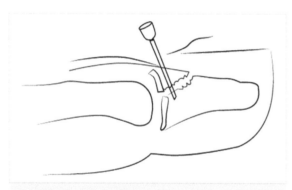

Fig. 19.5 23-gauge needle passed through reduced fragment to mark the opposing fracture surface, so holes are lined up.

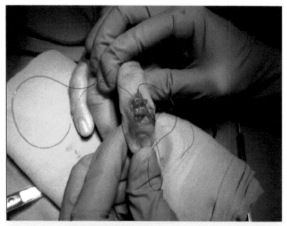

Fig. 19.7 Prolene suture passed through both fragment and phalanx.

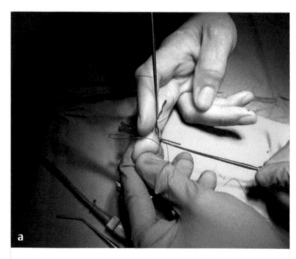

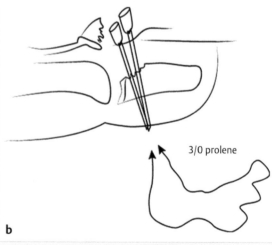

3/0 prolene

Fig. 19.6 (a, b) 23-gauge needles are passed through bone and exit volar. 3/0 prolene passed through two needles and must lie flush on periosteum.

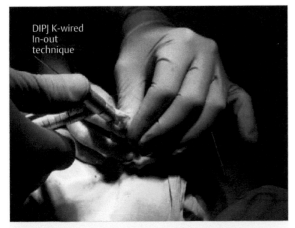

Fig. 19.8 DIPJ K-wired prograde—retrograde technique.

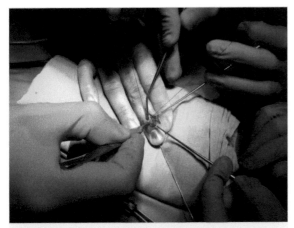

Fig. 19.10 Wire in situ. Fracture reduced and suture tied snugly.

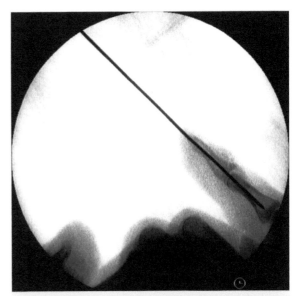

Fig. 19.9 Use fluoroscopy to confirm reduction prior to tying suture.

Prognosis

The prognosis for 4B fractures with no joint subluxation is good. Even moderately displaced fragments will unite and there will be some joint remodeling. Long-term arthrosis is rare.

Surgery to correct the subluxed joint has the inherent risks of all periarticular hand surgery—stiffness. Patients can expect a lag of 5 to 10 degrees with approximately 50 degrees of flexion. Long-term arthrosis is rarely a problem.

19.1.2 Boutonniere Fractures

A boutonniere injury associated with a dorsal fracture is relatively rare. We recognize two patterns:

1. The small avulsion fragment that represents a tiny piece of bone attached to the tendon. Where a purely tendinous injury is often managed nonoperatively with a splint because the tendon is difficult to suture, this injury with a small bone fragment affords the surgeon an opportunity to reattach firmly and start earlier range of motion exercises. We have used suture anchors and tension band nonabsorbable sutures passed through a drill hole in the base of the middle phalanx.
2. The large fracture fragment amenable to direct screw fixation.

19.1.3 Extensor Carpi Radialis Longus Avulsion Fractures

An extremely uncommon injury. Recently reviewed by Najefi et al.[11] They identified 18 cases in the literature.

separate needles through the dorsal fracture fragment, the same two ends of the prolene are now passed from volar to dorsal through the fracture fragment (▶Fig. 19.6). It is now time to reduce the fracture. The fracture is reduced and held. An image intensifier is used to confirm perfect reduction (▶Fig. 19.9).

Once the reduction is confirmed, the K-wire is driven across the fragment and the suture is carefully tied (▶Fig. 19.10).

The technique of this is illustrated (▶Fig. 19.11).

Hemostasis is achieved and the wound is closed with interrupted 5–0 nylon.

Because of the fact that there is a K-wire across the joint, no external splint is necessary. A bulky dressing is applied with removal of sutures at 10 days. The wire is normally kept in position for a minimum of 4 weeks and then the patient is carefully mobilized with a removable thermoplastic mallet splint. Active motion only is allowed for the first 2 weeks after wire removal with gentle passive motion starting at 6 weeks following wire removal.

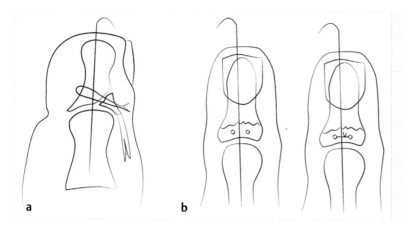

Fig. 19.11 Diagrammatic illustration of the technique.

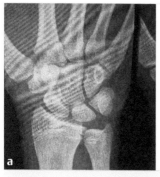
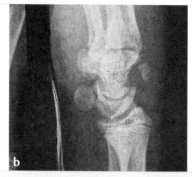
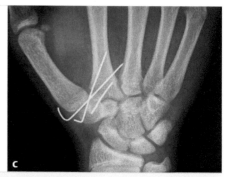

Fig. 19.12 (a–c) Avulsion extensor carpi radialis longus (ECRL) off base index metacarpal fixed with K-wires.

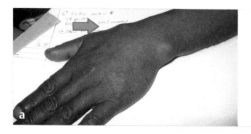
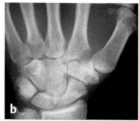

Fig. 19.13 (a, b) Clinical and radiological picture of second case of ECRL avulsion fracture. *Blue arrow* points to swelling and tenderness.

The general feeling is that it is best to perform an anatomical reduction and secure fixation to allow graduated movements ▶Fig. 19.12 and ▶Fig. 19.13.

19.2 Flexor Avulsion Fractures

19.2.1 FDP Avulsion Fractures

Trauma Mechanism

The classic description for this injury is "jersey finger" and it can occur in American Football, Soccer, and especially Rugby. Any activity that causes forced extension of the fully flexed finger can be implicated. Dog leash, surfboard leash, and horse reins are all well described causative mechanisms. The ring finger assumes the longest position in flexion and therefor is subjected to the highest force. We have seen very few cases of "jersey finger" that involve any finger other than the ring finger.

Classification

Leddy and Packer[12] classified avulsions of the FDP into three groups (▶Table 19.3). This is one of the few classifications in orthopaedics where a 1 is more difficult and more urgent than a 3!

The first group is where the tendon avulses of the bone, tears the long and short vincula, and retracts all the way into the palm. The muscle and tendon shorten and the pulley structure narrows rapidly. Time is of the essence and these injuries are best treated within 3 to 7 days.

The second group is where there is a small bony avulsion and the tendon retracts until the bone fragment is

Table 19.3 Classification of FDP avulsion injuries

Leddy and Packer classification of FDP avulsion 1977	
Type 1	Avulsion of tendon, ruptures short and long vincula, retracts into palm
Type 2	Avulses with small bone fragment. Holds up at FDS chiasm
Type 3	Avulses with large bone fragment. Holds up at A5 pulley
Type 4	Tendon pulls off of avulsed bone fragment and is situated more proximal than bone fragment suggests
Type 5	Large avulsion fracture (type 3) but with other fracture of P3
Type 5A	Extra-articular
Type 5B	Intra-articular

Abbreviation: FDS, flexor digitorum profundus.

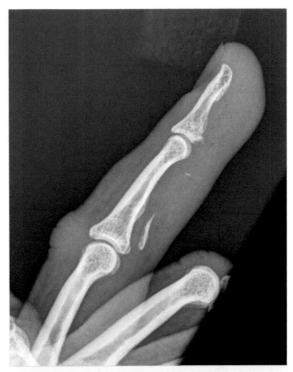

Fig. 19.14 Type 2 avulsion fracture held up at flexor digitorum profundus (FDS) chiasm at level of PIP joint.

held up by the FDS chiasm. The tendon end sits under or immediately proximal to the A3 pulley. Obviously, there is less shortening but passage of the tendon and small fragment under the collapsed A4 pulley can be tricky. A useful trick is to have pulley dilators (or urethral dilators) available (▶Fig. 19.14).

Type 3 involves a large piece of bone that is avulsed off the terminal phalanx with the tendon of FDP. Because of its size, it cannot pass through the A5 pulley and remains at the DIP joint.

Very uncommonly, we see injuries where there is a large bone fragment suggesting a type 3, but at surgery (or preoperative ultrasound) it is revealed that the tendon avulses off this bone fragment and sits in the type 1 or 2 position. These injuries are exceptionally rare and are usually managed as type 3 injuries.

Clinical Picture

The most striking feature is inability to flex the DIP joint of the affected finger. As stated above, it is almost always the ring finger. The final resting position of the avulsed tendon dictates further signs and symptoms. If it retracts into the palm (type 1), then it can often be a very tender lump palpable at or proximal to the A1 pulley. If it holds up at the PIPJ, then flexion of this joint might be painful and limited.

Surgical Options

Type 2 injuries are almost always managed as pure avulsions (type 1). A strong core suture is placed into the tendon end and incorporates the small bone fragment. This is then attached to the terminal phalanx by a pull-through suture over a button or a bone anchor.

Type 3 management depends on the size of the bone fragment.

A single large fragment can be fixed with a single small lag screw (1.5 or 2 mm).

If the fragment is smaller or there is any comminution, a core suture is woven through the tendon and passed through the fragment and through the P3 and tied over a button.

Some authors have used a plate. Access to the bone is limited by the flexor insertion covering most or all of the proximal volar aspect of the P3.

Author's Favored Techniques

We do not believe that the forces applied to the avulsed fracture attached to the FDP can be resisted by a single cortical screw. We prefer a standard pullout suture even for large fragments.

A 3/0 prolene is passed through a drill hole made with a 23-gauge needle from dorsal to volar through the fragment.

A double row of locked whip stitch incorporating three whips on each side is performed. The needle is then passed through the fragment from volar to dorsal exiting in the fracture site. The needle is removed leaving long suture ends. Fresh 23-gauge needles are used as "hand drills" to make two holes through P3 to exit dorsally through the nail bed distal to the lunula. Two fresh 23-gauge needles are railroaded over the first two needles from dorsal to volar. The 2/0 prolene is now threaded through these to exit the nail plate. A standard tie over a button is performed.

Postoperatively, the wrist and hand are protected in a dorsal slab plaster of Paris. The wrist is flexed 30 degrees and the metacarpophalangeal joints (MPJs)

60 degrees. Full active flexion is initiated with no resisted flexion and attention to active extension of all joints. At 4 weeks, the plaster is removed and the button is removed after a further 2 weeks. Because there is bone-to-bone healing we allow full resisted flexion at 8 weeks.

Prognosis

This very much depends on the time to surgery. After 3 days, the retracted FDP is both swollen and shortened which makes surgery difficult. A fixed flexion deformity is a common development and needs to be vigilantly monitored and addressed with splints and physiotherapy. After 10 days, the likelihood of a favorable outcome in a type 1 avulsion is substantially diminished and a detailed discussion regarding pros and cons needs to be engaged with the patient. Despite this we have operated in selected cases up to 6 weeks with satisfactory results. Obviously type 2 and 3 injuries are amenable to much later correction as the distance to restore is much less.

References

[1]   Doyle JR. Extensor tendons—acute injuries. In: Green DP, Hotchkiss RN, Pederson WC, eds. Green's Operative Hand Surgery. 4th ed. Philadelphia, PA: Churchill Livingstone; 1999:1962–1971

[2]   Husain SN, Dietz JF, Kalainov DM, Lautenschlager EP. A biomechanical study of distal interphalangeal joint subluxation after mallet fracture injury. J Hand Surg Am. 2008; 33(1):26–30

[3]   Kim JK, Kim DJ. The risk factors associated with subluxation of the distal interphalangeal joint in mallet fracture. J Hand Surg Eur Vol. 2015; 40(1):63–67

[4]   Lange RH, Engber WD. Hyperextension mallet finger. Orthopedics. 1983; 6(11):1426–1431

[5]   Handoll HH, Vaghela MV. Interventions for treating mallet finger injuries. Cochrane Database Syst Rev. 2004(3):CD004574

[6]   Ishiguro T, Itoh Y, Yabe Y, Hashizume N. Extension block with Kirschner wire for fracture dislocation of the distal interphalangeal joint. Tech Hand Up Extrem Surg. 1997; 1(2):95–102

[7]   Jupiter JB, Sheppard JE. Tension wire fixation of avulsion fractures in the hand. Clin Orthop Relat Res. 1987(214):113–120

[8]   Damron TA, Engber WD. Surgical treatment of mallet finger fractures by tension band technique. Clin Orthop Relat Res. 1994(300):133–140

[9]   Bauze A, Bain GI. Internal suture for mallet finger fracture. J Hand Surg [Br]. 1999; 24(6):688–692

[10] Ulusoy MG, Karalezli N, Koçer U, et al. Pull-in suture technique for the treatment of mallet finger. Plast Reconstr Surg. 2006; 118(3):696–702

[11] Najefi A, Jeyaseelan L, Patel A, Kapoor A, Auplish S. Avulsion fractures at the base of the 2(nd) metacarpal due to the extensor carpi radialis longus tendon: a case report and review of the literature. Arch Trauma Res. 2016; 5(1):e32872

[12] Leddy JP, Packer JW. Avulsion of the profundus tendon insertion in athletes. J Hand Surg Am. 1977; 2(1):66–69

Section III

Metacarpal Fractures

20 Intra-articular Fractures
and Dislocations at the Base
of Metacarpals 2 to 5   *195*

21 Intra-articular Fractures at
the Base of the First Metacarpal   *205*

22 Diaphyseal Fractures of the
Metacarpals   *213*

23 Metacarpal Neck Fractures   *223*

24 Correction of Malunion in
Metacarpal and Phalangeal
Fractures   *233*

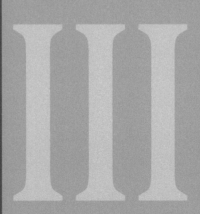

20 Intra-articular Fractures and Dislocations at the Base of Metacarpals 2 to 5

Michael Schädel-Höpfner

Abstract

Fractures and fracture dislocations of the base of the metacarpals 2 to 5 are rare but meaningful injuries. Anatomy and function of the carpometacarpal (CMC) joints differ from the second through the fifth ray, with little mobility radial and rather high mobility ulnar. Clinical signs of fractures and dislocations may be discreet. The extent of these injuries is regularly underestimated in the initial radiographical evaluation of the hand. Computed tomography (CT) is generally recommended to reveal the whole extent of the damage to bones and joints. Accurate restoration of bony and articular anatomy is required to preserve hand function and to prevent painful osteoarthritis. Best results are achieved by early surgical intervention. Depending on the extent of injury, different and individual treatment strategies should be applied. The operative concept includes closed or open reduction techniques and fixation by Kirschner's wires (K-wires), screws, or plates. If treated properly, good results can be expected in the medium and long term.

Keywords: metacarpal, carpometacarpal joint, fracture, fracture dislocation, reduction, fixation

20.1 Introduction

Fractures of the base of the metacarpals 2 to 5 and CMC fracture dislocations are rare injuries that may affect in addition the corresponding carpal bones and the attached ligaments. CMC fracture dislocations have been described first in 1844 by Blandin.[1] Dobyns et al found only three cases of these injuries in 1,621 fractures of the hand, that is, less than 0.2%.[2] CMC fracture dislocations can occur as well in the first ray, where they are rather common and known as Bennett's and Winterstein's fractures.[3]

For the metacarpals 2 to 5, the spectrum of injury extends from simple, nondisplaced fractures of the base of the one or several metacarpals to severe injuries with CMC fracture dislocations and considerable damage to soft tissues. Stable, isolated fractures are uncommon, whereas unstable fracture dislocations prevail. The challenges of these injuries are manifold and concern accurate diagnosis, treatment strategy, precise reduction, and stable fixation.

20.2 Trauma Mechanism and Anatomy

CMC injuries of the fingers 2 to 5 mostly result from high-energy injury trauma such as axial compression due to punch (54%), traffic injury (23%), and fall (14%).[4]

More than half of these injuries affect the fifth ray due to its exposed position at the ulnar side of the hand and because of its higher mobility.[5] However, there exists no single, reproducible pathomechanism that generally causes CMC injuries.[5,6] Even under controlled laboratory conditions, different fracture patterns have been produced in this area of the hand.[4]

In contrast to the thumb CMC joint, the metacarpals 2 to 5 are fixed to the distal carpal row by stable ligamentous attachments. Stability increases from ulnar to radial, supported by the shape of the base of the metacarpals 2 and 3 that fit exactly to the corresponding surfaces of trapezoid and capitate.[7,8] The metacarpal bones are fixed to the distal carpal row by dorsal and palmar carpometacarpal ligaments. In addition, stability is increased by intermetacarpal ligaments. Most rigid is the fixation of the base of the second metacarpal that holds a curved articular surface to the trapezoid and strong ligaments to the surrounding bones. Furthermore, the second metacarpal offers a radial and ulnar condyle to articulate with the trapezium and the base of the third metacarpal, respectively.[9] Stability is also added by the insertion of the tendon of the extensor carpi radialis longus on the base of the second metacarpal. For this reason, the second CMC joint is rarely affected by fractures, and fracture dislocations are seen only on very rare occasions (▶Fig. 20.1).

Nevertheless, CMC joints exhibit some mobility, especially for the fifth and fourth finger. El-Shennawy et al[8] examined the mobility of these joints within a three-dimensional kinematic analysis on cadaver wrist. They found a considerable range of motion for extension–flexion of the little finger with up to 44 degrees, and up to 20 degrees for the ring finger. This rather high mobility allows a powerful grip, particularly when encompassing objects, as well as forming a mold, for example, for scooping water. In contrast, mobility for extension–flexion is small for the second and third CMC joint with only 11 and 20 degrees, respectively.[8] Thus, the second and third CMC joints have a more stabilizing function and are recognized as central column of the hand.[7] As a consequence of these biomechanical considerations, for injuries of the fifth and fourth CMC joint, due to their high mobility and importance for grip function, best possible reconstruction of the articular anatomy should be aimed at.

20.3 Classification

The typical injury pattern of CMC fracture dislocations includes a proximal–dorsal displacement of the shaft of the involved metacarpal, with one or more fragments of the base being retained on the palmar side. In addition, there may be fractures of the distal carpal row,

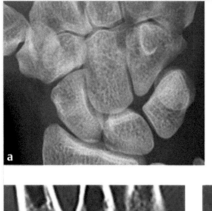
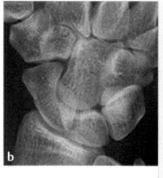
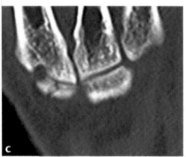
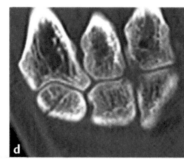

Fig. 20.1 Injury of the carpometacarpal joint of the second ray with nondisplaced fracture of the trapezoid that should be treated nonoperatively. **(a, b)** Plain radiographs being slightly suspicious of a trapezoid fracture. **(c, d)** Computed tomography confirms a fracture of the trapezoid with no displacement.

most frequent shear or avulsion fractures of the dorsal cortex of the hamate. The whole extent of fractures, displacement, and dislocation can be best demonstrated by CT.

There exists no generally accepted and helpful classification of fractures and fracture dislocations of the base of metacarpals 2 to 5. Although metacarpal and carpal fractures are included in the AO/OTA classification for fracture of the hand,[10] this classification is not sufficient to respect all features of the specific injuries. All classifications lack an adequate consideration of possible fracture dislocations and carpal fractures.

Thus, in the clinical routine it has been established to describe the following major issues of the injury:

- Number and position of the involved metacarpals (mostly fifth and fourth)
- Simple fracture, simple dislocation, or fracture dislocation of the metacarpal (mostly fracture dislocation)
- Direction of dislocation of the metacarpal (mostly dorsally)
- Additional fracture of the distal carpal row (mostly hamate)

Only for the fractures of the base of the fifth metacarpal, there exists a specific classification. On the base of an analysis of 64 cases, Kjaer-Petersen et al[11] have described four typical fracture patterns.[11,12] However, this classification is not being routinely used because it has only little impact on decision making.

Nevertheless, injuries of the base of the fifth metacarpal display some particularities. Displacements and dislocations occur as a general rule due to the force exerted by the tendon of the extensor carpi ulnaris muscle. This leads to a typical proximal displacement of the distal shaft fragment, whereas basal fragments may be retained palmar and radial when their ligamentous attachments are intact.[13] In analogy to the fractures of the base of the first metacarpal, these injuries have been named baby Bennet[14] or mirrored Bennett's fracture.[15] Further, radial displacement of the shaft fragment is caused by the hypothenar muscles. The avulsion fracture of the extensor carpi radialis tendon presents another unstable situation.[16,17] Consequently, the majority of injuries of the base of the fifth metacarpal requires reduction and fixation.

20.4 Clinical Signs and Tests

Usually, the patient reports some sort of injury, particularly if there was a severe blunt force impact to the hand resulting from a fall or traffic injury. In case of a punch, the history may be disguised, and some patients appear at the doctor with a significant delay.

Fractures of the base of metacarpals 2 to 5 and even fracture dislocations can be easily overlooked during clinical examination and on plain radiographs.[18–20] Clinical symptoms may be mild in injuries with no displacement, but even with distinct displacement. Local tenderness and swelling at the base of the respective metacarpal or the whole back of the hand are suggesting a fracture. A restricted and painful mobility of the CMC joints and a loss of grip power should be considered as indicative. Displacement may be palpable if swelling is not pronounced. A "dinner-fork deformity" with a step on the dorsal contour of the hand, similar to the "fourchette displacement" in distal radius fractures, can be found especially in serial fracture dislocations.[6] Open injuries are rare but implicate an immediate operative treatment (▶ Fig. 20.2).

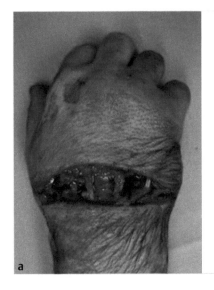
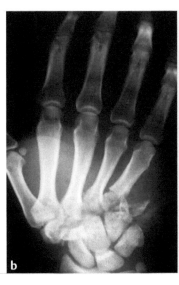

Fig. 20.2 Open carpometacarpal fracture dislocation of the second to fifth ray with considerable soft tissue damage. **(a)** Clinical image. **(b)** Plain radiograph showing severe displacement.

20.5 Investigatory Examinations

Radiographical examination is mandatory if an injury of bones or joints of the hand is suspected by medical history and clinical examination. For CMC injuries, it should be kept in mind that fractures and displacement are not obvious in all cases. On the one hand, this results from the uncommonness of these injuries. On the other hand, they are difficult to detect in oblique and lateral projections because of superpositions of the metacarpal bases. Nonetheless, a complete radiographical examination should be done including three standard projections of wrist and metacarpus:

- Dorsopalmar
- Strict lateral
- Oblique: semisupination for fourth and fifth ray, semipronation for second and third ray

In the radiographical analysis of dorsopalmar views, the parallel course of the corresponding joint planes of the carpal and metacarpal bone should be carefully considered (▶Fig. 20.3). Fisher at al[5] have emphasized the importance of these joint lines that will overlap in case of CMC joint dislocations. However, this requires an ideal dorsopalmar projection which may be difficult to gain due to pain during the diagnostic procedure.

In general, if a CMC injury is suspected, when being already proved by plain radiographs, a CT should be performed.[21] CT will allow both, that is, to exclude or verify an injury and to reveal the extent of bony and articular lesions. This is relevant for carpal fractures as well, which are common in CMC injuries. The CT should be done with thin slices (≤ 1 mm) and multiplanar reconstructions.

20.6 Treatment

All main treatment decisions should be rested on an exact diagnosis which, in turn, should be based on the analysis of the injury pattern by CT. First of all, it should be decided whether the injury can be treated nonoperatively (usually not). If operative treatment is mandatory, the results of CT should be considered for approach and selection of implants too.

20.6.1 Nonoperative Treatment

As injuries to the base of the metacarpals 2 to 5 are usually unstable lesions, conservative treatment represents a rare exception. Stable and nondisplaced base fractures can be treated nonoperatively (▶Fig. 20.4). In these uncommon cases, a plaster cast or splint is applied first, with the fingers not necessarily being included. Not later than swelling and initial pain have been decreased, that is, after 1 week, a mid-hand brace should be applied (▶Fig. 20.5). Because of the fact that the fracture is stable, immobilization should not exceed 3 weeks. Physical therapy is recommended only in rare cases when finger joints have been unnecessarily immobilized and/or the patient has neglected independent exercises. Generally, complete recovery can be expected.

Even more unusual would be the case of closed reduction of a CMC dislocation that results in a stable joint without the necessity of fixation (▶Fig. 20.6). Immobilization should then be prolonged to 4 to 6 weeks with a cast allowing unrestricted movement of all finger joints.

20.6.2 Operative Treatment

For injuries of the CMC joints and the metacarpal bases 2 to 5, operative treatment is essential in most cases. This may be required by displacement, dislocation, instability, soft tissue conditions, or combinations of these.

By a thorough analysis of plain radiographs and CT, the extent of bony and articular injury can be recognized. This determines the operative concept including approach and choice of implants. K-wires are used to fix small fragments and for transfixation of CMC and intermetacarpal joints. Screws are helpful

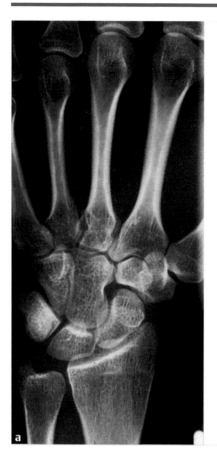
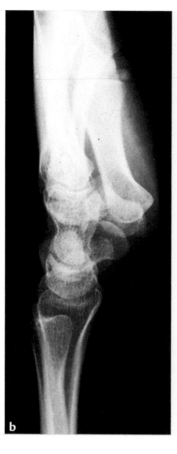

Fig. 20.3 Plain radiographs with correct views showing no fracture or displacement at the base of the metacarpals 2 to 5.
(a) Normal course of the carpal and metacarpal joint lines which should be parallel on the dorsopalmar view.
(b) In the lateral view, the dorsal parts of metacarpals 2 to 5 are in one line with the dorsal cortex of capitate and hamate.

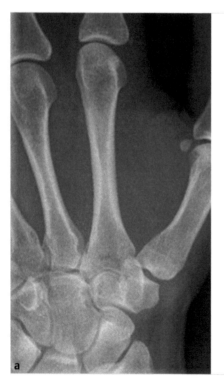
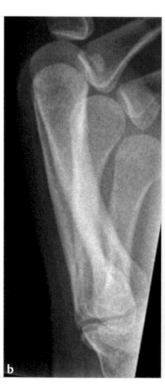

Fig. 20.4 Stable and nondisplaced fracture of the base of metacarpal 2 that needs only short-time immobilization. **(a)** Dorsopalmar view. **(b)** Lateral view.

especially for carpal fractures. Plates are indicated if metacarpal fracture lines extend more distally or—in rare exceptions—for temporary or definite CMC joint fixation.

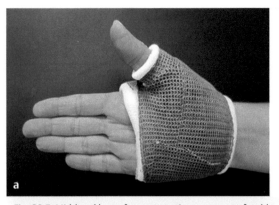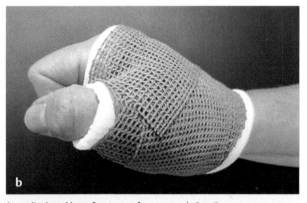

Fig. 20.5 Mid-hand brace for conservative treatment of stable and nondisplaced base fractures of metacarpals 2 to 5.

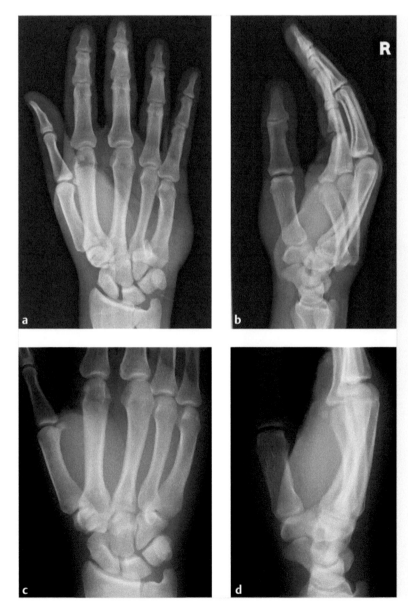

Fig. 20.6 Successful closed reduction and nonoperative treatment of isolated carpometacarpal dislocation of third and fourth ray. (a, b) Complete dislocation following axial trauma as a result of a punch. (c, d) Normal articular anatomy and stable condition after closed reduction.

Isolated CMC dislocations are uncommon. Usually, there are accompanying fractures leading to instability.

Closed reduction can be performed by pulling the respective finger distally and exerting dorsal pressure on the metacarpal base. Although this might be successful, retention by cast or splint will usually fail to be stable. Because of the high tendency for redislocation, primary reduction and secondary fixation are disputed. If the definitive treatment with anatomical fixation cannot be performed initially, painful maneuvers for reduction can be postponed until the requirements for an ideal therapy are met. Prerequisite is the absence of critical soft tissue conditions and compartment syndrome. Operative treatment with closed or open reduction and anatomical fixation should not be delayed for more than 48 hours.

Closed reduction and fixation by K-wires is favored if an anatomical articulation can be achieved, and if no or only small carpal fragments exist. Under such conditions K-wires can be placed percutaneously for CMC joint fixation and/or to fix one metacarpal to another (▶ Fig. 20.7). Preferred diameters for the wires are 1 to 1.4 mm. Attention should be paid to avoid heat damage to the bones that could result in necrosis and fracture, especially in the thin shaft of the metacarpals.

Position and number of wires depend on the injury pattern, the particular intraoperative situation, and the experience of the surgeon.

Open reduction is recommended whenever closed reduction results in an unsatisfactory result and relevant carpal fractures are present. Fragments and joint lines are easily exposed using a dorsal longitudinal or curved approach. Superficial sensory nerves (ramus dorsalis nervi ulnaris) and extensor tendons must be protected. Open reduction might be demanding in unstable conditions. Careful attention should be paid to avoid maltorsion of the metacarpals that inevitably will lead to impaired hand function by scissoring or divergence of the fingers. Greater fragments of the metacarpal base or the adjacent carpal bones (in most cases the hamate) can be fixed by small screws to restore articular anatomy (▶ Fig. 20.8). Plates can be applied for metacarpal fractures that involve more distal parts of the metacarpal (▶ Fig. 20.9). In complete unstable situations, plates may also be used to bridge a comminuted base of a metacarpal that allows no direct fixation.

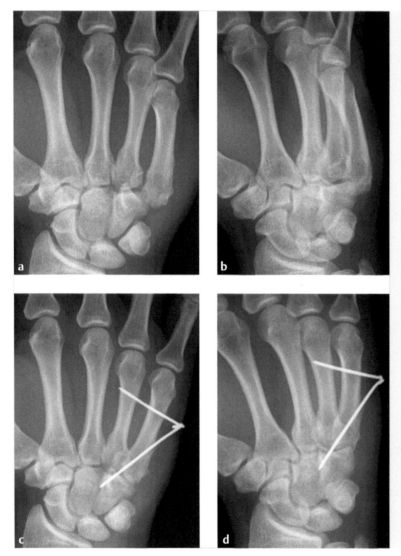

Fig. 20.7 Closed reduction and percutaneous fixation by K-wires for carpometacarpal dislocation of the fifth metacarpal. **(a, b)** Injury. **(c, d)** Postoperatively.

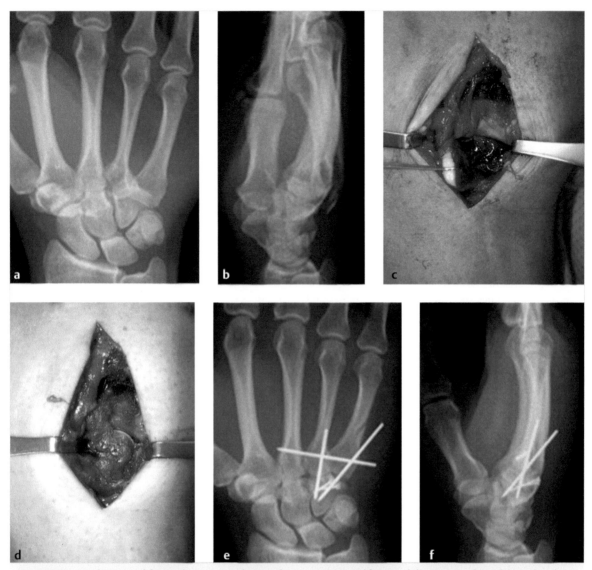

Fig. 20.8 Open reduction and fixation by K-wires and screws for carpometacarpal fracture dislocation 4 and 5 with large dorsal shear fragment of the hamate. **(a, b)** Injury. **(c, d)** Intraoperative situation before and after screw fixation of the hamate. **(e, f)** Postoperatively.

Postoperative treatment implies immobilization of the CMC joints for 6 weeks. All finger joints including CMC joints should be exercised as soon as possible to avoid stiffening. After healing of the bones and ligaments, all bridging implants should be removed to allow mobility, particularly of the important CMC joint of the little finger. K-wires can routinely be removed after 6 weeks. If not disturbing, screws can be left in place.

20.7 Evidence

There is no sufficient evidence to support specific methods in the diagnosis and especially the treatment of injuries of the CMC joints of the second to fifth fingers. Most publications are case reports that present special variants of these injuries concerning kind and number of the involved bones and joints, type of dislocation, and the respective way of treatment. However, even the small case series that exist are characterized by a considerable heterogeneity of the included injuries. As a result of the variety of these injuries, comparative studies are missing and prospective randomized controlled trials would be extremely difficult to conduct. Thus, the given recommendations are based on best clinical practice.

20.8 Author's Favored Treatment Option

As most of the fractures and fracture dislocations of the base of the metacarpals 2 to 5 are closed injuries, treatment can be planned thoroughly. This always requires

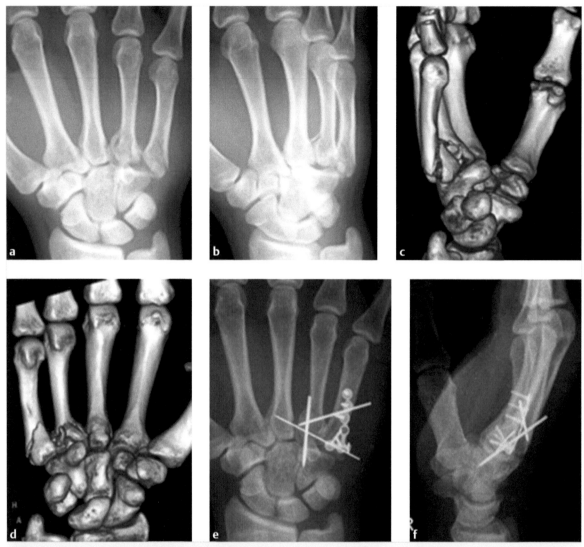

Fig. 20.9 Carpometacarpal fracture dislocation of the fourth and fifth ray treated by open reduction and fixation by K-wires and plate. **(a, b)** Injury. **(c, d)** Computed tomography showing the dorsal displacement of metacarpal 4 and 5 and the comminution of their bases. **(e, f)** Postoperatively.

CT to analyze the injury pattern and to plan the operative procedure. Usually, definitive treatment can be performed within 48 hours after the injury. Until then, to reduce the swelling, the hand is immobilized and kept in a raised position. Only in cases of severe displacement/dislocation, open injuries, or compartment syndrome, immediate treatment is required.

Closed reduction and percutaneous fixation by K-wires is the first choice in cases with CMC displacement and only small fragments. If in these cases, reduction under fluoroscopic control is successful and clinical examination shows no rotational deformity, the concerned metacarpals are fixed by 1.2 to 1.4 mm K-wires. For these transfixations, the wires are placed in a retrograde fashion from the proximal third of the respective metacarpal into the adjacent carpal bone (i.e., mostly the hamate) by crossing the CMC joint. It might be difficult to find the correct flat angle for the wires, but repeated drilling and

heat necrosis must be necessarily avoided. For the fifth metacarpal, one or two wires are used, for all the other metacarpals, one wire is generally enough. Additional stability can be achieved by a wire placed from ulnar to radial through the bases of the metacarpals parallel to the CMC joint line. This wire may also be difficult to place correctly because of the arched alignment of the metacarpal bases.

Open reduction and fixation is indicated if there are major fragments of the carpal or metacarpal bones and if closed reduction turns out unsatisfactory. An open procedure allows direct visualization of the fracture lines and joint lines. However, reduction and fixation of small fragments might be more difficult because they are denuded of their soft tissue attachments that would otherwise allow reduction by ligamentotaxis. First of all, open surgery must guarantee exact reduction, and in addition a stable fixation. Therefore, I prefer screws for fixation of carpal and metacarpal fragments. I use K-wires for additional transfixation, which is necessary in most cases, and to fix very small fragments. Plates are an option for fractures that extend more distally in the metacarpals.

20.9 Tips and Tricks

- Radiographical examination must include X-rays in three plains.
- Computed tomography is mandatory.
- Operative treatment is essential in most cases.
- Closed reduction and fixation by K-wires is preferred for dislocations with small fragments.
- Open reduction and fixation by screws/plates is favored for larger fragments and/orunsatisfactory results after closed reduction.
- Transfixation by K-wires is recommended for all unstable injuries.

20.10 Prognosis

Two major reasons for unsatisfactory results after intra-articular fractures and dislocations at the base of metacarpal 2 to 5 are missed diagnosis and ignored secondary displacement.[22] On the other hand, if the injury pattern has been carefully analyzed, especially by applying CT, and all components of the injury are addressed properly within an individual treatment concept, good and reproducible results can be expected. Surgical experience and individual concepts are the key to meet the target of treatment—pain-free function of the hand and prevention of osteoarthritis. Secondary joint fusions, especially those of the fifth and fourth CMC joints, can generally be avoided.

References

[1] Blandin N. Luxation incomplète du troisième métacarpien en haut. J des Connaissances Méd.- Chir. 1844; 12:177–179

[2] Dobyns JH, Linscheid RL, Cooney WP, III. Fractures and dislocations of the wrist and hand, then and now. J Hand Surg Am. 1983; 8(5 Pt 2):687–690

[3] Windolf J, Rueger JM, Werber KD, Eisenschenk A, Siebert H, Schädel-Höpfner M. Behandlung von Mittelhandfrakturen. Empfehlungen der Sektion Handchirurgie der Deutschen Gesellschaft für Unfallchirurgie. Unfallchirurg. 2009; 112(6):577–588, quiz 589

[4] Yoshida R, Shah MA, Patterson RM, Buford WL, Jr, Knighten J, Viegas SF. Anatomy and pathomechanics of ring and small finger carpometacarpal joint injuries. J Hand Surg Am. 2003; 28(6):1035–1043

[5] Fisher MR, Rogers LF, Hendrix RW. Systematic approach to identifying fourth and fifth carpometacarpal joint dislocations. AJR Am J Roentgenol. 1983; 140(2):319–324

[6] Waugh RL, Yancey AG. Carpometacarpal dislocations with particular reference to simultaneous dislocation of the bases of the fourth and fifth metacarpals. J Bone Joint Surg Am. 1948; 30A(2):397–404

[7] Carroll RE, Carlson E. Diagnosis and treatment of injury to the second and third carpometacarpal joints. J Hand Surg Am. 1989; 14(1):102–107

[8] El-Shennawy M, Nakamura K, Patterson RM, Viegas SF. Three-dimensional kinematic analysis of the second through fifth carpometacarpal joints. J Hand Surg Am. 2001; 26(6):1030–1035

[9] Takami H, Takahashi S, Ando M. Isolated volar displaced fracture of the ulnar condyle at the base of the index metacarpal: a case report. J Hand Surg Am. 1997; 22(6):1064–1066

[10] Petracić B, Siebert H. AO-Klassifikation der Frakturen des Handskeletts. Handchir Mikrochir Plast Chir. 1998; 30(1):40–44

[11] Kjaer-Petersen K, Jurik AG, Petersen LK. Intra-articular fractures at the base of the fifth metacarpal. A clinical and radiographical study of 64 cases. J Hand Surg [Br]. 1992; 17(2):144–147

[12] Lundeen JM, Shin AY. Clinical results of intraarticular fractures of the base of the fifth metacarpal treated by closed reduction and cast immobilization. J Hand Surg [Br]. 2000; 25(3):258–261

[13] Niechajev I. Dislocated intra-articular fracture of the base of the fifth metacarpal: a clinical study of 23 patients. Plast Reconstr Surg. 1985; 75(3):406–410

[14] Bushnell BD, Draeger RW, Crosby CG, Bynum DK. Management of intra-articular metacarpal base fractures of the second through fifth metacarpals. J Hand Surg Am. 2008; 33(4):573–583

[15] Goedkoop AY, van Onselen EB, Karim RB, Hage JJ. The 'mirrored' Bennett fracture of the base of the fifth metacarpal. Arch Orthop Trauma Surg. 2000; 120(10):592–593

[16] DeLee JC. Avulsion fracture of the base of the second metacarpal by the extensor carpi radialis longus. A case report. J Bone Joint Surg Am. 1979; 61(3):445–446

[17] Treble N, Arif S. Avulsion fracture of the index metacarpal. J Hand Surg [Br]. 1987; 12(1):38–39

[18] Crichlow TP, Hoskinson J. Avulsion fracture of the index metacarpal base: three case reports. J Hand Surg [Br]. 1988; 13(2):212–214

[19] Jena D, Giannikas KA, Din R. Avulsion fracture of the extensor carpi radialis longus in a rugby player: a case report. Br J Sports Med. 2001; 35(2):133–135

[20] Thomas WO, Gottliebson WM, D'Amore TF, Harris CN, Parry SW. Isolated palmar displaced fracture of the base of the index metacarpal: a case report. J Hand Surg Am. 1994; 19(3):455–456

[21] Eichhorn-Sens J, Katzer A, Meenen NM, Rueger JM. Karpometakarpale Luxationsverletzungen. Handchir Mikrochir Plast Chir. 2001; 33(3):189

[22] Petrie PW, Lamb DW. Fracture-subluxation of base of fifth metacarpal. Hand. 1974; 6(1):82–86

21 Intra-articular Fractures at the Base of the First Metacarpal

Yuka Igeta, Sybille Facca, Philippe A. Liverneaux

Abstract

Intra-articular fractures at the base of the first metacarpal are frequent and their consequences can affect the opposition of the thumb. They usually occur after trauma in compression along the axis of the thumb in flexion. Restoring the anatomy and biomechanics of the trapeziometacarpal joint is essential when treating these injuries, hence why surgical treatment is usually indicated. We distinguish small-fragment and large-fragment Bennett's fractures, articular three-fragment Rolando's and comminutive fractures of the base of the first metacarpal. All carry the risk of narrowing of the first web. Recent studies have described poor results with conservative treatment. Surgical techniques are varied: percutaneous surgery, open surgery, and arthroscopic surgery. The techniques of osteosynthesis are various: locking plates, and direct or indirect screw fixation or pinning. The prognosis depends on the quality of the restoration of the mobility of the trapeziometacarpal joint.

Keywords: first metacarpal, fracture, Bennett, Rolando

21.1 Trauma Mechanism

Intra-articular fractures at the base of the first metacarpal generally occur after trauma by compression along the axis of the thumb in flexion. It is estimated to occur in 4% of hand fractures.[1]

21.2 Classification

Intra-articular fractures can be divided into Bennett's fractures, Rolando's fractures, and comminuted fractures[2,3] (► Fig. 21.1).

Described by Edward H. Bennett in 1882,[4] fracture dislocation of the base of the thumb metacarpal is remarkable for its frequency and the extensive literature on its description and treatment.[5] They are similar to the pure trapeziometacarpal dislocations. They differ by the presence of a distinct separate fracture of a variable size. The smallest fragment comprises the anteromedial corner of the base of the thumb metacarpal, and stays in place (► Fig. 21.1), attached to the trapezium, because of the attachment of the oblique posteromedial ligament. The largest fragment of the bulk of the thumb metacarpal undergoes a double movement, first a dorsoradial trapeziometacarpal subluxation, under the effect of abductor pollicis longus and then adduction, narrowing the first web, under the effect of the medial thenar muscles. Depending on the size of the small anteromedial fragment, there are two types of Bennett's fractures according to Gedda: the ones with a large-fracture fragment (type I), and the others with a small-fracture fragment (type II).[6]

Rolando's fractures differ from Bennett's fractures by direction, number, and displacement of the fracture lines (► Fig. 21.1). An extra-articular fracture line,

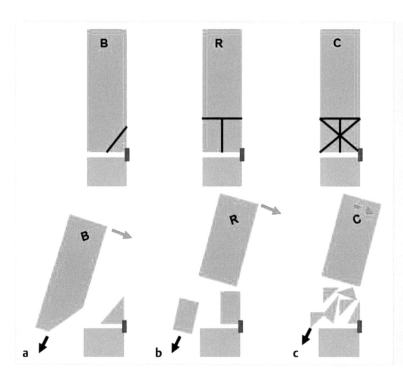

Fig. 21.1 (a–c) Classification of the fractures of the base of the first metacarpal. Above fracture lines: Bennett (B), Rolando (R), comminuted (C). The little red line represents the oblique posteromedial ligament. Below displacements under the effect of the abductor pollicis longus *(black arrow)*, and internal thenar muscles *(green arrow)*.

generally transverse, separates diaphysis and epiphysis. A second vertical intra-articular fracture line splits the epiphysis into two fragments. A central joint depression is often present. Each of these fragments undergoes a specific displacement. The large distal diaphyseal fragment is pulled in adduction, thus closing the first web under the effect of medial thenar muscles. The lateral epiphyseal fragment is drawn upward and outward, under the effect of the long abductor of the thumb. The medial epiphyseal fragment remains in place, attached to the trapezium, because of the oblique posteromedial ligament.

Comminuted fractures can be regarded as Rolando's fractures, of which they represent the worse stage (▶ Fig. 21.1).

21.3 Clinical Signs and Tests

The actions of the adductor pollicis and abductor pollicis longus tend to tilt the distal fragment causing adduction (varus) and shortening (dorsal subdislocation) of the first web.[3,7]

21.4 Investigatory Examinations

The diagnosis is confirmed by standard posteroanterior (PA) or lateral radiographs. Further information can be obtained with computed tomography (CT) scans, 3D reconstructions, or by a series of six radiographic projections[8] (▶ Fig. 21.2).

21.5 Possible Concurrent Lesions of Bone and Soft Tissue

None.

21.6 Evidence

Treatment remains controversial. Although historical reports have noted satisfactory results with conservative treatments until the 1980s,[9] recent studies have described poor results with closed reduction and casting alone for fractures of the base of the thumb metacarpal.[10–12] Most acute injuries of intra-articular fractures at the base of the first metacarpal are unstable and have similar risks of major complications if treated nonoperatively particularly narrowing of the first web.[13,14] Many osteosynthesis techniques have been described, including percutaneous pinning,[15] open screw fixation,[16] locking plates,[17,18] or arthroscopic techniques.[19]

Surgical indications depend on the size of the anteromedial fragment. For most authors, Bennett's fractures with large fragment and Rolando's fractures are usually treated by open reduction and internal fixation.[20] A step-off of greater than 1 mm increases the risk of posttraumatic arthrosis.[10] Leclere et al[16] reported their long-term results of treating 21 Bennett's fractures with large

fragment by open screw osteosyntheses. After 4 years, the overall strength of the hand was 89% of that of the contralateral side, but one patient had a secondary subluxation 9 weeks after surgery. Lutz et al[21] reported results at a mean of 7 years comparing open screw fixation to percutaneous transarticular pinning in 32 Bennett's fractures with large fragments. Although the percutaneous pinning group had a significantly higher incidence of adducted thumb deformities, the type of treatment did not influence the final clinical outcome nor the prevalence of posttraumatic radiological arthrosis. Postoperatively, a removable commissural splint is usually necessary for about 4 weeks, allowing early mobilization if the strength of the fixation permits it. We have developed a technique of percutaneous screw fixation under arthroscopy.[19]

If, the anteromedial fragment is too small to be fixed directly, reduction by external manipulation and percutaneous pinning is recommended by most authors.[20] Authors who recommend percutaneous pinning suggest various sites for the wires either through the trapezometacarpal joint[22,23] or extra-articular through the intermetacarpal spacing.[24] Intra-articular pins can cause further damage to the articular surface. Some authors have reported their results at a mean of 18 months after transarticular percutaneous pinning. Although the average strength was 80% of that of the contralateral side and the opposition of the thumb was complete in all patients, 16 of 21 patients presented at last follow with a thinning of the trapeziometacarpal joint indicating posttraumatic arthrosis.[25] The Iselin technique can also lead to complications. For example, if the distal pin protrudes from the dorsum of the second intermetacarpal space, it can cause irritation of the extensor apparatus of the index finger. In a series of 25 patients operated for fractures of the base of the first metacarpal with a mean follow-up of 24 months, there were three infections along the pin tracks and one notable cosmetic abnormality.[15]

21.7 Authors' Favored Treatment Option

After manual closed reduction (axial traction on the thumb and pressure on the first metacarpal base), two 18-mm K-wires are used to maintain maximal first web opening (▶ Fig. 21.3, ▶ Fig. 21.4). The proximal K-wire is placed so that it runs obliquely distally and medially, crossing the two cortices of the base of the first metacarpal and only the first cortex of the second metacarpal, sparing the second cortex as described by Iselin in his original technique[24] (▶ Fig. 21.2). For Bennett's fractures, the proximal pin is distal to the fracture fragment. The distal K-wire, unlike in the original technique, is made to cross obliquely proximally and medially, first the two cortices of the head of the first metacarpal then the first cortex of the second metacarpal without breaching the second. Good position of the two pins is checked by fluoroscopy. Unlike the original technique, both pins are externalized 1 to 2 cm beyond the skin, bent at 90 degrees, and fixed together externally by a connector (HK2, Arex, Palaiseau, France),

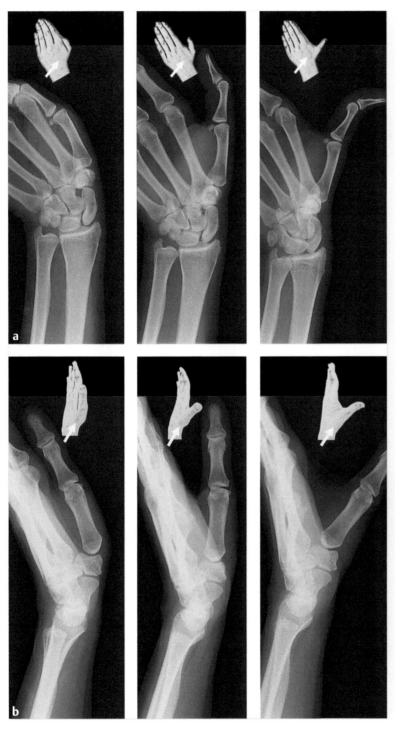

Fig. 21.2 Radiological projections of the trapezometacarpal according to Kapandji. The *arrow* represents the direction of ionizing radiation. **(a)** Three radiographs from the front (A = static, B = dynamic flexion, C = dynamic extension). **(b)** Three radiographs from the profile (D = static, E = dynamic retroposition, F = dynamic anteposition).

resembling an external fixator. The pins are then spread apart or brought closer together according to the required opening of the first web. The connector is then locked by pressure using specialized pliers (Manotte, Arex, Palaiseau, France). After locking, the two pins are cut at the connector level to prevent crowding of the system.

A simple dressing is placed at pin exit and immediate mobilization is encouraged without force. The patient was reviewed in 1 week, then at 2- week intervals with radiographical evaluation for secondary displacement.

K-wires were removed in clinic 6 weeks postoperatively and force grip was allowed at 8 weeks.

21.8 Alternative Treatment Options

All techniques—including arthroscopic and percutaneous approaches—risk neurovascular damage and secondary displacement.[26] The palmar cutaneous branch of

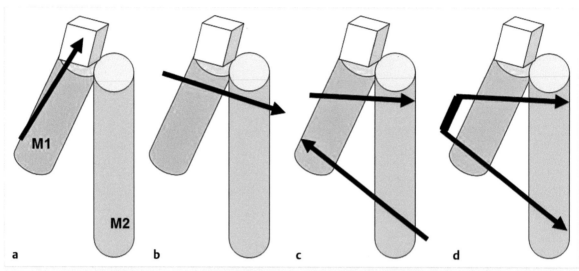

Fig. 21.3 Four examples of indirect pinning in Bennett's fractures. **(a)** Metacarpotrapezial pinning according to Wiggins–Budens, where a single pin goes from the distal portion of the first metacarpal, transfixes the trapezometacarpal joint, and ends in the trapezium. **(b)** Intermetacarpal simple pinning according to Wagner, to avoid crossing the trapeziometacarpal joint **(c)** Intermetacarpal double pinning, according to Iselin, to improve the mounting stability. A first proximal pin goes from the first to the second metacarpal without perforating the medial cortex, and wherein a second pin, oblique to the first, comes from the second to the first metacarpal without perforating the lateral cortex. **(d)** Double intermetacarpal blocked pinning, according to Adi, to improve the mounting stability and to prevent irritation of the extensor apparatus of the index. A first proximal pin goes from the first to second metacarpal without perforating the medial cortex, a second pin, oblique to the first, goes from the first to the second metacarpal without perforating the medial cortex, and where the two are joined by an external connector.

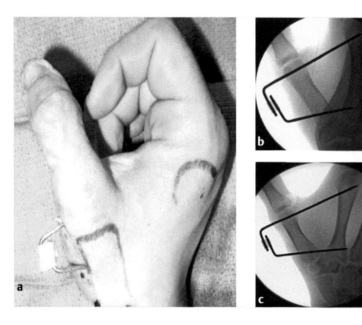

Fig. 21.4 (a–c) Clinical example of indirect pinning in Bennett's fracture, according to Adi, our preferred technique.

the median nerve must be protected during the anterior approach of Gedda–Moberg along the outer edge of the thumb metacarpal. Sensory branches of the radial nerve are vulnerable with more dorsal approaches: the postero-external approach; the dorsal approach of Cantero which goes between the tendons of the long abductor and short extensor of the thumb; and the transverse approach of Neidhart. Radial artery injury is a major risk of plate fixation. Pin tract infection is a common complication of closed reduction with percutaneous K-wire fixation.[27]

Loss of fracture reduction may cause an adduction malunion. This is probably more common with percutaneous K-wiring than plating. Nevertheless, this deformity generally does not influence clinical results.[21]

Concerning Bennett's fracture dislocations, the first stage is the reduction of the thumb metacarpal. The reduction of the "dislocation" is generally obtained by external manipulation, first moving the thumb into abduction to correct the narrowing of the first web and to relax the abductor pollicis longus, and secondly by direct pressure on the base of the thumb metacarpal in the anatomical snuffbox, under fluoroscopic control. The reduction is typically easy. The reduction of this articular fracture should be perfect, in order to avoid articular incongruence. The second stage is to maintain the reduction. More than 20 different methods have been identified[28] from conservative treatment with early mobilization to open reduction and internal fixation, passing through multiple closed pinning techniques. This lack of consensus demonstrates that there is no completely satisfactory therapeutic solution. Although the relationship between articular malunion and poor functional outcome remains debated,[28] the quality of the articular reduction remains the main objective.[29] Conservative treatment even with immobilization with a plaster is usually unable to maintain the reduction of this unstable injury.[11] Continuous traction with external fixation is difficult to achieve, uncomfortable, and requires very close monitoring. Surgical treatment is usually capable of restoring congruence and joint stability.

Osteosynthesis of Bennett's fracture dislocations can be performed by percutaneous fixation,[15,30] open surgery,[16,21] or under arthroscopy.[19,31] There are various reported means of fixation: pins,[15,21,30,31] screws,[16,32–34] or plates.[35]

Percutaneous osteosynthesis techniques mostly use pins for direct[29,31] or indirect fixation,[15,30] with or without crossing the fracture site. Percutaneous pins (▶ Fig. 21.3) are widely used because they reduce the risk of adhesions of the extensor tendons.[22–24] Among these techniques, the Iselin method, which consists of a double intermetacarpal extra-articular pinning,[24] is considered one of the most reliable treatments.[30] However, it can lead to complications such as secondary displacement, pseudarthrosis, malunion, posttraumatic arthrosis, superficial and deep infections, limitation of mobility of the thumb and narrowing of the first web.[25,36,37] The latter is most often linked to the migration of the pins. To avoid this issue, we have proposed interconnecting the pins with a connector.[38] Some use percutaneous screws.[34] All the percutaneous osteosynthesis techniques are at risk of infection or nerve injury[39] and all those which cross the trapeziometacarpal joint are at risk of joint stiffness, septic arthritis, or posttraumatic osteoarthritis.[29,40]

Open reduction and internal fixation (ORIF) offers the advantage of extracting the ligament or capsular interposition, anatomically reduce a joint fracture under direct vision and finally perform the osteosynthesis. The surgical approach can be dorsal (Cantero's approach), or palmar (Gedda–Moberg approach). As for percutaneous techniques, one can use pins but the exposure of the fracture facilitates the establishment of more stable techniques such as plates[2] or screws,[21] which may be simple[16,35] or compression screws[31] and may be cannulated.[33]

Arthroscopic reduction and internal fixation (ARIF) seems the most successful for two reasons.[31] First, it is a minimaly invasive technique, minimising damage to the soft tissues and vascularization of the bone fragments so theoretically limiting the risk of tendon adhesions and bone necrosis. Second, it allows direct visual control

of the joint surface reduction, which is theoretically inversely proportional to the appearance of posttraumatic arthrosis. It also helps to extrate any ligament or capsular interposition. The major drawback of this technique is that a single K-wire is unstable and does not prevent the occurrence of secondary displacement. We replaced the single K-wire by double screw fixation, assuming that two compression screws improve the stability of the assembly and prevent rotation of the small fragment.[19] Some consider the inability to reduce the fracture by closed manipulations is a limitations of the technique of percutaneous screw fixation.[34] We reduce them using intrafocal pins without surgically approaching the fracture,[19] in the manner of tibial plateau fractures fixed by cannulated compression screws.[41,42] In Bennett's fractures type I according to Gedda, as in tibial plateau fractures type I,[43] joint reduction is obtained by traction causing ligamentotaxis and the reduction of the gap between the fragments is obtained by compression of the fracture site by the screws. In Bennett's fractures type II according to Gedda, as in tibial plateau fractures type III, joint reduction is obtained by disimpaction of the fragments using a pin or an intrafocal spatula, followed by the introduction of a screw into a subchondral position which precludes the depression of the fragment in the manner of a forestay. The disadvantages of ARIF in Bennett's fractures are the complications associated with the learning curve, extended setup time and tourniquet time, and financial cost. These drawbacks are heavily outweighed by the benefits of ARIF: reduction facilitated by traction in the axis of the thumb; and a better control of the quality of the articular reduction.

Concerning Rolando's fracture, being a three-fragment articular fracture the reduction must be perfect in order to avoid articular incongruence which is arthrogenic. Reduction by external manipulation is usually impossible, because of the complexity of the fracture. Conservative treatment and direct percutaneous osteosynthesis usually do not give a good result. Some authors have shown that trapezometacarpal joint pinning does not give a satisfactory reduction as well as causing further iatrogenic joint damage.[44]

An articular approach is recommended to restore joint congruity and stability, either by open surgery or for us by arthroscopy.[19] Whatever the technique, the articular approach allows removal of any ligament or capsular interposition, identification of a possible joint depression, and anatomical reduction of the fracture under visual control, and temporary K-wire fixation and then fixation of the epiphysis to the diaphysis either by pins or miniplates. Postoperatively, a removable commissural splint is put in place for 4 weeks. We recommend immediate mobilization if the strength of the construct permits it.[3]

Concerning comminuted fractures, surgical treatment depends on the degree of comminution. There is no consensus, but the major challenge is to maintain the opening of the first web, at best indirectly by intermetacarpal blocked pinning,[38] at worst by external fixation.[16,45,4,6]

Additional trapeziometacarpal arthroscopy may be useful for the resection of a free osteochondral fragment or to perform a ligament repair.

21.9 Prognosis

The prognosis of Bennett's fracture dislocations treated in the acute stage is favorable, especially with small-fragment fractures.[2] A persisting step in the articular surface greater than 1 to 2 mm is a poor prognostic factor in fractures with large fragments.[47]

Restoration of the opposition function of the thumb is essential. In our experience, this often requires surgical rather than conservative treatment. Restoration of the first carpometacarpal joint mobility remains the major objective.

21.10 Tips and Tricks

Intra-articular fractures at the base of the first metacarpal are common; their sequelae may affect the opposition of the thumb.

Their treatment varies according to their proximity to the trapeziometacarpal joint. Unlike lesions of the finger metacarpal, articular fractures of the base of the first metacarpal tolerate moderate malunion in rotation or inclination in the frontal and sagittal planes due to the compensatory effects of the adjacent joints.[48] Narrowing of the first web, due to shortening and varus angulation of the metacarpal of less than 30 degrees, can be compensated by the metacarpophalangeal (MCP) joint hyperextension.[13] However, imperfectly reduced articular fractures are sources of joint stiffness and instability in the short term and arthrosis in the long term.

Conflicts of interest: Philippe Liverneaux has conflicts of interest with Newclip Technics, Argomedical, Biomodex, Zimmer Biomet. None of the other authors has conflicts of interest.

References

[1] Stanton JS, Dias JJ, Burke FD. Fractures of the tubular bones of the hand. J Hand Surg Eur Vol. 2007; 32(6):626–636

[2] Surzur P, Rigault M, Charissoux JL, Mabit C, Arnaud JP. [Recent fractures of the base of the 1st metacarpal bone. A study of a series of 138 cases] Ann Chir Main Memb Super. 1994; 13(2):122–134

[3] Liverneaux PA, Ichihara S, Hendriks S, Facca S, Bodin F. Fractures and dislocation of the base of the thumb metacarpal. J Hand Surg Eur Vol. 2015; 40(1):42–50

[4] Bennett EH. Fractures of metacarpal bone of the thumb. BMJ. 1886; 2(1331):12–13

[5] Hove LM. Fractures of the hand. Distribution and relative incidence. Scand J Plast Reconstr Surg Hand Surg. 1993; 27(4):317–319

[6] Gedda KO, Moberg E. Open reduction and osteosynthesis of the so-called Bennett's fracture in the carpo-metacarpal joint of the thumb. Acta Orthop Scand. 1952; 22(1–4):249–257

[7] Edmunds I, Trevithick B, Honner R. Fusion of the first metacarpophalangeal joint for post-traumatic conditions. Aust N Z J Surg. 1994; 64(11):771–774

[8] Kapandji A, Moatti E, Raab C. [Specific radiography of the trapezo-metacarpal joint and its technique (author's transl)] Ann Chir. 1980; 34(9):719–726

[9] Cannon SR, Dowd GS, Williams DH, Scott JM. A long-term study following Bennett's fracture. J Hand Surg [Br]. 1986; 11(3):426–431

[10] Kjaer-Petersen K, Langhoff O, Andersen K. Bennett's fracture. J Hand Surg [Br]. 1990; 15(1):58–61

[11] Oosterbos CJ, de Boer HH. Nonoperative treatment of Bennett's fracture: a 13-year follow-up. J Orthop Trauma. 1995; 9(1):23–27

[12] Livesley PJ. The conservative management of Bennett's fracture-dislocation: a 26-year follow-up. J Hand Surg [Br]. 1990; 15(3):291–294

[13] Foucher G. [Injuries of the trapezo-metacarpal joint] Ann Chir Main. 1982; 1(2):168–179

[14] Stern PJ. Fractures of the metacarpals and phalanges. In: Hotchkiss G, Pederson, WC, eds. Green's Operative Hand Surgery, 5th ed. Philadelphia, PA: Elsevier Churchill Livingstone; 2005; 277–341

[15] Greeven AP, Alta TD, Scholtens RE, de Heer P, van der Linden FM. Closed reduction intermetacarpal Kirschner wire fixation in the treatment of unstable fractures of the base of the first metacarpal. Injury. 2012; 43(2):246–251

[16] Leclère FM, Jenzer A, Hüsler R, et al. 7-year follow-up after open reduction and internal screw fixation in Bennett fractures. Arch Orthop Trauma Surg. 2012; 132(7):1045–1051

[17] Diaconu M, Facca S, Gouzou S, Liverneaux P. Locking plates for fixation of extra-articular fractures of the first metacarpal base: a series of 15 cases. Chir Main. 2011; 30(1):26–30

[18] Soyer AD. Fractures of the base of the first metacarpal: current treatment options. J Am Acad Orthop Surg. 1999; 7(6):403–412

[19] Zemirline A, Lebailly F, Taleb C, Facca S, Liverneaux P. Arthroscopic assisted percutaneous screw fixation of Bennett's fracture. Hand Surg. 2014; 19(2):281–286

[20] van Niekerk JL, Ouwens R. Fractures of the base of the first metacarpal bone: results of surgical treatment. Injury. 1989; 20(6):359–362

[21] Lutz M, Sailer R, Zimmermann R, Gabl M, Ulmer H, Pechlaner S. Closed reduction transarticular Kirschner wire fixation versus open reduction internal fixation in the treatment of Bennett's fracture dislocation. J Hand Surg [Br]. 2003; 28(2):142–147

[22] Wagner CJ. Method of treatment of Bennett's fracture dislocation. Am J Surg. 1950; 80(2):230–231

[23] Wiggins HE, Bundens WD, Jr, Park BJ. A method of treatment of fracture dislocations of the first metacarpal bone. J Bone Joint Surg Am. 1954; 36-A(4):810–819

[24] Iselin M, Blanguernon S, Benoist D. First metacarpal base fracture. Mem Acad Chir (Paris). 1956; 82:771–774

[25] Brüske J, Bednarski M, Niedźwiedź Z, Zyluk A, Grzeszewski S. The results of operative treatment of fractures of the thumb metacarpal base. Acta Orthop Belg. 2001; 67(4):368–373

[26] Foster RJ, Hastings H, II. Treatment of Bennett, Rolando, and vertical intraarticular trapezial fractures. Clin Orthop Relat Res. 1987(214):121–129

[27] Proubasta IR. Rolando's fracture of the first metacarpal. Treatment by external fixation. J Bone Joint Surg Br. 1992; 74(3):416–417

[28] Cullen JP, Parentis MA, Chinchilli VM, Pellegrini VD, Jr. Simulated Bennett fracture treated with closed reduction and percutaneous pinning. A biomechanical analysis of residual incongruity of the joint. J Bone Joint Surg Am. 1997; 79(3):413–420

[29] Capo JT, Kinchelow T, Orillaza NS, Rossy W. Accuracy of fluoroscopy in closed reduction and percutaneous fixation of simulated Bennett's fracture. J Hand Surg Am. 2009; 34(4):637–641

[30] Bennani A, Zizah S, Benabid M, et al. [The intermetacarpal double pinning in the surgical treatment of Bennett fracture (report of 24 cases)] Chir Main. 2012; 31(3):157–162

[31] Culp RW, Johnson JW. Arthroscopically assisted percutaneous fixation of Bennett fractures. J Hand Surg Am. 2010; 35(1):137–140

[32] Strömberg L. Compression fixation of Bennett's fracture. Acta Orthop Scand. 1977; 48(6):586–591

[33] Tourne Y, Moutet F, Lebrun C, Massart P, Butel J. [The value of compression screws in Bennett fractures. Apropos of a series of 44 case reports] Rev Chir Orthop Repar Appar Mot. 1988; 74(suppl 2):153–155

[34] Meyer C, Hartmann B, Böhringer G, Horas U, Schnettler R. [Minimal invasive cannulated screw osteosynthesis of Bennett's fractures] Zentralbl Chir. 2003; 128(6):529–533

[35] Uludag S, Ataker Y, Seyahi A, Tetik O, Gudemez E. Early rehabilitation after stable osteosynthesis of intra-articular fractures of the metacarpal base of the thumb. J Hand Surg Eur Vol. 2015; 40(4):370–373

[36] Page SM, Stern PJ. Complications and range of motion following plate fixation of metacarpal and phalangeal fractures. J Hand Surg Am. 1998; 23(5):827–832

[37] Huang JI, Fernandez DL. Fractures of the base of the thumb metacarpal. Instr Course Lect. 2010; 59:343–356

[38] Adi M, Miyamoto H, Taleb C, et al. Percutaneous fixation of first metacarpal base fractures using locked K-wires: a series of 14 cases. Tech Hand Up Extrem Surg. 2014; 18(2):77–81

[39] Sidharthan S, Shetty SK, Hanna AW. Median nerve injury following K-wire fixation of Bennett's fracture-lessons learned. Hand (NY). 2010; 5(4):440–443

[40] Sawaizumi T, Nanno M, Nanbu A, Ito H. Percutaneous leverage pinning in the treatment of Bennett's fracture. J Orthop Sci. 2005; 10(1):27–31

[41] Holzach P, Matter P, Minter J. Arthroscopically assisted treatment of lateral tibial plateau fractures in skiers: use of a cannulated reduction system. J Orthop Trauma. 1994; 8(4):273–281

[42] Burdin G. Arthroscopic management of tibial plateau fractures: surgical technique. Orthop Traumatol Surg Res. 2013; 99(suppl 1):S208–S218

[43] Schatzker J, McBroom R, Bruce D. The tibial plateau fracture. The Toronto experience 1968–1975. Clin Orthop Relat Res. 1979(138):94–104

[44] Vichard P, Tropet Y, Nicolet F. Longitudinal pinning of fractures of the base of the first metacarpal. Ann Chir Main. 1982; 1(4):301–306

[45] Keramidas EG, Miller G. The Suzuki frame for complex intraarticular fractures of the thumb. Plast Reconstr Surg. 2005; 116(5):1326–1331

[46] Giesen T, Cardell M, Calcagni M. Modified Suzuki frame for the treatment of a difficult Rolando's fracture. J Hand Surg Eur Vol. 2012; 37(9):905–907

[47] Moutet F, Bellon-Champel P, Guinard D, Gérard P. [Synthetic ligament reconstruction of the thumb metacarpophalangeal joint. 21 cases] Ann Chir Main Memb Super. 1993; 12(3):196–199

[48] Ozer K, Gillani S, Williams A, Peterson SL, Morgan S. Comparison of intramedullary nailing versus plate-screw fixation of extra-articular metacarpal fractures. J Hand Surg Am. 2008; 33(10):1724–1731

22 Diaphyseal Fractures of the Metacarpals

Pierluigi Tos, Simona Odella, Ugo Dacatra, Jane Messina, Emilio Pedrini

Abstract

The purpose of this chapter is to understand when surgical treatment is necessary in case of diaphyseal metacarpal fractures and which is the best surgical technique when it's necessary. Metacarpal fractures account for 30% of hand fractures, and non-thumb fractures for 88%. Most patients (70%) are in the second and third decade of life. The bone shaft is affected in injuries involving axial loading, torsion, direct falls, or crushing. The initial evaluation focuses on fracture stability to establish whether surgical or conservative treatment is required; the deformity that is less tolerated is malrotation because it causes overlapping finger. Our favorite technique is pinning and intramedullary fixation to obtain a good stability avoiding soft tissue damage during dissection. In case of long spiral fracture, an open reduction and an internal fixation by screws can be performed, only in case of transverse or oblique or multiple metacarpal fracture, we perform an open reduction and internal fixation using plate and screws.

Metacarpal fractures have a good prognosis if treated conservatively or surgically, complications are generally related to nonunion, shortening, and malrotation in case of incorrect indication to the nonsurgical treatment; when surgery is performed, stiffness, tendon adhesion, loss of range of motion, and superficial infections are the most common complications.

None of the available operative methods have proved superior in treating of metacarpal fractures. Also in this context, a number of studies have documented the value and reported good long-term outcomes of various operative approaches.

Keywords: metacarpal fractures, metacarpal fractures treatment, plate or screw fixation metacarpals, external fixation metacarpals

22.1 Trauma Mechanism

Metacarpal fractures account for 30% of hand fractures, and non-thumb fractures for 88%. Most patients (70%) are in the second and third decade of life. The bone shaft is affected in injuries involving axial loading, torsion, direct falls, or crushing. Metacarpal fractures can be classified as transverse, oblique, spiral, and comminuted. If the trauma involves directly the hand, the fracture pattern is usually transverse or comminuted, whereas a fall on an outstretched arm mostly causes spiral or oblique fractures. The majority of metacarpal fractures are isolated, simple, and stable and can be managed without surgery. The most common event affecting the thumb shaft is a spiral or oblique fracture.

22.2 Classification

Metacarpal fractures can be classified in relation to anatomical region. This chapter examines diaphyseal fractures. There are four major types of metacarpal fractures: transverse, oblique, spiral, and comminuted. The AO classification identifies six major patterns: head subcapital, head intra-articular, shaft oblique, shaft transverse, shaft multifragmentary, and base fracture.

22.3 Clinical Signs

The initial evaluation focuses on fracture stability to establish whether surgical or conservative treatment is required.

Fractured metacarpal bones, from the first to the fifth, are characterized by edema and deformity; in oblique or spiral fractures, the finger may be malrotated and shortened. In the case of the thumb, the misalignment is more difficult to detect because it cannot be directly compared to a finger.

On examination, the hand presents swelling and dorsal deformity; when the patient is asked to close the hand into a fist, the interosseous muscles depress the metacarpal head and the knuckle disappears (dropped knuckle). A rotation problem is easily identified by having the patient flex the fingers into a fist, which demonstrates overlapping fingers or malrotation of the nail apparatus. If the patient cannot flex the fingers, local anesthesia at the fracture site is required to assess them for malrotation.

Shortening is detected by X-rays, it is more common in the little and index finger and in case of multiple fractures. The intermetacarpal ligaments prevent shortening by more than 3 to 4 mm in the central digits; shortening exceeding 5 mm reduces the efficiency of intrinsic muscle contraction and extension is impaired.[1,2]

22.4 Investigatory Examination

Three radiographical views, posteroanterior, lateral, and oblique, are required for diagnosis. Semipronated oblique views allow evaluating the index and middle finger; semisupinated oblique views enable evaluation of the ring and little finger. Computed tomography (CT) is rarely indicated and should be used in complex fractures.

22.5 Possible Concurrent Lesions of Bone and Soft Tissue

If soft tissue is involved and the fracture is open, the standard approach includes debridement, irrigation, and antibiotic administration. Extensive soft tissue loss requires coverage with local tissue if possible or else with a free flap. A wound requires surgical exploration and examination (and repair as needed) of the extensor tendon. Kirschner (K)-wire or intramedullary fixation is preferred in open fractures where soft tissue healing is a cause for concern. In open fractures with bone loss and inpatients with multiple metacarpal fractures, we feel that locking plate fixation is more effective in preserving length and alignment, if the soft tissue envelope permits. In patients with bone loss and/or soft tissue damage, external fixation is to be preferred. Dorsal fasciotomy is required in crush injury if compartment syndrome is to be prevented. In severely comminuted fractures with bone loss, cement application to replace the bone loss followed by use of secondary bone chips (induced membrane technique) or by a bone graft has been reported.[3]

22.6 Evidence and Anatomical Considerations

A lack of randomized control trials and nonrandomized comparative studies is reported by Daniel Winston in the FESSH Instructional Courses 2017 chapter "Metacarpal shaft fractures" (Evidence-based data in hand surgery and therapy—FESSH IC book).[4] There is robust evidence for conservative treatment options in two randomized control trials. According to the literature, the application of a functional cast to manage transverse metacarpal fractures significantly improves outcomes. Selection of the treatment option for metacarpal fractures requiring fixation is less straightforward, and there is no significant advantage in using any one fixation technique.

The goals of treatment are to restore length, correct rotational deformity, and enable early mobilization to prevent stiffness.

A detailed anatomical knowledge is essential to understand local biomechanics and select the correct treatment; the index and the middle finger are fixed to the carpus whereas the ring and the small finger are mobile, with a flexion arc of 15 to 20 degrees at the carpometacarpal (CMC) joint.

Collateral ligaments of the metacarpophalangeal (MCP) joint are lax in extension and the joints may deviate in ulnar and radial direction; in flexion, the ligaments are taut and only minimal lateral motion is allowed; increased stability provides greater grip strength and key stability. The intermetacarpal ligaments connect the volar plate between adjacent digits and stabilize the fingers, minimizing shortening and rotation in case of fracture; the volar plate stabilizes the MCP joint in extension. The interosseous muscles arise from the metacarpal bones and insert into the extensor

expansion and proximal phalanx; proximally, the extensor carpi radialis longus and brevis insert into the base of the middle and index finger; the extensor carpi ulnaris attaches to the base of the metacarpal of the little finger. The ring finger is the only finger lacking tendon attachment and is therefore less prone to deformation forces in case of fracture. The metacarpal bones form a volar concave arc and provide a stable platform for the phalanges and neurovascular structures. The sagittal bands stabilize the extensor tendon over the head of the metacarpal and unite the collateral ligaments and the intermetacarpal ligaments of the volar plate.

When using a dorsal surgical approach, the complexity of hand anatomy should always be kept in mind to prevent impairment/loss of extension or stiffness.

The *majority of metacarpal fractures can be managed without surgery*. The fibrocartilage volar plate and the intermetacarpal ligaments form a strong structure between the bones and prevent shortening in case of fracture of a single metacarpal bone. Transverse fractures show a dorsal angulation, due to the unequal traction of the interosseous muscles and the force exerted by the extrinsic extensor tendons on the distal fracture segment.

22.7 Indications for Surgery

The tolerance to dorsal angulation is different in each metacarpal bone: 10 degrees are the maximum in the index finger and 20 degrees in the middle finger, owing to the poor mobility of these metacarpal bones; 30 and 40 degrees are the maximum in the ring and little finger, respectively, due to the greater mobility of the CMC joints. Each 2 mm of shortening results in 7 degrees of extensor lag. Since the MCP joints are endowed with 20 degrees of natural hyperextension, a shortening up to 6 mm is tolerable with a neutral MCP joint, although it results in inadequate force to the proximal interphalangeal (PIP) joint, leading to extensor lag (pseudoclawing). In spiral or oblique fractures, the rotational deformity is the most obvious problem and the one tolerated least: 1 mm causes 5 degrees of malrotation, which results in 1.5 finger overlap in flexion.[5] Considering that most metacarpal fractures are stable, they can be managed conservatively with a variety of splint and cast techniques. Often, thumb shaft fractures can also be managed conservatively; malrotation and angular deformity are rarely a functional problem, because the CMC joint that can compensate for the lack of motion. Up to 30 degrees of angulation can be tolerated. Patients with 75% bony apposition of the thumb shaft may have aesthetic concerns. After 30 degrees of dorsal angulation, the MCP joint compensates for the volar plate stretch, allowing hyperextension.

Several approaches are available to restore normal anatomy and provide stability. The use of intramedullary fixation, external fixation, screws, and plates is determined by fracture type, the number of metacarpals involved, and the finger affected.

Different shaft fractures are managed with different hardware.

Transverse fractures are managed with intramedullary techniques, either anterograde or retrograde (nails, K-wires, headless screws), which involve minimal dissection. These techniques can also be used to treat multiple transverse shaft fractures. Sometimes these fractures require open reduction and internal fixation because of the disruption of surrounding support structures, especially the intermetacarpal ligaments.

In patients with shaft fracture of the fourth and fifth metacarpal, and sometimes also those with fracture of other metacarpal shafts, external fixation with K-wires, and/or external fixation (Joshi or others) is an optimal solution that avoids soft tissue damage and bone devascularization and provides stable reduction and early mobilization.

In case of a *long oblique fracture line*, the use of interfragmentary compression screws is indicated if the fracture length is double in length of the bone diameter; this permits the positioning of at least two screws. Soft tissue dissection is required for anatomical reduction, and achieving compression is technically demanding.

In *short, oblique fractures* or transverse fractures, plate and screws can provide stable fixation and ensure early mobilization. A variety of plates and screws are available; titanium and locking plates have been the most widely used in the past few years. This technique also involves soft tissue dissection. Complication rates up to 35% have been reported in some series due to hardware failure, infection, and poor fracture healing.[1]

The use of cast for immobilization does not induce stiffness; immobilization for the first few weeks to support soft tissue and bone healing after K-wire fixation has been reported to induce no functional impairment, whereas reoperation due to functional impairment was required when the cast was not applied following open reduction and internal fixation.

First metacarpal extra-articular fractures can generally be managed conservatively,[6] although screw and plate fixation also enable early mobilization.[7] An angulation exceeding 30 degrees usually requires closed reduction and K-wire fixation, which provides stabilization through the trapezoid bone or external fixation. The main concern with shaft fractures of the first metacarpal is the possible loss of the first web space due to adduction deformity determined by the flexor and extensor pollicis muscles, which reduces both pinch and grip strength of the hand.

22.8 Authors' Favored Treatment Option

We always try to reduce and treat conservatively all metacarpal fractures, also in patients where two metacarpals are involved. In stable fractures, we suggest a cast where the involved ray is splinted, with the MCP flexed to 30 to 40 degrees; in unstable fractures, or when shortening is

possible, continuous finger traction is applied in addition to the cast (see below).

If misalignment or rotational deformity cannot be managed conservatively, we favor intermetacarpal pinning and intramedullary techniques to provide fracture stability without affecting the extensor tendons or other soft tissues during dissection. Long spiral fractures can be managed by open reduction and screw fixation; plate fixation is reserved for transverse/short oblique, comminuted fractures, or for multiple metacarpal fractures where other methods are not practicable. In patients with severe trauma and multiple fractures where fasciotomy is indicated, external or internal fixation is performed depending on tissue condition.

These methods are described briefly below.

22.8.1 Nonsurgical Treatment

Whenever possible, we treat metacarpal shaft fractures conservatively to preserve the complex anatomy of the extensor mechanism and prevent stiffness or lack of extension; immobilization does not induce stiffness.[7]

Closed reduction of metacarpal shaft fractures involves local anesthesia (5 mL of 1% lidocaine injected into the fracture line and in subcutaneous tissue), with longitudinal finger trap traction, dorsal pressure at the fracture site, and correction of rotation with MCP joint flexion as needed. Three-point molding—dorsal pressure at the fracture site and palmar pressure proximally and distally—is important in transverse fractures.

Several different splint and cast techniques have been devised. We describe five major approaches[8]:
1. MCP joint flexion with full range of motion of IP joints (▶ Fig. 22.1a).
2. MCP joint extension with full range of motion of IP joints (▶ Fig. 22.1b).
3. Intrinsic-plus position with MCP joint flexion and IP joint immobilization in extension (▶ Fig. 22.1c).
4. Same as above, but with "continuous traction" applied with a tubular finger bandage and glue (▶ Fig. 22.1e) that is our favored treatment.
5. Functional treatment with a small "metacarpal cast" and syndactyly[9] (▶ Fig. 22.1d).

The immobilization period is 5 weeks.

The potential for secondary displacement is so high that X-rays should be taken weekly for at least 3 weeks. Any displacement should be treated with repeat reduction and cast or surgery if necessary.

Tavassoli et al[8] reported that MCP joint position and the absence/presence of IP joint motion during immobilization had little effect on motion, grip strength, and fracture alignment. These findings contradict the common notion that the MCP joint must be immobilized in flexion to prevent long-term loss of extension. Such outcomes are probably due to the young age of the patient population typically affected by these fractures, where tissues are smooth and less prone to develop stiffness.

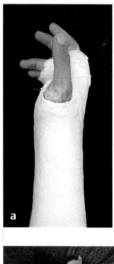
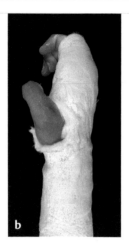
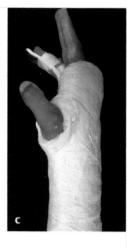
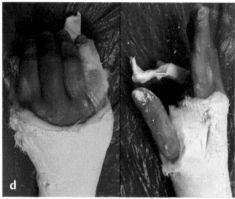
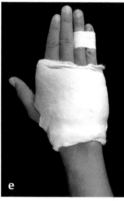

Fig. 22.1 Different cast immobilization. **(a)** The metacarpophalangeal joints are flexed, and a full range of motion of the proximal interphalangeal joints is permitted. **(b)** The metacarpophalangeal joints are in extension, and a full range of motion of the proximal interphalangeal joints is permitted. **(c)** The metacarpophalangeal joints are immobilized in flexion, and the proximal interphalangeal joints are immobilized in extension. **(d)** The metacarpophalangeal joints are immobilized in flexion, and the proximal interphalangeal joints are immobilized in extension, a tubiton bandage is fixed with glue (Mastisol) to the skin and a "continuous traction" is provided by the aluminum digital splint. **(e)** Functional splintage of a metacarpal fracture allowing the wrist and digits a free range of motion.

▶Fig. 22.2 shows results of a fourth metacarpal fracture healed with 3-mm shortening in professional piano player treated conservatively with "continuous traction" method.

22.8.2 Surgical Treatment

Intramedullary Approaches

Pinning

Simple pinning, antegrade or retrograde, with one or two wires/nails applied in a crossed fashion has been used for many years and is still applied to fix metacarpal fractures. The advantages of this technique are that it avoids stripping the periosteum, involving minimal devascularization and enabling very early motion. It is still possible to use pins alone (K-wires/nails 1, 1.2, 1.4 up to 1.6 mm in diameter). Two to four prebent K-wires (1 mm) can be inserted into the medullary canal though multiple drill holes in an anterograde fashion. Filling the medullary canal by the wires confers greater stability. Pins can be bent and cut outside the skin or buried under the skin and are removed later under local anesthesia. Retrograde application is less favored because it may damage the extensor apparatus and may leave some residual MCP joint stiffness. A plaster cast can be used if stability is not achieved.

K-wires or external fixation are optimal solutions for transverse fractures of the first metacarpal.

Intramedullary Locking Nails

A novel device enabling locking of the proximal part of the nail can be applied to enhance stability. It can also be used in unstable fractures and in patients with fracture of several metacarpal bones.[10] The nails are introduced under fluoroscopy, and a cortical window is made at the metacarpal base, 1 cm distal to the CMC joint. The dorsal cortex is perforated to introduce the nail. The nail is then introduced under fluoroscopic guidance into the intramedullary canal, to fix the fracture site. At the end of the procedure, the locking system is introduced perpendicular to the nail at the base of the metacarpal and cut. Its end is covered with a cap that covers the metal part. The nail is then removed under local anesthesia when the fracture has healed (▶Fig. 22.3).

Intramedullary Screws

Retrograde intramedullary fixation can also be performed with headless screws.[11,12]

The proximal phalanx is maximally flexed to expose the head of the metacarpal. A transverse incision (1 cm) is made, and the extensor tendon is also cut along the midline. A 1-mm guidewire is inserted along the longitudinal axis of the metacarpal under fluoroscopic guidance. Screw length is calculated on preoperative images. A screw diameter of 3 mm is suitable in most fractures of the metacarpals except the fifth (▶Fig. 22.4).

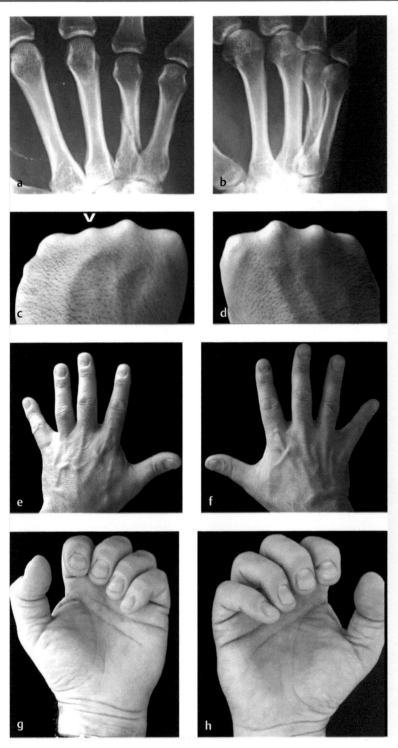

Fig. 22.2 (a-h) Results of a fourth metacarpal spiroid fracture with 3-mm shortening in professional piano player treated conservatively with "continuous traction" method. Dropped knuckle is visible (*white arrow head*) but any functional deficit is not visible.

External Fixation

External fixation is usually advocated to treat comminuted fractures of the metacarpal shaft with or without soft tissue injury. It may also be used in some cases managed conservatively, when it is difficult to achieve optimal digit rotation and length. Pins or K-wires are inserted transversely from the ulnar side of the fifth metacarpal to fix the fifth, fourth, and third metacarpal (▶Fig. 22.5). It can also be used for the second and third metacarpal bone and for the second metacarpal bone, it is inserted from the radial side; it can be useful also in the first metacarpal fracture treatment (▶Fig. 22.6). The technique is easy, safe, and fast to apply, and is therefore frequently used also in patients with simple closed fractures with little comminution.[13]

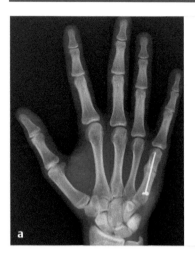
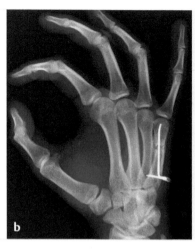

Fig. 22.3 (a, b) Intramedullary proximally blocked nail.

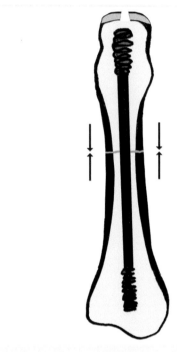

Fig. 22.4 Headless retrograde screw.

External fixation can also be used after open fracture reduction. However, it should not be applied to fix transverse fractures with a gap, where compression at the fracture site is needed; in such cases, plate and screw fixation is more indicated. Stability is commonly achieved leaving the MCP joints and fingers free to move. The most frequent possible complication is pin tract infection; the patient should be warned that getting the fixator wet should be avoided. Removal of K-wire or pins is at 5 weeks as in cases managed conservatively.

Open Reduction and Internal Fixation

Screws

Two or three screws are indicated in long oblique uncomminuted fractures. The fracture is exposed as described below, carefully avoiding soft tissue damage. The reduction is achieved and maintained with a fracture-reduction forceps or K-wires. After a fluoroscopic check, the compression screws are inserted. To withstand axial and torsional loading, the screws should be placed transversely to the fracture plane. Two 2.4-mm screws or three 2-mm screws can be used. There is no tolerance of technical error with this technique. If 2-mm screws are used, the bicortical drill hole will be measured 1.5 mm. The near hole is countersunk to accept the screw head, avoiding protrusion. Screw length is measured with a depth gauge. The near "gliding hole" is over drilled with a 2-mm drill bit. The screw is then inserted engaging the far hole and achieving fracture compression. The technique allows early finger mobilization, but a volar splint is required for 4 weeks, maintaining free MCP joint, until initial healing is detected by an X-ray (▶Fig. 22.7).

Plates

Internal fixation has evolved rapidly in recent years. Plate fixation enables optimal fracture stabilization, early mobilization of the fingers and wrist, and a prompt return to light activities, with reliable results. A number of different internal fixation systems are available and have been used with very low profiles to avoid conflict with the extensor tendons. A dorsal skin incision is performed along the longitudinal axis of the fractured metacarpal. If two metacarpals are involved, the incision is made between them to gain access to both of them and leave one single scar. Care is taken to isolate the superficial sensory nerves and to spare the paratenon of the extensor tendons. Occasionally, the division of the *juncturae tendinum* is required for better fracture identification and management. Fixation should precede repair of *junctura*. The dorsal interosseous muscles are gently dissected from the periosteum, which is respected as much as possible. The fracture fragments are isolated and freed from hematoma, adhesions, and the initial fibrous callus. Fragment reduction is performed by longitudinal traction maneuvers. Provisional

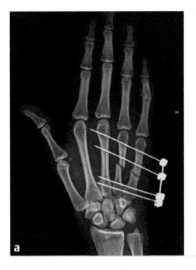
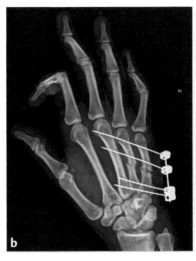

Fig. 22.5 (a, b) External fixation in transverse fashion for IV and V metacarpal fractures.

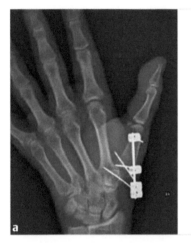
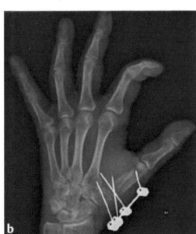

Fig. 22.6 (a, b) External fixation for first metacarpal fracture.

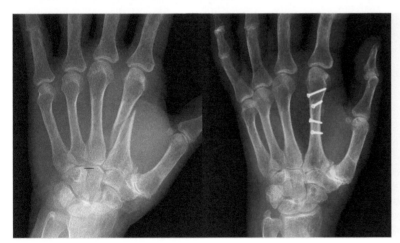

Fig. 22.7 Screw fixation.

stabilization with K-wires or fracture reduction forceps can be done. After a fluoroscopic check, the plate is positioned with the K-wires or the reduction forceps. Modern internal fixation systems allow pin fixation through the plate, thus facilitating subsequent screw fixation to the plate. Screws are inserted according to the AO technique[14] (▶ Fig. 22.8). In patients with a transverse fracture line, compression can be obtained with the oval plate hole, whereas if the fracture is comminuted, the plate is placed in neutralization mode (without compression, which would displace the fracture). In case of an oblique/spiral fracture line, fixation can be with interfragmentary screws and a plate in neutralization mode. The plate can be secured with locking or nonlocking, usually bicortical screws; unicortical screws must be locking screws, to avoid implant failure.[15]

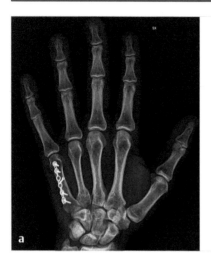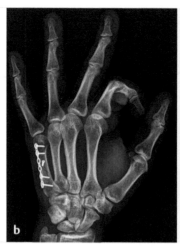

Fig. 22.8 (a, b) Plate and screw fixation.

The plate sometimes needs to be removed afterward, whereas the screws do not require removal.

22.9 Alternative Treatment Options

A fixation technique that is often employed in patients with partial or complete amputation and in those with a long oblique/spiral fracture is cerclage wiring. The method is practical, achieves stable fixation, and in patients with transverse fractures permits gentle mobilization after a neat lesion. Spiral fractures can also be treated with or without unicortical interosseous wiring.[16]

Absorbable plates are popular tools used in craniofacial surgery. Preliminary studies of animal and cadaveric models for application to hand surgery have yielded encouraging results. The plates are thicker than the usual metal plates, to provide extra strength. Absorbable intramedullary rods ensure stable fixation of metacarpal shaft fractures, avoid tendon irritation, and reduce the scope for additional surgery to remove the implant.[17]

22.10 Prognosis

These fractures commonly have a good prognosis whether they are treated conservatively or surgically. Complications are rare in patients with isolated fractures treated conservatively. Malunion (abnormal rotation, shortening, flexion) is the most frequent complication and is often related to an incorrect follow-up (weekly X-rays) or incorrect indication (instability, malrotation, shortening).

When surgery is required, internal or external stabilization avoids dissection and respects the biology of bone healing, reducing the complications related to the hardware and the surgical procedure. If a plate is required, the most common complications are tendon adhesion (extensor tenosynovitis) and limited MCP joint flexion/extension, which are usually solved by hardware removal and tenolysis or arthrolysis. Stiffness is due to anterograde stabilization with K-wires, to limit MCP joint function (the joint should consistently be flexed). Other complications related to K-wires include superficial wound infections, which are managed with oral antibiotics.

Several studies support the value of the different methods and report satisfactory long-term outcomes. Early active range of motion after operative fixation is recommended by most authors; however, conservative treatment and 5-week immobilization do not induce MCP joint stiffness.

Since high-level comparative studies are not available, fracture management is largely based on surgeon training and experience.[18,19]

According to several recent reviews of evidence-based treatment,[4,20,21] none of the available operative methods have proved superior in treating of metacarpal fractures. Also in this context, a number of studies have documented the value and reported good long-term outcomes of various operative approaches.

22.11 Tips and Tricks

Nonsurgical treatment
- Local anesthesia for reduction and to test length and rotation.
- Transverse fractures need traction for reduction and a three-point molding cast.
- *Continuous traction* prevents shortening.
- Weekly X-rays for 3 weeks are recommended for not perfectly stable fractures.

External fixator or pinning
- Avoids extensor apparatus, permits movement.

Intramedullary stabilization
- Retrograde or internal fixation is preferable.
- The medullary canal should be filled with thick wires/nails for stability.
- Fractures fixed with anterograde K-wires require MCP joint flexion.

Screws
• No less than two screws.
• Sliding hole in the first cortex.

Plates
• Avoids soft tissue damage.
• Low profile, good stability for early active motion.

References

[1] Diaz-Garcia R, Waljee JF. Current management of metacarpal fractures. Hand Clin. 2013; 29(4):507–518

[2] Loryn PW, Hanel DP. Metacarpal fractures J Am Soc Surg Hand. 2002; 4(2):168–180

[3] Moris V, Guillier D, Rizzi P, et al. Complex reconstruction of the dorsal hand using the induced membrane technique associated with bone substitute: a case report. JPRAS Open. 2015; 6:31–39

[4] Giddins G, Leblebicioğlu G. Evidence based data in hand surgery and therapy. In: Winston D, ed. Metacarpal Shaft Fractures. Budapest: FESSH; 2017

[5] Ben-Amotz O, Sammer DM. Practical management of metacarpal fractures. Plast Reconstr Surg. 2015; 136(3):370e–379e

[6] Kahler DM. Fractures and dislocations of the base of the thumb. J South Orthop Assoc. 1995; 4(1):69–76

[7] Haughton D, Jordan D, Malahias M, Hindocha S, Khan W. Principles of hand fracture management. Open Orthop J. 2012; 6:43–53

[8] Tavassoli J, Ruland RT, Hogan CJ, Cannon DL. Three cast techniques for the treatment of extra-articular metacarpal fractures. Comparison of short-term outcomes and final fracture alignments. J Bone Joint Surg Am. 2005; 87(10):2196–2201

[9] Konradsen L, Nielsen PT, Albrecht-Beste E. Functional treatment of metacarpal fractures 100 randomized cases with or without fixation. Acta Orthop Scand. 1990; 61(6):531–534

[10] Orbay JL, Touhami A. The treatment of unstable metacarpal and phalangeal shaft fractures with flexible nonlocking and locking intramedullary nails. Hand Clin. 2006; 22(3):279–286

[11] Ruchelsman DE, Puri S, Feinberg-Zadek N, Leibman MI, Belsky MR. Clinical outcomes of limited-open retrograde intramedullary headless screw fixation of metacarpal fractures. J Hand Surg Am. 2014; 39(12):2390–2395

[12] del Piñal F, Moraleda E, Rúas JS, de Piero GH, Cerezal L. Minimally invasive fixation of fractures of the phalanges and metacarpals with intramedullary cannulated headless compression screws. J Hand Surg Am. 2015; 40(4):692–700

[13] Pennig D, Gausepohl T, Mader K, Wulke A. The use of minimally invasive fixation in fractures of the hand—the minifixator concept. Injury. 2000; 31(suppl 1):102–112

[14] Jupiter J, Ring DC. Manual of Fracture Management—Hand. New York, NY:Thieme; 2016:67–97

[15] Ochman S, Doht S, Paletta J, Langer M, Raschke MJ, Meffert RH. Comparison between locking and non-locking plates for fixation of metacarpal fractures in an animal model. J Hand Surg Am. 2010; 35(4):597–603

[16] Al-Qattan MM, Al-Lazzam A. Long oblique/spiral mid-shaft metacarpal fractures of the fingers: treatment with cerclage wire fixation and immediate post-operative finger mobilisation in a wrist splint. J Hand Surg Eur Vol. 2007; 32(6):637–640

[17] Dumont C, Fuchs M, Burchhardt H, Appelt D, Bohr S, Stürmer KM. Clinical results of absorbable plates for displaced metacarpal fractures. J Hand Surg Am. 2007; 32(4):491–496

[18] Kollitz KM, Hammert WC, Vedder NB, Huang JI. Metacarpal fractures: treatment and complications. Hand (NY). 2014; 9(1):16–23

[19] Bannasch H, Heermann AK, Iblher N, Momeni A, Schulte-Mönting J, Stark GB. Ten years stable internal fixation of metacarpal and phalangeal hand fractures-risk factor and outcome analysis show no increase of complications in the treatment of open compared with closed fractures. J Trauma. 2010; 68(3):624–628

[20] Bloom JM, Hammert WC. Evidence-based medicine: metacarpal fractures. Plast Reconstr Surg. 2014; 133(5):1252–1260

[21] Wong VW, Higgins JP. Evidence-based medicine: management of metacarpal Fractures. Plast Reconstr Surg. 2017; 140(1):140e–151e

23 Metacarpal Neck Fractures

Hebe Désirée Kvernmo

Abstract

Fractures of the metacarpal neck are common injuries. The small finger metacarpals are most frequently involved, and account for around one-fourth to one-third of all metacarpal fractures. Controversy exists regarding choice of treatment, but majority of metacarpal neck fractures respond well to conservative management. The degree of acceptable deformity depends on which metacarpal is involved. The literature suggests that fractures of small finger metacarpal neck of less than 50 to 70 degrees of volar angulation may be best treated conservatively with early mobilization, although there is weakness in existing literature due to heterogeneity of the data. Using functional treatment, no reduction should be performed, as the mobilization depends on the stability of an impacted fracture. The initial treatment may, however, be in a cast for a few days until pain settles, and then followed by mobilization with a buddy strap to the ring finger. Fractures with angulation of more than 50 to 70 degrees are few. Operative treatment should be considered for fractures with rotational malalignment or pseudo-clawing of the small finger. Antegrade intramedullary (bouquet) pinning is a good method of choice, and allows for immediate mobilization. Less angulation is accepted for the other metacarpal necks, with as less as 15 to 20 degrees for the second and third metacarpal to as much as 30 to 40 degrees for the forth metacarpal.

Keywords: metacarpal neck fracture, boxer's fracture, definition of metacarpal neck, measurement of angulation and shortening, conservative treatment, operative treatment, evidence

23.1 Trauma Mechanism

Metacarpal neck fractures are common fractures. They occur most often in the small finger metacarpals, which account for 10% of all hand fractures[1] and 25 to 36% of all metacarpal fractures.[1–3] The index, middle, and ring finger metacarpal neck fractures account for 6, 2, and 5% of all metacarpal fractures, respectively.[1] The small finger metacarpal neck fracture is often called boxer's fracture. This is a misnomer, as fractures in professional boxers usually occur in the metacarpal neck of the index finger. The small finger metacarpal neck fractures occur most often in brawlers, who impulsively hit a solid object or another person with a closed fist. The direct blow is causing a longitudinal compression through the knuckle, resulting in a fracture of the neck of the metacarpal (▶Fig. 23.1). The injury usually occurs in association with alcohol intake and violence.[3]

23.2 Classification

There are no definitions commonly used in the literature for metacarpal neck fractures. Although angulation of the metacarpal neck results in less shortening than angulation of the metacarpal shaft (▶Fig. 23.2), the transition zone between the shaft and the distal segment has not been uniformly defined and used. This may have contributed to difficulties in comparing results of different studies. The Orthopaedic Trauma Association (OTA) divides the metacarpals into distal, shaft, and proximal segments.[4] The implementation of this definition in metacarpal neck fractures is, however, difficult. In a study of Sletten et al,[5] the validity and reliability of nine different neck fracture definitions were tested against expert opinion, using a logistic regression and inter- and intraobserver coefficient. Based on this study, the authors showed that the metacarpal neck area is best defined as the squared distance between the insertions of the collateral ligaments in the metacarpal head (▶Fig. 23.3) and that 75% or more of the fracture line should be distal to the proximal border of the neck area. This definition is used in the authors' later randomized controlled trial (RCT) where a functional treatment is compared with bouquet pinning.[6]

23.3 Clinical Signs and Tests

The typical symptoms of a metacarpal neck fracture are pain and tenderness localized around the knuckle. There may be pain with movement of the fingers. The hand may swell, and a discoloration and/or bruising of the affected area may be seen. The metacarpals are concave in the sagittal plane and relatively flat on the dorsal side. The

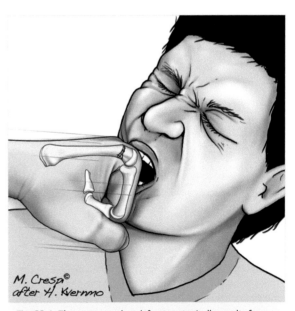

Fig. 23.1 The metacarpal neck fracture typically results from striking an object or another person with a closed fist, causing longitudinal compression through the knuckle. (Copyright Hebe Désirée Kvernmo and Massimiliano Crespi.)

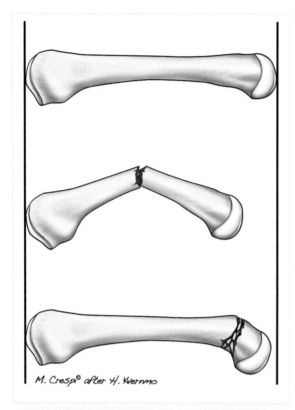

Fig. 23.2 The figure illustrates shortening of the metacarpal bone, which is more pronounced when the shaft fracture is angulated rather than the neck. (Copyright Hebe Désirée Kvernmo and Massimiliano Crespi.)

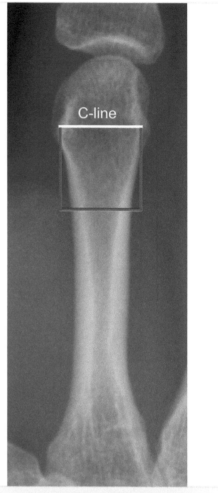

Fig. 23.3 The metacarpal neck is defined as the squared distance of the C-line, which represents the line between the tuberosities of the metacarpal head at the broadest part. (Sletten et al 2011)

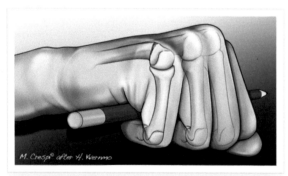

Fig. 23.4 Typical clinical appearance of a boxer's fracture with loss of the knuckle. (Copyright Hebe Désirée Kvernmo and Massimiliano Crespi.)

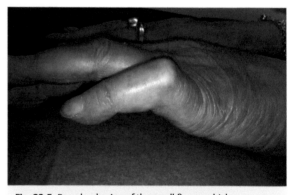

Fig. 23.5 Pseudo-clawing of the small finger, which is a compensatory metacarpophalangeal (MCP) joint hyperextension and proximal interphalangeal (PIP) joint flexion.

neck of the metacarpals has a normal volar angulation of 14 degrees.[7] The direct blow causing the fracture results in an additionally volarly flexed position of the metacarpal neck. The knuckle disappears (▶Fig. 23.4), and a hard lump may be felt in the palm. Because of shortening of the metacarpal bone (▶Fig. 23.2), a weakness of flexion force may result as the flexors become relatively too long for the finger.[8] The extension may also be affected, with development of a compensatory metacarpophalangeal (MCP) joint hyperextension and proximal interphalangeal (PIP) joint flexion, called a pseudo-clawing of the finger (▶Fig. 23.5). However, pseudo-clawing is seldom

seen. The fracture may also result in a malrotation of the fracture, leading to scissoring or overlap of the fingers on flexion. This may lead to discomfort, decreased grip, and cosmetic complaints. Also, a laceration of the skin may be seen. This indicates a more serious type of a metacarpal neck fracture.

23.3.1 Investigatory Examination

Imaging helps in assessment of angulation, shortening, possible metacarpal head involvement, and possible associated fractures.

23.4 Radiographs

Standard radiographs for evaluation of metacarpal fractures include anteroposterior (AP) (▶Fig. 23.6), lateral (▶Fig. 23.7), and oblique views. The AP view is better than the posteroanterior (PA) view as it gives better and more symmetrical frontal projection of the small finger metacarpal.[9] Volar angulation and shortening of the neck fracture are two important determinates in assessment of indication for operative treatment. The measurements of these determinates differ extensively in the existing literature.

23.4.1 Measurement of Angulation

It is difficult to measure the degree of angulation in the metacarpal neck fractures consistently.[10] The measurements have been performed on either the lateral view or oblique views, by measuring lines that pass through the center of the metacarpal head and the shaft on the dorsal aspect of the bone, in the mid-medullary canal or on the volar aspect. In a cadaveric study, the mid-medullary canal measurement in the lateral view was proven to be most valid.[11] This result is supported by a recent clinical RCT,[6] in which study, inter- and intraobserver reliability of four different methods for evaluation of angulation were performed. The measurement of the mid-medullary canal on the lateral view (▶Fig. 23.7) was shown to be both most reliable and valid.

23.4.2 Measurement of Shortening

The angulation of the metacarpal neck fracture causes a shortening of the metacarpal neck (▶Fig. 23.2). This shortening may be evaluated by two different methods.[12] First, the length may be evaluated by measurements on the contralateral hand radiograph. Another method, which only requires a radiograph of the injured hand,

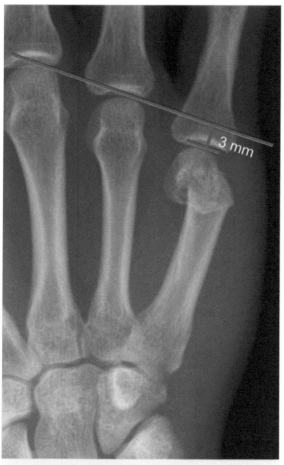

Fig. 23.6 Metacarpal shortening for small finger metacarpal fracture is best measured as the distance between the line going through the neighboring middle finger and ring finger metacarpal head and the small finger metacarpal head, both lines going at the most distal point of the heads.

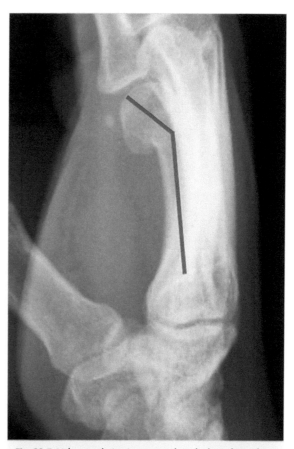

Fig. 23.7 Volar angulation is measured on the lateral view by measuring the angle between the line that passes through the center of the metacarpal head and a line in the mid-medullary canal.

is to make a stipulation of shortening by drawing a line through the most distal point of the heads of two neighboring fingers (▶Fig. 23.6).

Computed Tomography Scan

A computed tomography (CT) scan may be necessary for inconclusive radiographs involving a complex metacarpal head fracture.

23.5 Possible Concurrent Lesions of Bone and Soft Tissue

High-energy injuries may result in a comminuted fracture or involvement of a metacarpal head fracture. There may also be a wound, indicating an open fracture and associated injuries. In these cases, this may result from a fight bite over the MCP joint (▶Fig. 23.8), where the injured person is hit by the opponent's teeth. This is a human bite. The cartilage of the metacarpal head may be injured and a remnant of the teeth may be seen. Human bites may result in septic arthritis due to the virulent microorganisms in the mouth, unless it is treated immediately. Also, the extensor tendon(s) may be injured and retracted, with loss of finger extension.

23.6 Evidence

A review of the evidence for treatment of metacarpal neck fractures was published in the FESSH Instructional Course book in 2017.[13] Thirteen existing RCT or pseudo-RCT concerning either conservative or operative treatment of metacarpal neck fractures were included. The outcome measures were not reported consistently, and a further meta-analysis was therefore not performed. Seven of the 13 RCT evaluated conservative treatment only, two compared operative to conservative techniques, and four compared the use of different operative techniques. Only four studies reported patient reported outcome measures.[6,14–16]

23.6.1 Conservative Treatment

The study of Yum Man and Trickett[13] concluded that most metacarpal neck fractures may be treated conservatively. Research effort has been focusing on identifying the optimal method of conservative treatment. A previous Cochrane review[2] on conservative treatment of small finger metacarpal neck fractures demonstrated that no conservative treatment strategy is statistically superior over others and that no definitive recommendations could be given due to the heterogeneity of the data. However, all seven studies comparing functional treatment with cast immobilization[16–22] favored functional treatment with neighbor strapping and early mobilization, with beneficial effects demonstrated for both range of motion (ROM) and grip strength. The study of van Aaken et al,[16] which included fractures of up to 70 degrees of volar flexion deformity, showed 11 days less of work for functional treatment compared to casting. The functional treatment consisted of no reduction and early mobilization, which depends on the stability of an impacted fracture as it gives less pain. Usually, a soft wrap is used to remind the patient of his/her fracture and a neighbor strapping prevents painful abduction of the finger. A reduced fracture will most likely redislocate, due to the flexion forces of the intrinsic muscles that are crossing the MCP joint since they lie volar to the axis of rotation.

23.6.2 Conservative versus Operative Treatment

The issue of conservative versus operative treatments is evaluated in two RCT, both comparing bouquet pinning to conservative treatment.[6,23] No statistical difference in

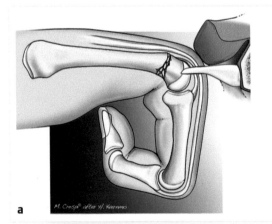
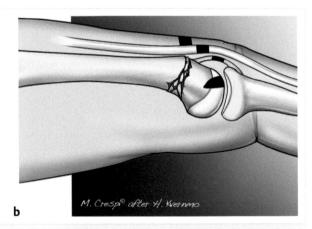

Fig. 23.8 **(a)** Fight bite resulting in a metacarpal neck fracture and a concomitant injury to the MCP joint. **(b)** Note how the soft tissue layers shift position when the MCP joint is extended. It is therefore important to put the joint into the same position as when the bone was injured (flexed position) when examining the patient. (Copyright Hebe Désirée Kvernmo and Massimiliano Crespi.)

ROM or grip strength was demonstrated. The first study also measured Quick-DASH, but found no significant difference between the groups. The study recommended conservative treatment with early mobilization for fractures up to 50 degrees of volar angulation. There was a trend toward better satisfaction with hand appearance in the operative group, but longer sick leave and more complications were seen. The latter study found that satisfaction and appearance were superior in the operative group, and concluded that operative treatment offers an aesthetic, but not functional advantage.

23.6.3 When to Consider Operative Treatment?

The thresholds for surgical intervention have not been firmly established.[13] The authors therefore concluded that it seems unlikely that surgical fixation of most of these fractures will offer additional benefits compared to conservative treatment. When deciding on which fracture that may benefit from operative treatment, these factors may be worth considering:

1. **The degree of angulation**
There has been a controversy to what extent radiological parameters as volar angulation and shortening can be tolerated. Acceptable limitations may be up to 70 degrees for the small finger and 30 to 40 degrees for the ring finger metacarpal neck fractures. The small- and ring finger metacarpals have up to 20 to 30 degrees of mobility in the carpometacarpal joints in the sagittal plane, and can better compensate for the fracture angulation than the index and middle finger metacarpals which have less mobility. The latter metacarpal neck fractures may tolerate as little as 15 to 20 degrees of volar angulation.

2. **The degree of shortening**
Shortening of the metacarpal of more than 3 mm has been proposed to influence the treatment, but there exists no guideline on acceptable metacarpal shortening. However, for every 2 mm of metacarpal shortening, the extension is reduced by 7 degrees.[24] As most MCP joints have the ability of 10 to 20 degrees of hyperextension, this may compensate for up to 2 to 4 mm of shortening.

3. **Presence of rotational deformity**
Malrotation is poorly tolerated, as the finger may be scissoring during flexion, and operative treatment should be considered.

4. **Open injuries with associated injuries** (e.g., fight bites, metacarpal head fractures, extensor tendon injuries)
Fractures with lacerations over the MCP joints are open fractures, and should be operated. There may be a concomitant metacarpal head fracture and/or an extensor tendon laceration, which most likely result in the need of operative treatment. An infection is likely to develop.

5. **Multiple injuries** (e.g., multi traumas)
High-energy injuries may result in multiple and/or complex fractures, and the indication for operation is stronger.

23.6.4 Operative Treatment

The issue of optimal surgical technique has also been evaluated.[13] Two studies compared bouquet (intramedullary) pinning with transverse pinning.[25,26] The first study showed better functional results for bouquet pinning, but the follow-up time was only 3 months. The bouquet pining was, however, more technically demanding and time consuming. The latter study, with a follow-up time of 24 months, showed both methods to be comparable, good, and safe operative techniques for metacarpal neck fractures of the small finger.

23.7 Author's Favored Treatment Option

The author uses the definition of metacarpal neck fracture defined as the squared distance between the insertions of the collateral ligaments in the metacarpal head and that 75% or more of the fracture line is distal to the proximal border of the neck area.[5] The volar angulation of the fracture is measured on the lateral view as the angle between a line that passes through the center of the metacarpal head and the shaft in the mid-medullary canal.[6,11]

23.7.1 Conservative Treatment

The author's preferred treatment is a conservative approach for neck fractures of the small finger metacarpal up to 50 to 70 degrees of volar angulation,[6,16] unless a rotational malalignment or a pseudo-clawing of the small finger is present. The author accepts a volar angulation of 15 to 20 degrees for index and middle finger and 30 to 40 degrees for ring finger metacarpal neck fractures. However, the acceptable degree of angulation may vary between patients, depending on occupation, avocation, and/or preferences. Although the deformity may not result in any functional limitations, the patient must be willing to accept the loss of appearance of the knuckles. As these injuries typically occur in young men, who have injured themselves by fighting or hitting a wall or door in frustration, they will probably tolerate considerable deformity.[27] If the patient understands this and consent to the conservative treatment, the patient is given a splint until pain settles, usually until a week after the injury. Thereafter, the patient is given a buddy strap (▶ Fig. 23.9) for 4 to 6 weeks or until the patient feels confident to stop using it. No follow-up is needed since patients report better satisfaction and a sick leave of only 2.7 weeks,[28] compared to 5 weeks if treated in a cast.

23.7.2 Operative Treatment

Indication

The author advocates operative treatment if the volar angulation exceeds 50 to 70 degrees, if the fracture is unstable, if there are any clinical important

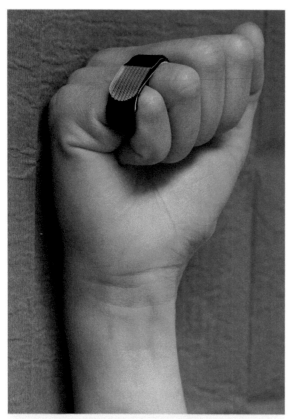

Fig. 23.9 Functional treatment with neighbor strapping of the small finger to the ring finger. An additional buddy strap may be added on the middle phalanx level.

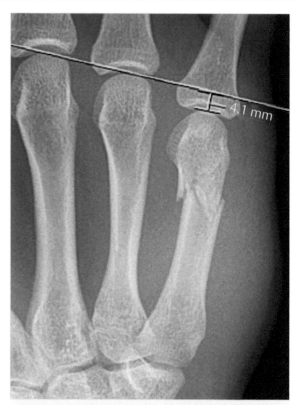

Fig. 23.10 A neck fracture close to the proximal border defined by the squared distance of the C-line is less impacted and therefore less stable, and the author prefer operative treatment for such borderline fractures.

malrotation, if pseudo-clawing is present, the fracture involves the metacarpal head, if there is an open fracture, fight bite, or cast immobilization is contraindicated (i.e., multitrauma). Also, if the fracture is a borderline neck fracture (▶Fig. 23.10), it is considered less impacted and less stable, and the author prefers operative treatment.

Positioning

The patient is placed in a supine position on the operating table. The hand is placed on a hand table in a prone position. A tourniquet is applied to the upper arm if not the wide-awake method is applied. As the hand is tilted ulnarly, the surgeon sits at the hand table adjacent to the patient's head for best visualization of the metacarpals.

Reduction

Closed reduction is performed and reduction is confirmed under fluoroscopy. The Jahss maneuver is applied,[28] with the fingers flexed into the palm with 90 degrees of MCP joint flexion. Then, a dorsally directed force through the proximal phalanx is applied, while stabilizing the metacarpal shaft (▶Fig. 23.11). This force is applied during the operative procedure until the K-wires are placed to keep the reduction. The correction of a possible rotational deformity and shortening is checked both clinically and fluoroscopically.

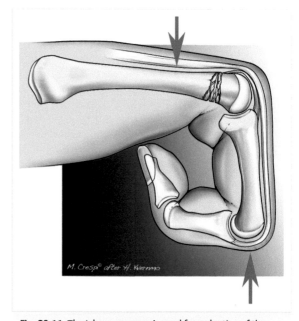

Fig. 23.11 The Jahss maneuver is used for reduction of the metacarpal neck fracture for operative cases. The *arrows* indicate where to put pressure to reduce the fracture. (Copyright Hebe Désirée Kvernmo and Massimiliano Crespi.)

Exposures

Bouquet Pinning

Neck fractures may be treated with bouquet intramedullary fixation with flexible pins (0.8–1.2 mm), placed antegrade in the base of the metacarpal bone (▶Fig. 23.12). For the small finger metacarpal, a 1 to 2 cm dorsoulnar incision over the base of the small finger is made. The dorsal sensory nerve branches are identified and protected. The starting point for the pins are best at the dorsoulnar side at the very proximal end of the small finger metacarpal. Open the cortex using

a 3.5 drill bit or an awl. Insert two to four K-wires which are slightly prebent at the tip, by gentle hammering the pins through the intramedullary canal into the metacarpal head, pointing in different directions into the metacarpal head (▶Fig. 23.12). Control reduction and K-wire position under fluoroscopy (▶Fig. 23.13). The pins are cut flush with the bone if they are planned to be there, but left outside the skin if planned to be removed. The patient is usually given a splint for a week, but may be mobilized immediately post-operatively. If the pins are planned to be removed, this is performed after approximately 4 to 6 weeks, depending on the radiographs and the clinical evaluation.

Open Reduction with Screw or Plate Fixation

Large, oblique neck fractures with involvement of the metacarpal head are unstable fractures as they have no bony support as the transverse fractures. These fractures are fixed with screws or a plate. A dorsal incision over the distal part of the metacarpal is made. The extensor apparatus is split with an incision between the extensor digit communis (EDC) and extensor digiti minimi (EDM) and the tendons are retracted to either side (▶Fig. 23.14). In some cases, an approach through the sagittal band is required. The capsule is incised longitudinally and peeled off the metacarpal head. The collateral ligaments are protected on exposure of the metacarpal head. The fragments are reduced and there may be a need of using a reduction clamp to secure the reduction as no degree of articular displacements is accepted. Multiple small screws in the collateral recess or countersinked in the head fragments or an angle stable plate may be used to retain the reduction. As stiffness is the most common complication when performing an open reduction, the ideal fixation should

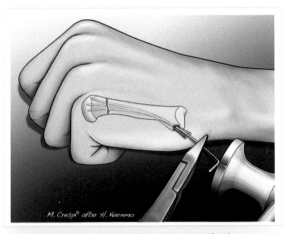

Fig. 23.12 Bouquet pinning. The starting point for the pins of a fifth metacarpal is best at the dorsoulnar side at the very proximal end of the metacarpal. Open the cortex using a 3.5 drill bit or an awl. Insert the slightly prebent K-wires (2–4 pins) by gently hammering the pins through the intramedullary canal into the metacarpal head, pointing in different directions. (Copyright Hebe Désirée Kvernmo and Massimiliano Crespi.)

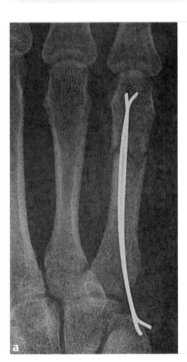
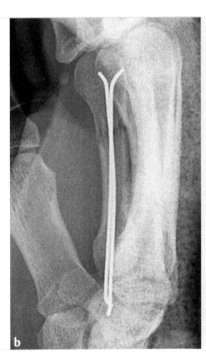

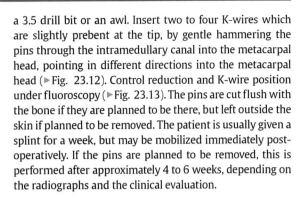

Fig. 23.13 Bouquet pinning. Postoperative radiographs after bouquet pinning a small finger borderline metacarpal neck fracture in (a) anteroposterior view and (b) lateral view.

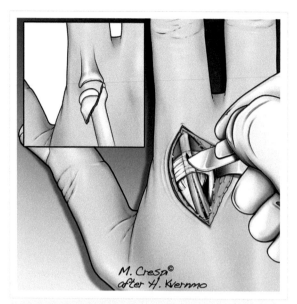

Fig. 23.14 Open reduction and internal fixation. The figure illustrates the approach to the neck and metacarpal neck in an index finger metacarpal neck. (Copyright Hebe Désirée Kvernmo and Massimiliano Crespi.)

allow for early mobilization. If the sagittal band is incised, it is repaired at the end of the procedure as it aids in stability of the extensor tendons. After internal fixation, the patient starts active ROM immediately under protection.

23.8 Alternative Treatment Options

Alternative pin placement may be applied, although controversies exist due to rate of complications. Transverse pinning of the fractures is less technically demanding than bouquet pinning. One pin is placed proximal to the fracture into the neighbor metacarpal bone and two pins are placed distally. Two RCT investigating operative techniques compared bouquet pinning with transverse pinning.[25,26] The study of the highest Coleman methodological analysis score[30] reported no statistical differences in ROM, grip strength and pain at 6 weeks and 3 months after surgery.[30] No RCT exist on the comparison of crossed retrograde K-wire fixation of the fracture to bouquet or transvers pinning. Both the crossed retrograde and transvers pinning techniques may result in stiffness of the MCP joint as the pins may be placed through the collateral ligaments to stabilize the fracture. It is therefore crucial to place the pins when the MCP joint is fully flexed. Otherwise the pins will cause pain when the hand is immobilized in a cast for 3 weeks with the MCP joints flexed, which is the safest position ensuring no joint contracture. The pins are usually removed after 3 to 4 weeks. The cast may leave the PIP joint free. PIP joint motion is encouraged.

23.9 Prognosis

Adequate short- and long-term results have been shown in several RCT, regardless of fracture angulation and treatment method applied. The fracture usually heals well within 4 to 6 weeks. Functional treatment using soft wrap and buddy strapping results in better MCP joint ROM, better strength and less swelling than treatment with reduction and splint immobilization. Some patients complain of dissatisfaction with the aesthetic appearance of a lost knuckle. In operatively treated fractures, stiffness may occur, and especially with retrograde and transverse pinning. Some heavy manual labors may need as much as 6 weeks off work. The bone may be vulnerable to repeat injuries in the early phase, and contact sports are best avoided for 3 to 6 months. Nonunion is uncommon. Malunion may occur, but it may not affect the functional result.

23.10 Tips and Tricks

Conservative treatment:
- Do not perform reduction of metacarpal neck fractures with an angulation of less than 50 to 70 degrees. Mobilize early by using a soft neighbor strapping.
- Inform the patient the following:
  - The fracture usually heals well within 4 to 6 weeks, with normal movement and grip strength, but there will be a loss of the prominence of the knuckle.
  - Most patients return to work at 3 weeks, but heavy works at around 6 weeks.
  - Contact sports are best avoided for 3 to 6 months, as the bone may be vulnerable to repeated injuries in the early phase.

Operative treatment:
- Patients with unacceptable fracture angulation or excessive shortening, malrotation, pseudo-clawing, or concomitant injuries are best treated operatively.
- The treatment of choice is bouquet pinning, as the patient may be mobilized early. However, for the third and fourth metacarpal, cast application may be necessary to avoid extensor tendon irritation.
- Be aware of the dorsal branch from the ulnar and radial nerves when making the incision. Prebend the K-wires at the tips, and insert these with the tips pointing in different directions in the metacarpal head. If there has been a fracture earlier, there may be a problem to cross this area. Transvers pinning may then be a better option.

References

[1] Hove LM. Fractures of the hand. Distribution and relative incidence. Scand J Plast Reconstr Surg Hand Surg. 1993; 27(4):317–319
[2] Poolman RW, Goslings JC, Lee JB, Statius Muller M, Steller EP, Struijs PA. Conservative treatment for closed fifth (small

finger) metacarpal neck fractures. Cochrane Database Syst Rev. 2005(3):CD003210

[3] Gudmundsen TE, Borgen L. Fractures of the fifth metacarpal. Acta Radiol. 2009; 50(3):296–300

[4] Marsh JL, Slongo TF, Agel J, et al. Fracture and dislocation classification compendium—2007: Orthopaedic Trauma Association classification, database and outcomes committee. J Orthop Trauma. 2007; 21(suppl 10):S1–S133

[5] Sletten IN, Nordsletten L, Holme I, Hellund JC, Hjorthaug GA, Kvernmo HD. Definisjon av collum metacarpale og collumfrakturer. En metodologisk studie. Høstmøteboken 2011, Abstract 37, 127

[6] Sletten IN, Hellund JC, Olsen B, Clementsen S, Kvernmo HD, Nordsletten L. Conservative treatment has comparable outcome with bouquet pinning of little finger metacarpal neck fractures: a multicentre randomized controlled study of 85 patients. J Hand Surg Eur Vol. 2015; 40(1):76–83

[7] Abdon P, Mühlow A, Stigsson L, Thorngren KG, Werner CO, Westman L. Subcapital fractures of the fifth metacarpal bone. Arch Orthop Trauma Surg. 1984; 103(4):231–234

[8] Ali A, Hamman J, Mass DP. The biomechanical effects of angulated boxer's fractures. J Hand Surg Am. 1999; 24(4):835–844

[9] Frere G, Hoel G, Moutet F, Ravet D. Fractures of the fifth metacarpal neck. Ann Chir Main. 1982; 1(3):221–226

[10] Leung YL, Beredjiklian PK, Monaghan BA, Bozentka DJ. Radiographic assessment of small finger metacarpal neck fractures. J Hand Surg Am. 2002; 27(3):443–448

[11] Lamraski G, Monsaert A, De Maeseneer M, Haentjens P. Reliability and validity of plain radiographs to assess angulation of small finger metacarpal neck fractures: human cadaveric study. J Orthop Res. 2006; 24(1):37–45

[12] Sletten IN, Nordsletten L, Husby T, Ødegaard RA, Hellund JC, Kvernmo HD. Isolated, extra-articular neck and shaft fractures of the 4th and 5th metacarpals: a comparison of transverse and bouquet (intra-medullary) pinning in 67 patients. J Hand Surg Eur Vol. 2012; 37(5):387–395

[13] Yum Man W, Trickett R. Metacarpal neck fractures. In: FESSH Instructional Course Book 2017. http://www.fessh2017.com/down/Evidence Based Data In Hand Surgery And Therapy.pdf. Accessed November 10, 2017

[14] Hofmeister EP, Kim J, Shin AY. Comparison of 2 methods of immobilization of fifth metacarpal neck fractures: a prospective randomized study. J Hand Surg Am. 2008; 33(8):1362–1368

[15] Kim JK, Kim DJ. Antegrade intramedullary pinning versus retrograde intramedullary pinning for displaced fifth metacarpal neck fractures. Clin Orthop Relat Res. 2015; 473(5):1747–1754

[16] van Aaken J, Fusetti C, Luchina S, et al. Fifth metacarpal neck fractures treated with soft wrap/buddy taping compared to reduction and casting: results of a prospective, multicenter, randomized trial. Arch Orthop Trauma Surg. 2016; 136(1):135–142

[17] Hansen PB, Hansen TB. The treatment of fractures of the ring and little metacarpal necks. A prospective randomized study of three different types of treatment. J Hand Surg [Br]. 1998; 23(2):245–247

[18] Harding IJ, Parry D, Barrington RL. The use of a moulded metacarpal brace versus neighbour strapping for fractures of the little finger metacarpal neck. J Hand Surg [Br]. 2001; 26(3):261–263

[19] Konradsen L, Nielsen PT, Albrecht-Beste E. Functional treatment of metacarpal fractures 100 randomized cases with or without fixation. Acta Orthop Scand. 1990; 61(6):531–534

[20] Kuokkanen HOM, Mulari-Keränen SK, Niskanen RO, Haapala JK, Korkala OL. Treatment of subcapital fractures of the fifth metacarpal bone, a prospective randomised comparison between functional treatment and reposition and splinting. J Plast Reconstr Surg Hand Surg. 1990; 33:315–317

[21] Statius Muller MG, Poolman RW, van Hoogstraten MJ, Steller EP. Immediate mobilization gives good results in boxer's fractures with volar angulation up to 70 degrees: a prospective randomized trial comparing immediate mobilization with cast immobilization. Arch Orthop Trauma Surg. 2003; 123(10):534–537

[22] Hofmeister EP, Kim J, Shin AY. Comparison of 2 methods of immobilization of fifth metacarpal neck fractures: a prospective randomized study. J Hand Surg Am. 2008; 33(8):1362–1368

[23] Strub B, Schindele S, Sonderegger J, Sproedt J, von Campe A, Gruenert JG. Intramedullary splinting or conservative treatment for displaced fractures of the little finger metacarpal neck? A prospective study. J Hand Surg Eur Vol. 2010; 35(9):725–729

[24] Strauch RJ, Rosenwasser MP, Lunt JG. Metacarpal shaft fractures: the effect of shortening on the extensor tendon mechanism. J Hand Surg Am. 1998; 23(3):519–523

[25] Winter M, Balaguer T, Bessière C, Carles M, Lebreton E. Surgical treatment of the boxer's fracture: transverse pinning versus intramedullary pinning. J Hand Surg Eur Vol. 2007; 32(6):709–713

[26] Wong TC, Ip FK, Yeung SH. Comparison between percutaneous transverse fixation and intramedullary K-wires in treating closed fractures of the metacarpal neck of the little finger. J Hand Surg [Br]. 2006; 31(1):61–65

[27] Westbrook AP, Davis TR, Armstrong D, Burke FD. The clinical significance of malunion of fractures of the neck and shaft of the little finger metacarpal. J Hand Surg Eur Vol. 2008; 33(6):732–739

[28] Bansal R, Craigen MA. Fifth metacarpal neck fractures: is follow-up required? J Hand Surg Eur Vol. 2007; 32(1):69–73

[29] Jahss P. Fractures of the metacarpals: a new method of reduction and immobilization. J Bone Joint Surg Am. 1938; 20:178–186

[30] Coleman BD, Khan KM, Maffulli N, Cook JL, Wark JD; Victorian Institute of Sport Tendon Study . Group. Studies of surgical outcome after patellar tendinopathy: clinical significance of methodological deficiencies and guidelines for future studies. Scand J Med Sci Sports. 2000; 10(1):2–11

24 Correction of Malunion in Metacarpal and Phalangeal Fractures

Hermann Krimmer

Abstract

We regard the technique for correction of rotational malalignment by using a special rotational plate as safe and reliable. It facilitates difficult surgery significantly. Precise surgery with premounting the plate, correct position of the osteotomy, and early rehabilitation are key points for good clinical outcome.

Keywords: malunion, metacarpal fractures, phalangeal fractures, correction osteotomy, rotational plate

24.1 Trauma Mechanism

Symptomatic malunited fractures of the metacarpals or phalanges can significantly affect hand function. Isolated fractures of metacarpals and phalanges are the commonest injuries of the upper extremity, which constitute about 10% of skeletal fractures in general and 40% of all upper extremity fractures. The failures include nonunion and malunion, which disturb hand function or are cosmetically unacceptable. Frequently, these failures are followed by reduction of finger movement, degenerative changes in neighbored joints, and algodystrophy. The management of nonunion and malunion in the metacarpals and phalanges is influenced by the multiple gliding structures and the propensity for stiffness making this kind of surgery challenging.[1]

Complications associated with these fractures are also prevalent, and can arise with both conservative and surgical treatment of hand fractures, making treatment of complications an essential part of caring for these injuries. Failed conservative treatment might be caused by just looking on the radiograph missing the clinical situation mostly in case of rotational malalignment. Complications of surgery are usually determined by fixing the fracture in a wrong position or with insufficient stability leading to secondary malalignment.[2]

24.2 Classification

Rotational and axial deformity are indications for correction osteotomy. Correction osteotomy should be performed in case of severe deformity leading to significant restriction of function. If only slight deformity is present, it depends on patients' complaints and profile.

24.3 Clinical Signs and Tests

Whereas axial deformity is obvious, rotational deformity needs precise clinical testing by examination of finger movement from extension to full flexion. Already

10 degrees of malrotation at the metacarpal site lead to 2-cm dislocation at the fingertip (▶Fig. 24.1).

24.4 Evidence

Correction of rotatory malunion of the proximal phalanx might be done either at the site of the malunion or the base of the metacarpal. An osteotomy at the site of the malunion offers the best condition for full correction of the deformity but involves an increased risk for tendon adhesions leading to contractures of the proximal interphalangeal (PIP) joint and even the metacarpophalangeal (MCP) joint.[3] Osteotomy at the metacarpal side provides less risk for tendon adhesions but can lead to imbalance of the intrinsic muscles and if additionally, axial deformity is present to some kind of Z-deformity. Nowadays with the low-profile implants, we absolutely recommend performing the osteotomy at the site of the malunion as full correction of the deformity only can be achieved by that.

24.5 Author's Favored Treatment Options

24.5.1 Time for Surgery

Early recreation of the fracture or osteotomy is more likely to be rewarded with favorable results than late operation. However, if severe swelling and restriction of motion at the MCP and PIP joint are present, one should initially go for physiotherapy to improve soft tissue conditions and wait for surgery. In case of additional nonunion, early surgery of course is necessary.

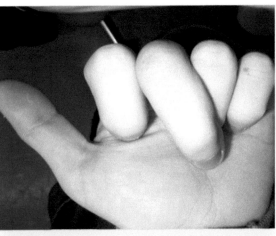

Fig. 24.1 Rotational malalignment at the ground phalanx of the middle finger.

24.5.2 Technique

For correction of malrotation, two important points are essential: first, premounting the plate before osteotomy and second, precise control of the amount of correction and the functioning result. A special rotational plate with an oblong hole in the distal part which allows a controlled correction after the osteotomy facilitates correction of malrotation (▶Fig. 24.2).

We prefer a dorsal approach splitting the extensor tendon in case of phalangeal correction with harvesting a periosteal flap from ulnar or radial for later covering, at least

partially, the implant (▶Fig. 24.3). In case of metacarpal correction, the extensor tendons are mobilized to one site.

Usually, a complete transverse osteotomy is performed. First, the plate is fixed with two screws in the proximal part and one screw in the oblong hole in a radial position if correction to the radial site is necessary or ulnar position vice versa. The plate has a mark where the osteotomy has to be done after removing the plate. When the osteotomy is completed, the plate is fixed again and by the screw in the oblong hole, the correction is guided till the correct position is reached (▶Fig. 24.4a, b).

For precise check of the rotation bending, the neighbor fingers in the palm is helpful (▶Fig. 24.5a, b). After tightening the screw, the other screws are inserted leading to three screws on each site (▶Fig. 24.6). The plate offers locking screws as well which are preferable in poor bone quality. For correction at the metacarpals, usually 2-mm screws are used and for phalangeal correction 1–5mm screws are

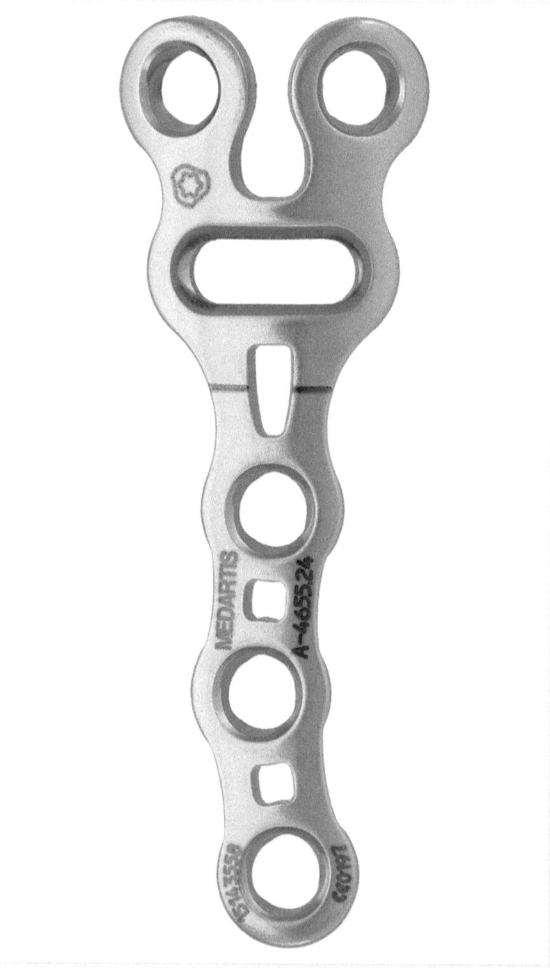

Fig. 24.2 Rotational plate with offset holes to prevent bone splitting and screw collision. Mark for the osteotomy, 1.5-mm plate thickness 0.8 mm for phalangeal correction, and 2 mm with plate thickness 1.3 mm, 1.5 and 2.0 Trilock screws polyaxial with 15 degrees of freedom. (Agreement by Medartis Basel, Switzerland)

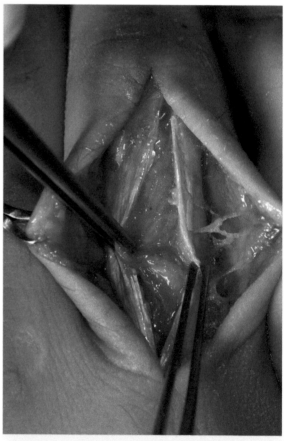

Fig. 24.3 Dorsal approach to the ground phalanx with tendon split and harvest of a periosteal flap.

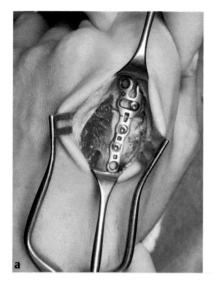
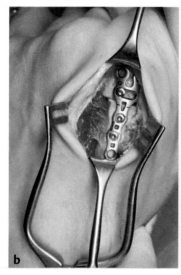

Fig. 24.4 Intraoperative view of rotational plate at the metacarpal **(a)** before and **(b)** after correction.

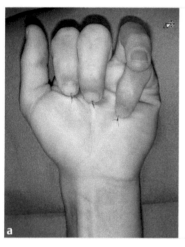
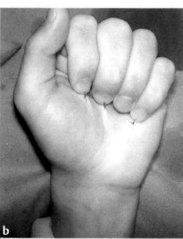

Fig. 24.5 **(a)** Neighbor fingers fixed to the palm. **(b)** Check for accuracy after correction.

used. It is essential to precisely check the screw length on a true lateral view to avoid flexor tendon laceration.

In case of axial deformity at the ground phalanx, it is even more important to perform the osteotomy at the site of the malunion to avoid Z-deformity. It might be done through a dorsal as well as a lateral approach using an opening wedge osteotomy by fixation with a small plate (▶ Fig. 24.7).

Postoperative protocol should start with immediate mobilization protecting the hand for 2 weeks in an intrinsic-plus position in case of phalangeal correction, whereas an ulnar-sided splint leaving finger motion free is sufficient in case of metacarpal correction.

24.6 Clinical Results

Using this technique with the rotational plate, all osteotomies out of seven united in a correct position and all patients were satisfied with the result. This confirms the data of the literature where the authors found a high satisfaction rate following correction of malunions at the hand.[4] If restriction of motion is present, hardware removal with tenolysis or even arthrolysis is necessary, however, prerequisites are solid bony union and at least a time interval of 6 months to the previous surgery.

24.7 Tips and Tricks

In case of combination of axial and rotational deformity, a dome (curved) osteotomy might be an alternative allowing correction in all planes. Anyway, whatever kind of technique is used, premounting the plate distal of the osteotomy should be performed.

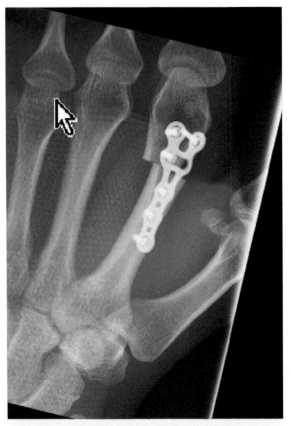

Fig. 24.6 Postoperative radiograph following correction osteotomy at the metacarpal.

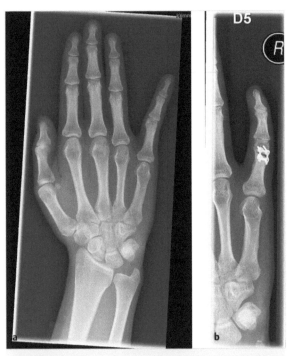

Fig. 24.7 (a, b) Correction of axial deformity at the ground phalanx by open wedge osteotomy and fixation with 1.5-mm grid plate.

References

[1] Freeland AE, Lindley SG. Malunions of the finger metacarpals and phalanges. Hand Clin. 2006; 22(3):341–355

[2] Balaram AK, Bednar MS. Complications after the fractures of metacarpal and phalanges. Hand Clin. 2010; 26(2):169–177

[3] Büchler U, Gupta A, Ruf S. Corrective osteotomy for post-traumatic malunion of the phalanges in the hand. J Hand Surg [Br]. 1996; 21(1):33–42

[4] Karthik K, Tahmassebi R, Khakha RS, Compson J. Corrective osteotomy for malunited metacarpal fractures: long-term results of a novel technique. J Hand Surg Eur Vol. 2015; 40(8):840–845

Section IV

Carpal Fractures

25 Acute Scaphoid Fractures 239

26 Nonunion of the Scaphoid 249

27 Other Carpal Fractures 261

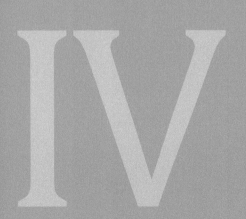

25 Acute Scaphoid Fractures

Joseph J. Dias, Lambros Athanatos

Abstract

This chapter describes the "care delivery value chain" for acute scaphoid fractures. The most common mechanism of injury is axial loading across a hyperextended and radially deviated wrist. A scaphoid fracture should be suspected if there is tenderness in the anatomical snuff box and/or on palpating the scaphoid tuberosity with radial sided pain increasing on radial or ulnar deviation and/or pain on longitudinal compression of the thumb. Adequate radiographic views, usually four or five, of the wrist are needed. The alternative is to investigate using a magnetic resonance imaging (MRI) scan or a fine-cut computed tomography (CT) scan. An undisplaced scaphoid fracture will heal anatomically when immobilized in a below-elbow plaster cast with the thumb free and may need this for only 4 weeks. We almost never immobilize a patient in a cast longer than 6 to 8 weeks. Should a fracture be minimally displaced (≤1 mm), the surgeon may also consider percutaneous screw fixation. The benefits of internal fixation are that the fracture is stabilized usually sufficiently to avoid external immobilization, but the patient is exposed to surgical risks. Fractures displaced ≥2 mm and proximal pole scaphoid fractures that have a high risk of nonunion (30%) or avascular necrosis may need internal fixation. The care delivery value chain describes the six clinical stages in managing such fractures.

Keywords: scaphoid fracture, diagnosis, treatment, outcome

25.1 Introduction

The word "scaphoid" derives from the Greek word "σκαφωιδες" meaning "boat shaped." It has an incidence of 12.4 to 43 in 100.000.[1-4] It is a wonder that a fracture of such a small bone can cause so much trouble. In the United Kingdom, injuries to the hand cost the tax payer over £100 million each year.[5]

▶Fig. 25.1 depicts the care delivery value chain for acute scaphoid fractures, which is an adaptation to Michael Porter's value chain for medical conditions.[6] This illustrates the "journey" through which the patient "travels" after sustaining an acute scaphoid fracture. It consists of six stages: preventing, diagnosing, preparing, intervening, recovering/rehabilitating, and finally monitoring/managing.

Each stage consists of the following: patient involvement (what patients need to be educated about), measures needed to be collected, patient care activities taking place, and finally delivery of care (what activities of care occur).

Porter emphasized:

The care delivery value chain highlights questions such as how each activity in the care cycle is best performed, and by whom; how the effectiveness of one activity is affected by others; what sets of activities are best performed within a single care center and which are shared; how the patient is best reached over time; how patients should be informed and engaged in their own care and what patient overall outcomes and risk factors need to be measured to guide care decisions.

This chapter will describe each of the stages of the care delivery value chain for the acute scaphoid fracture.

25.2 Trauma Mechanism

The most common mechanism of injury is axial loading across a hyperextended and radially deviated wrist.[7] This is best illustrated by fractures occurring in sport with the incidence of wrist injuries constituting 3 to 9% of all sport injuries.[8] The scaphoid fracture is a common injury particularly in American football and basketball and it is estimated that 1 in 100 college football players will sustain a fracture of the scaphoid.[9] Recent studies show that the use of wrist braces has reduced the incidence of carpal fractures.[10,11] Various "landing strategies" used in martial arts have a significant effect on reducing impact load during a fall and may be effective in preventing carpal injuries.[12] Contact sport athletes should probably receive education on injury prevention.

25.3 Clinical Signs and Tests

Having sustained the injury, the patient attends the emergency department (ED) where a careful history is taken and examination performed by a doctor or a non-medically qualified but trained clinician. The first question that needs to be answered is how severe the injury is. The more severe it is, the likelier that there will be a bony injury. The second question is whether there is radial-sided wrist pain. Third, where is the pain precisely situated? Young patients often underestimate an injury and assume it is a "sprain" that will settle quickly. The salient features of examining a scaphoid fracture include tenderness in the anatomical snuff box (ASB) and/or on palpating the scaphoid tuberosity (ST) with radial-sided pain increasing on radial-ulnar deviation and/or pain on longitudinal compression (LC) of the thumb. These clinical signs are "inadequate indicators" of scaphoid fractures when used alone and should be combined to achieve a more accurate clinical diagnosis.[13]

Parvizi et al[13] showed that at the initial assessment, within 24 hours of injury, all cases with a scaphoid fracture have ASB and ST tenderness and pain on longitudinal compression, a sensitivity of 100%. The corresponding specificities for these signs at the initial examination were 19, 30, and 48% for ASB, ST, and LC, respectively.

When all three signs are positive at the initial examination, the specificity improves to 74%, so three out of four patients will have a fracture.

The care delivery value chain: acute scaphoid fracture

PATIENT PATHWAY	PREVENTING	DIAGNOSING	PREPARING	INTERVENING	REHABBING	MONITORING MANAGING
INFORMING & ENGAGING — What do patients need to be educated about?	• Importance of being careful during sporting activities • Wearing wrist protectors	• Meaning of diagnosis • Short/long term prognosis • Smoking cessation • Treatment: Cast vs. surgery (Benefits/risks)	• Patient Information leaflets • Set expectations • Explain preoperative planning • Take consent-1st stage (Benefits/Risks)	• Written instructions for cast • Reconfirm consent-2nd stage • Discharge summary • Instructions on wound care ADL • Postop recovery/rehab	• Advise return to activity and work as able • Hand exercises • Smoking cessation • Change health lifestyle	• Advise on pain expectation and OA after injury
MEASURING — What measures need to be collected?	• Rate of scaphoid fracture	• Presence of fracture • Location • Displacement • Overall health	• Health status • Fit for surgery (ASA)	• Fluoroscopy exposure • Operative time • Complications • Length of Stay	• Infection • PROM score • Return to normal activity/sports	• PROM score • Hand function • State of union (Partial or non-union) • OA
ACCESSING — Where do patient care activities take place?	• Sport/Health club • Workplace	• Emergency Department • Fracture clinic • Radiology	• Fracture clinic • Pre-op clinic (if available)	• Plaster room • Operating Theatres • Recovery • Day ward	• Fracture clinic • Physiotherapy • Home	• Fracture clinic at final visit • Sport/Health club • Workplace
CARE DELIVERY — What activities are performed at each stage? (Trauma & Orthopaedic Team)	**MONITOR** • Sport/Health club **PREVENT** • Wear wrist protectors • Safe landing strategies	**CLINICAL EVALUATION** • Q1: Injury severity • Q2: Is the pain radial • Q3: Examination **RADIOLOGY** • Q4: Perform & evaluate adequate scaphoid X-rays • Fracture presence • Location • Displacement • Ligament injury	**FRACTURE CLINIC** • Discussion (Prognosis) • Consenting **PREOP ASSESSMENT** • PMHx • Anaesthetic review • Bloods/ECG/Spirometry	**PLASTER ROOM** • Casting • Discussing cast care/hygiene • Advice on what to look out for • Access and advice **ANAESTHESIA** • Administer GA/Regional block **SURGERY** • Determine approach (e.g. percutaneous) • Insert Screw +/- grafting • Apply cast or splint **PAIN MANAGEMENT** • Prescribe WHO analgesic ladder	**SURGERY** • Return to OR for • Infection • Implant inadequate • Implant misplaced or too long **PHYSIOTHERAPY** • Exercise regime	**MONITOR** • Partial union • Non-union • OA **RADIOLOGY** • Perform & evaluate X-ray/CT/MRI **MANAGE** • Revision surgery for • Non-union • SNAC

FLOW DIAGRAM

Injury → Review / Investigate / Discharge → Fracture / No Fracture → Undisplaced / Displaced / Proximal → Cast / Fix / Graft → Splint / Free → United / Partial / Not United → Observe / Fix / Graft

Fig. 25.1 The care delivery value chain for acute scaphoid fractures is shown with a corresponding decision flow diagram for each aspect of this chain.

25.4 Investigatory Examinations

The fourth question is what imaging is needed. When assessing the imaging for a scaphoid injury, the following questions must be answered by the clinician. First, is the scaphoid fractured? This is verified with adequate views, usually four or five, of the wrist (▶Fig. 25.2; posteroanterior [PA] and/or an elongated scaphoid view, usually obtained with ulnar deviation of the pronated hand; lateral; semipronated oblique; and semisupinated oblique views). Second, what is the "state" of the fracture? Is it undisplaced, displaced, or complicated? Third, what is the cause of the complicated fracture? Is it a ligamentous injury or is it associated with another bony injury, and, fourth, if so, is it associated with subluxation or dislocation? The fracture dislocation should be promptly reduced in the ED after being given appropriate analgesia and a local anesthetic block if needed. This injury will not be dealt with in this chapter.

The answers to the four questions on imaging confirm the presence or absence of a scaphoid fracture. In patients who do not have a fracture, the decision is then to either discharge, image further, or review again (if a scaphoid fracture is clinically suspected, defined as a patient with (1) an appropriate injury, (2) pain on the radial side of the wrist, (3) tenderness or pain on the tests mentioned earlier, and (4) no obvious fracture seen on at least four good-quality radiographic views).

Strong clinical suspicion of a scaphoid fracture should include more than one of the signs mentioned earlier.[13]

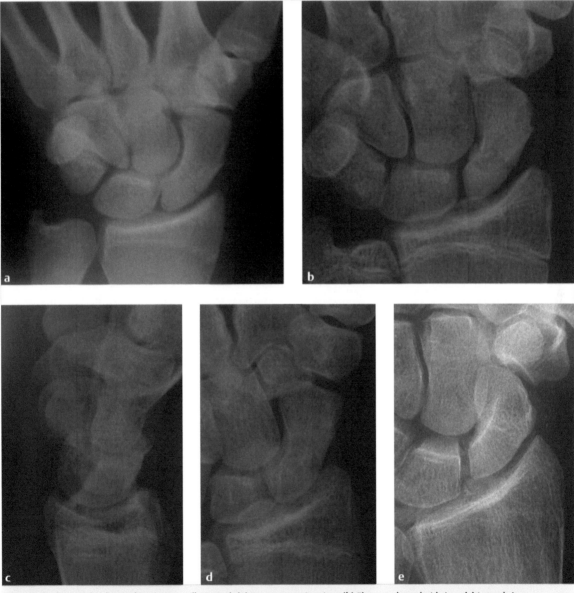

Fig. 25.2 The usual radiographic views are illustrated. (a) Posteroanterior view. (b) Elongated scaphoid view. (c) Lateral view. (d) Semiprone view. (e) Semisupine radiographic view.

In patients that do have a fracture, the location and amount of displacement needs to be quantified as this will determine the treatment pathway. A fracture is defined as displaced if the step or gap is ≥1 mm and the gap is usually seen at the radial or dorsal cortical surface on an elongated scaphoid, the PA, or oblique radiographic views.[14] Only parts of classifications, such as the Herbert classification, apply to the acute fracture. Types A and B describe some of the attributes discussed earlier. Types B1 and B2 are based on the line of the fracture, while proximal fractures (B3), fracture–dislocations (B4), and comminution (B5) account for the other types.[15] These descriptions do not clearly assist in decision making.

25.5 Alternative Treatment Options

The cornerstone of scaphoid fracture management is stabilization. This can be achieved either with a plaster cast or with screw fixation. The objective is to limit movement at the fracture site so that it can heal.

25.5.1 Clinically Suspected Scaphoid Fracture

After being reviewed in the ED, if a scaphoid fracture is clinically suspected (defined earlier), the patient should be informed about the possibility of a fracture, placed in a removable splint, and be given a follow-up appointment in an appropriate clinic. The alternative is to image further using either a MRI scan or a fine-cut CT scan to resolve the question on whether there is a fracture. After an interval of around a couple of weeks, a thorough examination and repeat scaphoid radiographs should be taken after removing the plaster to identify those with persistent symptoms and signs. If radiographs do not explain the pain, further imaging may be required.

In the absence of a fracture, either the patient can be treated as a soft-tissue injury of the wrist and be discharged with wrist exercises or a follow-up appointment can be arranged in 6 weeks to ensure a significant soft-tissue injury is not missed. We usually discharge patients with advice if there is no clinical indication of a ligament injury. Patient information leaflets should be provided for further education of the possibility of a fracture and what to look out for in the first few weeks with the patient provided with direct access back to the treating team if symptoms persist.

25.5.2 Cast

When the patient with a fracture is reviewed in fracture clinic, a more detailed history should include handedness, past medical history, medication taken (including steroids), past injury/fracture/surgery to the affected wrist, social history (smoking status, alcohol consumption, hobbies), occupation, and finally level of sporting activity. Smoking cessation should be re-emphasized due to higher risk of nonunion in all fractures.[11]

An undisplaced scaphoid fracture will heal anatomically when immobilized in a below-elbow plaster cast with the thumb free and may need this for only 4 weeks.[16] About 50% of units in the United Kingdom (including the authors') use a below-elbow cast,[17] which leaves the thumb free and, by permitting pinch, allows better function,[18] whereas the other 50% continue to use a traditional scaphoid plaster that immobilizes the thumb.

With the thumb immobilized, the additional restriction of movement of the scaphoid is very small, so not much is gained, but patient disability is increased. The thumb can be immobilized in two positions. A functional position is when the thumb is kept in a position of opposition to allow pulp pinch and tripod pinch. A dysfunctional position is when the thumb is placed so pinch is not possible. This only permits the hand to be used to assist or to hook a bag. This position does not allow prehension and the patient has very limited capacity to perform even activities of daily living. There are two groups of patients who may require restricting the function of the thumb: patients in whom compliance is uncertain and those with marked ligamentous laxity in whom even light pinch may cause scaphoid movement.

In summary, hand function is "good" in a below-elbow cast with the thumb left free, "adequate" in a scaphoid cast in functional position, "restricted" in a scaphoid cast in a dysfunctional position, and "hugely compromised" in an above-elbow cast (▶ Fig. 25.3). That is why there is no place for an above-elbow cast as this disables the patient.

A discussion regarding cast care/hygiene and possible problems should take place and written instructions provided. In particular, we ask patients to return if the cast softens enough to allow wrist movement and explain that this may permit wrist and scaphoid movement and could result in a breakdown of the healing process.

Proximal pole scaphoid fractures have a high risk of nonunion (30%)[18] or avascular necrosis (AVN).

25.5.3 Fix

An unstable scaphoid fracture is defined as one with displacement of the fracture fragments ≥1 mm on any view[17] and the surgeon may want to discuss with the patient regarding treating this in a cast or operatively.

Immobilization in a cast for 6 weeks will result in union of 80 to 85% of displaced fractures of the scaphoid.[18]

For some fractures, internal fixation is considered appropriate and the decision making must be agreed with the patient. The procedure must be explained and the patient should understand the benefits and risks of surgery and clearly know the alternative to surgery. The benefits are that the fracture is stabilized usually sufficiently to avoid external immobilization. Many patients assume that fixing the fracture means that they can resume activity, regardless of its demands on the wrist, as if the fracture has "healed" and do not appreciate that

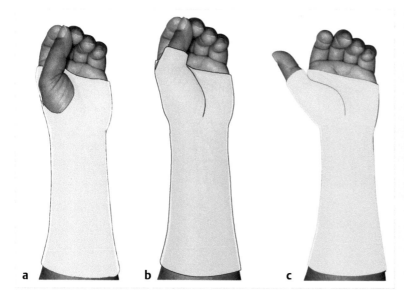

Fig. 25.3 Below-elbow casts used for acute scaphoid fractures. **(a)** The below-elbow cast with the thumb left free. This permits early restoration of hand function. Restricting wrist movement, particularly radioulnar deviation, restricts scaphoid movement. **(b)** The scaphoid cast with the thumb metacarpophalangeal joint incorporated. This is more restrictive but permits some function as pulp pinch and tripod pinch are preserved. **(c)** The thumb metacarpal is in abduction, so no pinch is now possible and the hand is effectively defunctioned.

fixation is only an internal splint that holds the alignment of bones as the normal processes of healing occur.

The risks of surgery include infection (1%[19]), the need for additional surgery (7.7%[19]), chronic regional pain syndrome (2%[19]), and osteoarthritis, if the approach damages joint cartilage (40%[20]). Delayed union and nonunion (3–7%[20, 21]) after internal fixation can occur if there is a loss of rigid fixation caused by screw malpositioning, fixation maintaining a gap, inadequate reduction, AVN of the proximal pole,[7] or implant loosening. Chondrolysis and implant-related problems can also occur especially if the hold was poor or the implant was long protruding into a joint.

Patients being treated surgically are reviewed on the ward on the day of the procedure. By this point, the surgeon will have determined the approach and method of treatment. The procedure of percutaneous reduction and techniques for reduction have been well described and are now commonly employed.

After the procedure is completed, the patient is either left free with only a bandage, are placed in a thumb spica splint, or placed in a below-elbow cast, based upon the security of fixation and the surgeons' judgment on patient compliance. The patient is discharged from hospital after being given appropriate analgesia and provided with a discharge summary with clear instructions regarding wound care and postoperative instructions. Activity is restricted to not lifting greater than 1 kg (around a bag of sugar) and the patient is advised to avoid repetitive movement of the wrist. Utilizing the hand for activities of daily living, personal hygiene,[22] and immediate return to light work activity are usually allowed and encouraged.

25.5.4 Rehabilitation

There are two objectives of recovering/rehabbing: first, to achieve union of the fracture and, second, to return the patient to function.

25.5.5 Cast

In patients who have been treated conservatively in a cast, a decision needs to be taken regarding duration of immobilization. As discussed in the previous section, depending on the fracture displacement this can vary between 4 weeks in undisplaced or minimally displaced fractures and 6 weeks, which is acceptable in most cases. We almost never immobilize a patient in a cast longer than 6 to 8 weeks. Once the cast is removed, the step-down process may involve using a wrist splint or allowing the wrist to be fully free, depending on the presence of partial union, which is discussed in the following section.

25.5.6 Fix

Patients treated surgically are followed up within 2 weeks of their procedure to ensure the wound has healed. Hand therapy is only needed if there is persistent, unexpected stiffness without any obvious structural cause. Should the patient develop a postoperative complication such as infection, he or she should be taken back to the theater to address the problem immediately, but this is rarely needed. Any malposition or incorrect length of the screw fixation must be immediately corrected. This aspect is important and needs a clear decision as cartilage is damaged irreversibly if a long implant is not immediately revised. It is not uncommon to see poor decision making when malposition, inadequate fixation, or protrusion of the implant used to fix the broken scaphoid is identified (▶Fig. 25.4).

Return to activity should be individualized to the personality of the fracture, the quality of stabilization, and the patient. The patient is usually advised against contact sports for 2 to 3 months and counseled about the risk of refracture.[23] The total time off work after being treated in a cast in one study has been reported to be as

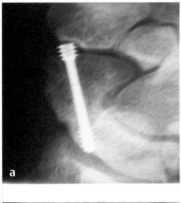
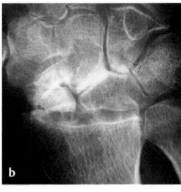
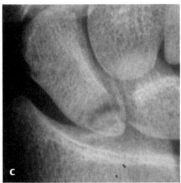
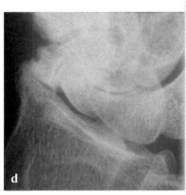

Fig. 25.4 Demonstration of some decisions to be taken during rehabbing and monitoring. **(a)** The distal screw is too long and needs immediate revision if the cartilage of the scaphotrapezium joint is to be protected. **(c)** The proximal pole is developing a nonunion and the fragment is tiny. **(b, d)** A scaphoid nonunion advanced collapse pattern with grade 3 osteoarthritis. Note the radiolunate joint cartilage and that between the proximal part of the scaphoid and the radius is maintained.

long as 144 days[24] compared to 33 days after surgery,[25] but this is not the experience reported in several studies[26] and does not reflect current practice.

25.6 Prognosis

After diagnosing a patient with a scaphoid fracture, the doctor needs to answer a set of questions. The first question is, does the fracture need to be reduced? The answer is "no," if it is minimally displaced (with a step or gap of ≤1 mm), "yes, possibly" if the step or gap is ≥1 mm, and "yes, probably" if the step or gap is ≥2 mm. Second, how will the fracture be stabilized? The fracture may be stabilized with a cast, a screw, or very rarely it may need bone graft to restore structure and stability. Should the fracture be minimally displaced (≤1 mm), the surgeon may still offer the alternative of percutaneous screw fixation. Or, if the fracture is displaced (especially ≥2 mm), the surgeon may offer reduction (closed, assisted, arthroscopic assisted, or open) with internal fixation (ORIF) with a headless compression screw (▶Fig. 25.5).

It is at this stage that the surgeon assesses other factors to determine the patients' suitability and schedules surgery, if agreed.

The next stage in the patient's journey is to prepare them for the intervention whether it is cast immobilization or surgery. This is an important phase as the surgeon needs to clarify expectations so that the surgeons' and patients' expectations coincide. The problem faced in scaphoid fractures is poor compliance, where patients think that this is a minor injury with little consequence. In fact, the

impact on disability-adjusted life years (DALY) is huge for scaphoid fractures. Raimbeau[27] investigated residual disability following injury in France. He reported "of all work injuries causing time off work of over one day, almost a third were injury to the worker's hand." He also reported that 18% of total days lost by work accidents and 18% of the costs of work accidents were due to hand injuries.

Most patients with a scaphoid fracture are young, active, and are expected to have had normal hand function prior to the injury. This needs to be established. In addition, the surgeon should establish whether the patient uses their hands regularly for dexterous tasks and especially tasks needing wrist movement. For assessment of preinjury hand function, the preoperative disabilities of the arm, shoulder, and hand (DASH) score,[28] Patient Evaluation Measure (PEM) score[29] or Patient-Rated Wrist Evaluation (PRWE) score[30] may be collected. The alternative is to document preinjury function in the records. The anesthetist may review the patient for a formal discussion and decision on the use of regional anesthetic block or general anesthesia.

The consent process ensures that the patient understands the procedure, the aftercare, the impact on their activities, and the possible complications. The surgeon should use plain language and incorporate the use of drawings or models to help the patient understand the procedure. It is important that the postoperative recovery and rehabilitation process is also discussed.

In all cases, the clinician should stress the importance of smoking cessation, given that it significantly increases the risk of nonunion of fractures overall[31] and its association with failure of operative treatment in established nonunion.[32,33]

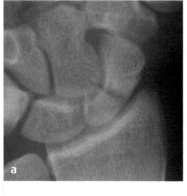
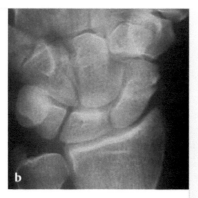
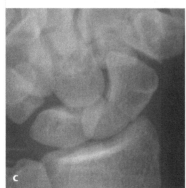
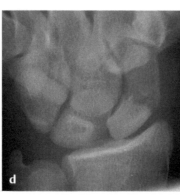

Fig. 25.5 Illustration of some decisions made when diagnosing the fracture. **(a)** A waist fracture of the scaphoid that is transverse with a clear gap across the scaphoid. **(b)** Sometimes the fracture is difficult to see on a posteroanterior view due to the oblique orientation of the scaphoid. **(c)** A scaphoid waist fracture with a step. **(d)** This demonstrates four features: (1) a waist scaphoid fracture; (2) a step at the fracture site, so the fracture is displaced; (3) radiodensity of the proximal fragment suggesting avascularity; and (4) a wide scapholunate interval suggesting either laxity or ligament disruption.

It is in this stage of the patient's "journey" that the surgeon can significantly influence the outcome of fracture healing by educating the patient about the impact of injury and its prognosis. Return to activities of daily living and work should also be discussed. We encourage patients to regain function and return to work as soon as possible regardless of the method of stabilization, but the rate of recovery is influenced by the proposed activity, the patient's occupation, and the characteristics of the fracture.

25.6.1 Outcome

The focus and attention at this stage is on answering the question "Has the fracture gone into nonunion?" as you can never be certain of whether it has united (i.e., bony bridging and remodeling has occurred) until around 6 months to a year later.

Union

Patients who have been treated in a cast for the past 6 weeks should have their cast removed and be examined for tenderness. Radiographic views of the scaphoid should be taken to confirm the absence of adverse radiological features such as a gap at the fracture site, displacement, and, very rarely, if an implant has been used, lucency or implant movement will suggest failure of union.[34] If these adverse features are absent, the wrist should be mobilized.

Radiographs taken 12 weeks after a scaphoid fracture do not provide reliable and reproducible evidence

of healing.[35] The usual advice is that radiological union is only considered to have occurred when "bridging trabeculae" are seen across the whole cross-section of the scaphoid on radiographs or a CT scan.[23] This is difficult to confirm so it is sensible to identify failure rather than assume that "no gap" means that the bone has united. In our clinical practice, CT scans are only indicated to identify nonunion and quantify significant partial union. We do not routinely use CT scans to confirm union due to cost, capacity, and availability.

Partial union is defined as presence of a visible gap across part of the fracture site associated with probable "trabecular bridging" in other areas identified on radiographs but quantified on CT scan.[36] It is common (reported in up to 42%) and with trabeculae bridging across more than 25% of the cross-section of the scaphoid, it progresses, in most patients, to full union without the need for further cast immobilization, although the wrist may need protection in a splint for heavy activity for a further 4- to 6-week period.[36]

Nonunion

Nonunion is the absence of radiographic signs of healing at 12 weeks with a clear gap on radiographs on any view and is again confirmed on a CT scan.[23] A high-quality CT scan (fine-cut, bone window) will help establish a diagnosis of nonunion, define the anatomy, and help with preoperative planning. At this point, the surgeon needs to have a discussion with the patient and explain the pros and cons of surgical treatment and the possible need for a bone graft. Patients with an established scaphoid nonunion (whether they are symptomatic or not) who decide to be treated nonoperatively should be advised that osteoarthritis is a very likely eventuality[37] that may be avoidable.

The aim of the operation is to treat the nonunion and prevent scaphoid nonunion advanced collapse (SNAC[7,37]; ►Fig. 25.4). The procedure recommended would be internal fixation with or without nonvascularized bone graft. It is very rare to need a vascularized bone graft at this time point. The nonunion rates following this procedure for all ununited scaphoid fractures are 6 to 23% for nonvascularized bone graft[38] compared to 12 to 20% for vascularized bone graft[38,39] depending on the type of nonunion and its location but are much higher when failure is identified and treated early.

Patients already treated with the procedure discussed earlier should have interval radiographs to confirm absence of nonunion or posttraumatic osteoarthritis. Patients should also have an assessment of function (either using the DASH/PEM/PRWE scores or an overall judgment recorded). Should they develop any complications, they may need revision surgery for which they need appropriate counseling.

25.7 Conclusion

The scaphoid is the most frequently fractured carpal bone.[40] Michael Porter's adapted care delivery value chain for scaphoid fractures illustrates the "journey" through which the patient "travels." Current controversies regarding scaphoid fractures include treating undisplaced fractures with cast immobilization versus with percutaneous screw fixation. Treatment decisions for acute scaphoid fractures should reflect the patients' needs. It is the surgeon's task to help their patient "negotiate" this journey and avoid the dangers. In addition, patient education regarding recovery of function is of paramount importance. Sir Francis Bacon once said, "knowledge is power." This was never so true as in the case of patients sustaining scaphoid fractures where the consequences of failure of union are profound and well understood.

References

[1] Larsen CF, Brøndum V, Skov O. Epidemiology of scaphoid fractures in Odense, Denmark. Acta Orthop Scand. 1992; 63(2):216–218

[2] Hove LM. Epidemiology of scaphoid fractures in Bergen, Norway. Scand J Plast Reconstr Surg Hand Surg. 1999; 33(4):423–426

[3] Duckworth AD, Jenkins PJ, Aitken SA, Clement ND, Court-Brown CM, McQueen MM. Scaphoid fracture epidemiology. J Trauma Acute Care Surg. 2012; 72(2):E41–E45

[4] Garala K, Taub NA, Dias JJ. The epidemiology of fractures of the scaphoid: impact of age, gender, deprivation and seasonality. Bone Joint J. 2016; 98-B(5):654–659

[5] Dias JJ, Garcia-Elias M. Hand injury costs. Injury. 2006; 37(11): 1071–1077

[6] Kim JY, Farmer P, Porter ME. Redefining global health-care delivery. Lancet. 2013; 382(9897):1060–1069

[7] Kawamura K, Chung KC. Treatment of scaphoid fractures and nonunions. J Hand Surg Am. 2008; 33(6):988–997

[8] Geissler WB. Carpal fractures in athletes. Clin Sports Med. 2001; 20(1):167–188

[9] Geissler WB. Arthroscopic management of scaphoid fractures in athletes. Hand Clin. 2009; 25(3):359–369

[10] Schieber RA, Branche-Dorsey CM, Ryan GW, Rutherford GW, Jr, Stevens JA, O'Neil J. Risk factors for injuries from in-line skating and the effectiveness of safety gear. N Engl J Med. 1996; 335(22):1630–1635

[11] Rønning R, Rønning I, Gerner T, Engebretsen L. The efficacy of wrist protectors in preventing snowboarding injuries. Am J Sports Med. 2001; 29(5):581–585

[12] Moon Y, Sosnoff JJ. Safe landing strategies during a fall: systematic review and meta-analysis. Arch Phys Med Rehabil. 2017; 98(4):783–794

[13] Parvizi J, Wayman J, Kelly P, Moran CG. Combining the clinical signs improves diagnosis of scaphoid fractures. A prospective study with follow-up. J Hand Surg [Br]. 1998; 23(3):324–327

[14] Cooney WP, Dobyns JH, Linscheid RL. Fractures of the scaphoid: a rational approach to management. Clin Orthop Relat Res. 1980(149):90–97

[15] Herbert TJ, Fisher WE. Management of the fractured scaphoid using a new bone screw. J Bone Joint Surg Br. 1984; 66(1): 114–123

[16] Geoghegan JM, Woodruff MJ, Bhatia R, et al. Undisplaced scaphoid waist fractures: is 4 weeks' immobilisation in a below-elbow cast sufficient if a week 4 CT scan suggests fracture union? J Hand Surg Eur Vol. 2009; 34(5):631–637

[17] Davis TRC. Prediction of outcome of non-operative treatment of acute scaphoid waist fracture. Ann R Coll Surg Engl. 2013; 95(3):171–176

[18] Clay NR, Dias JJ, Costigan PS, Gregg PJ, Barton NJ. Need the thumb be immobilised in scaphoid fractures? A randomised prospective trial. J Bone Joint Surg Br. 1991; 73(5):828–832

[19] Buijze GA, Doornberg JN, Ham JS, Ring D, Bhandari M, Poolman RW. Surgical compared with conservative treatment for acute nondisplaced or minimally displaced scaphoid fractures: a systematic review and meta-analysis of randomized controlled trials. J Bone Joint Surg Am. 2010; 92(6):1534–1544

[20] Saedén B, Törnkvist H, Ponzer S, Höglund M. Fracture of the carpal scaphoid. A prospective, randomised 12-year follow-up comparing operative and conservative treatment. J Bone Joint Surg Br. 2001; 83(2):230–234

[21] Rettig ME, Kozin SH, Cooney WP. Open reduction and internal fixation of acute displaced scaphoid waist fractures. J Hand Surg Am. 2001; 26(2):271–276

[22] Steinmann SP, Adams JE. Scaphoid fractures and nonunions: diagnosis and treatment. J Orthop Sci. 2006; 11(4):424–431

[23] Singh HP, Dias JJ. Focus on scaphoid fractures J Bone Joint Surg Br. 2011:1–7

[24] van der Molen AB, Groothoff JW, Visser GJ, Robinson PH, Eisma WH. Time off work due to scaphoid fractures and other carpal injuries in The Netherlands in the period 1990 to 1993. J Hand Surg [Br]. 1999; 24(2):193–198

[25] Filan SL, Herbert TJ. Herbert screw fixation of scaphoid fractures. J Bone Joint Surg Br. 1996; 78(4):519–529

[26] Dias JJ, Wildin CJ, Bhowal B, Thompson JR. Should acute scaphoid fractures be fixed? A randomized controlled trial. J Bone Joint Surg Am. 2005; 87(10):2160–2168

[27] Raimbeau G. Coûts des urgences mains. Chir Main. 2003; 22(5):258–263

[28] Hudak PL, Amadio PC, Bombardier C; The Upper Extremity Collaborative Group (UECG). Development of an upper extremity outcome measure: the DASH (disabilities of the arm, shoulder and hand) [corrected]. Am J Ind Med. 1996; 29(6):602–608

[29] Macey AC, Burke FD, Abbott K, et al; British Society for Surgery of the Hand. Outcomes of hand surgery. J Hand Surg [Br]. 1995; 20(6):841–855

[30] MacDermid JC, Turgeon T, Richards RS, Beadle M, Roth JH. Patient rating of wrist pain and disability: a reliable and valid measurement tool. J Orthop Trauma. 1998; 12(8):577–586

[31] Scolaro JA, Schenker ML, Yannascoli S, Baldwin K, Mehta S, Ahn J. Cigarette smoking increases complications following fracture: a systematic review. J Bone Joint Surg Am. 2014; 96(8):674–681

[32] Dinah AF, Vickers RH. Smoking increases failure rate of operation for established non-union of the scaphoid bone. Int Orthop. 2007; 31(4):503–505

[33] Little CP, Burston BJ, Hopkinson-Woolley J, Burge P. Failure of surgery for scaphoid non-union is associated with smoking. J Hand Surg [Br]. 2006; 31(3):252–255

[34] Dias JJ. Definition of union after acute fracture and surgery for fracture nonunion of the scaphoid. J Hand Surg [Br]. 2001; 26(4):321–325

[35] Dias JJ, Taylor M, Thompson J, Brenkel IJ, Gregg PJ. Radiographic signs of union of scaphoid fractures. An analysis of inter-observer agreement and reproducibility. J Bone Joint Surg Br. 1988; 70(2):299–301

[36] Singh HP, Forward D, Davis TRC, Dawson JS, Oni JA, Downing ND. Partial union of acute scaphoid fractures. J Hand Surg [Br]. 2005; 30(5):440–445

[37] Ruby LK, Stinson J, Belsky MR. The natural history of scaphoid non-union. A review of fifty-five cases. J Bone Joint Surg Am. 1985; 67(3):428–432

[38] Merrell GA, Wolfe SW, Slade JF, III. Treatment of scaphoid non-unions: quantitative meta-analysis of the literature. J Hand Surg Am. 2002; 27(4):685–691

[39] Tambe AD, Cutler L, Murali SR, Trail IA, Stanley JK. In scaphoid non-union, does the source of graft affect outcome? Iliac crest versus distal end of radius bone graft. J Hand Surg [Br]. 2006; 31(1):47–51

[40] Dias J, Kantharuban S. Treatment of scaphoid fractures: European approaches. Hand Clin. 2017; 33(3):501–509

26 Nonunion of the Scaphoid

Susanne Roberts, Scott W. Wolfe

Abstract

Scaphoid nonunion refers to a spectrum of failed healing, each of which requires a tailored approach. Rigid internal fixation is key to achieving good outcomes, regardless of nonunion type. However, dorsal or volar approaches may be used depending on the fracture location. Autogenous bone grafting is used in most cases of scaphoid nonunion. Correction of deformity should be addressed during the same surgical procedure. Dysvascular nonunions are often treated with vascularized bone grafts. If traditional treatments fail, a number of salvage treatment options still remain.

Keywords: proximal pole, scaphoid waist, humpback deformity, vascularized bone graft, scaphoid, nonunion, internal fixation

26.1 Trauma Mechanism

The oft-quoted definition of scaphoid nonunion is a scaphoid fracture that has failed to heal radiographically 6 months after cast immobilization or surgical intervention. However, delay in diagnosis is a leading cause of scaphoid nonunion. Many scaphoid fractures are either dismissed by the patient or family as a sprain or may be missed on early evaluation and radiographs by the primary care provider. Adequate radiographs and thorough examination may be insufficient to diagnose an acute scaphoid fracture. Many of these missed scaphoid fractures present as nonunions months to years after injury. Initial providers should have a high index of suspicion in patients with a fall on an outstretched hand or, less commonly, a high impact to a closed fist.

The unusual vascularity of the scaphoid has been investigated as a primary cause of nonunion. The proximal 70 to 80% of scaphoid vascularity is based on retrograde blood flow from radial artery branches entering through the narrow, oblique dorsal ridge. The distal portion of the blood supply comes from direct radial artery branches entering the volar tubercle. The volar and dorsal branches of the anterior interosseous artery anastomose with the radial artery branches to provide collateral blood flow. The proximal pole of the scaphoid is covered almost entirely with articular cartilage and few perforating vessels. Therefore, it is not surprising that, while only 30% of middle third fractures have been associated with avascular necrosis, nearly 100% of proximal pole fractures are rendered avascular as a result of poor retrograde blood flow.[1]

Fracture displacement, angulation, and comminution also increase the likelihood of scaphoid nonunion. Scaphoid fractures with ≥1.0 mm of displacement,

intrascaphoid angle of greater than 45 degrees, or height-to-length ratio of greater than 0.65 have been shown to have higher incidence of malunion and nonunion.[2]

Even among nondisplaced fractures, inadequate immobilization or poor compliance has also been cited as an important but difficult-to-quantify cause of scaphoid union. Some fracture patterns such as distal pole and tubercle fractures have excellent vascularity and are highly amenable to a short period of casting. In nondisplaced proximal pole and waist fractures, the precise method of immobilization has not been shown to influence outcomes.[3] However, young, active patients are less likely to tolerate prolonged immobilization and may have better outcomes with early surgical management.[4]

26.1.1 Natural History of Scaphoid Nonunion

In a long-term study of nonoperatively treated scaphoid fractures, the rate of nonunion was found to be 10%.[5] In its early stages, scaphoid nonunion is often asymptomatic.[6] Because the scaphoid serves as a critical link between the proximal and distal rows of the carpus, a disruption of this link can be expected to have a profound effect on carpal mechanics. Under normal circumstances, the scapholunate interosseous ligament pulls the lunate into flexion as the wrist and hand move from ulnar to radial deviation. However, with loss of scaphoid integrity, the scaphoid is rendered incapable of coordinating proximal row mechanics (▶Fig. 26.1). With time, the volar waist of the scaphoid erodes, the distal scaphoid collapses into flexion, and the proximal scaphoid extends, resulting in a "humpback deformity" of the scaphoid. This frequent collapse pattern of scaphoid nonunion is usually associated with lunate instability and dorsal intercalated segment instability (DISI; ▶Fig. 26.2).[7] The natural history of untreated scaphoid nonunions is continued carpal collapse and osteoarthritis.[8] In a 30-year study of scaphoid fractures, osteoarthritis was seen in 56% of patients with nonunion as compared to 2% of healed scaphoid fractures.[5]

The characteristic pattern of posttraumatic arthritis is known as scaphoid nonunion advanced collapse (SNAC). Arthritic changes originate in the radial styloid articulation and are followed by a degenerative cascade into the midcarpal joint, first at the distal scaphocapitate joint, and subsequently at the capitolunate joint.[9] The radiolunate joint is relatively spared until late in the disease, given the nearly perfect concentricity of the proximal lunate articular surface and the lunate facet of the distal radius.

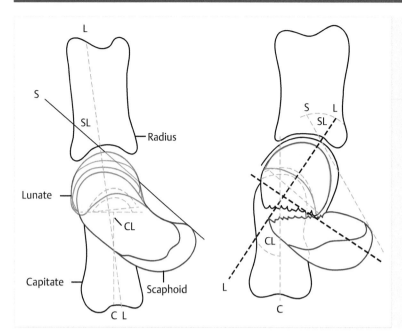

Fig. 26.1 Disruption of the link between the scaphoid and lunate through the nonunion site results in altered carpal mechanics and instability whereby the distal portion of the scaphoid collapses into flexion as the proximal portion extends with the lunate.

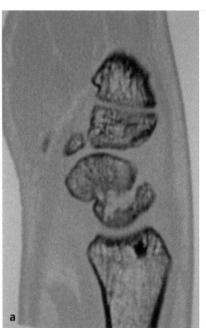

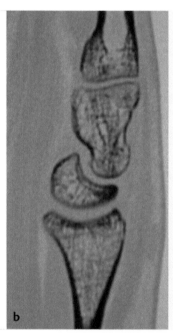

Fig. 26.2 (a) Characteristic humpback deformity with resorption of the scaphoid waist and collapse. (b) Corresponding dorsal intercalated segment instability deformity with dorsal tilt of the lunate. (Copyright © Scott W. Wolfe, MD.)

26.1.2 Classification

Both Herbert and Fisher[10] and Slade and Geissler[11] advanced classification systems intended to guide treatment of scaphoid fractures and nonunion, but it is difficult to build consensus around a classification system given the wide variety of anatomy, chronicity, and vascularity. For the purposes of intervention, four main characteristics of scaphoid nonunion guide treatment; within these broad categories, there is variation of fragment size and fracture orientation. Some nonunions may have more than one factor to consider. The most straightforward group are nonunions without deformity. Such fractures appear to have some element of stability and may be fibrous nonunions.

They do not have evidence of bone loss, by either resorption or cyst formation that portends mechanical instability and can be managed with a more limited approach. The second class relates to those that have lost inherent stability as demonstrated by humpback or DISI deformity, which is the result of displacement and bone loss. Treatment of these fractures focuses on correction of mechanical malalignment, restoration of deficient bone, and provision of stability. The third class of scaphoid nonunions are those with impaired poor blood supply as determined by imaging or by direct operative inspection. Restoration of vascular flow to the proximal pole is critical to healing. The final characteristic is the presence of degenerative arthritis, which may redirect treatment toward a salvage procedure.

26.2 Diagnostic Techniques and Criteria

26.2.1 Clinical Signs and Tests

When evaluating a patient with scaphoid nonunion, it is important to keep in mind that the term scaphoid nonunion actually applies to a spectrum of failed healing, each of which requires a different approach to treatment. The primary patient factors that should be considered in evaluation of a scaphoid nonunion include time from injury, patient age, patient activity level, and amount of pain or disability. Not surprisingly, increased time from injury is associated with increased incidence and severity of osteoarthritis.[8] Younger patients with higher activity levels and minimal arthritic change may be amenable to more aggressive treatment, while older or low-demand patients may favor nonoperative treatment until more severe functional impairment demands a salvage procedure. Other patient factors that should be considered include tobacco use and an assessment of compliance, which can derail even the best efforts at treatment. Patient comorbidities such as inflammatory arthritis or steroid dependency will also pose challenges to healing.

As an acute fracture may be missed, and early scaphoid nonunions may be asymptomatic, patients may present with an insidious onset of pain and without a recollection of trauma. Most commonly, patients complain of vague wrist discomfort and loss of motion. On examination, there is often localized swelling on the dorsoradial aspect of the wrist. Tenderness is usually localized to the anatomic snuffbox, and pressure over the scaphoid tubercle or performance of a "scaphoid shift" test is generally painful. Depending on the degree of arthritis that may be present, sharp radial deviation may elicit pain, and there may be tenderness, swelling, or synovitis at the midcarpal joint.

26.2.2 Imaging

If history and physical examination suggests scaphoid nonunion, diagnostic radiographs should include the following: posteroanterior (PA), lateral, and scaphoid views (partly supinated PA in ulnar deviation), and oblique pronation views. The primary goal is to identify the location of the fracture and to note displacement. Most nonunions occur either in the scaphoid waist or in the proximal pole, and the optimal approach differs depending on location. Deformity such as the characteristic "humpback" should be noted, as this will need to be corrected surgically. Any comminution or cyst formation will require additional bone grafting. Attention should be paid to overall carpal alignment and the presence of DISI deformity, as defined by a radiolunate angle of greater than 15 degrees and generally accompanied by scaphoid collapse and humpback. If carpal malalignment is present and is long-standing, it is important to note the presence of SNAC osteoarthritis at the radiocarpal and/or midcarpal joints.

When plain radiographs are equivocal, and especially when planning surgery, advanced imaging with computed tomography (CT) should be obtained. CT provides more precise visualization of osseous anatomy. This allows not only confirmation of suspected scaphoid nonunion, but also more exact determination of bone loss and precise measurement of intrascaphoid angles. Carpal collapse can be quantified using either the intrascaphoid angle or the height-to-length ratio on sagittal CT. An intrascaphoid angle of greater than 45 degrees is associated with an increased rate of functional impairment.[7] Height-to-length ratio of greater than 0.65 correlates with increased carpal collapse. While the latter measurement has excellent interobserver reliability, it has yet to be correlated to outcomes.[2] CT is ideal for visualizing the degree of comminution or cavitation present. This aids in determining the type and location of bone graft, and the type of fixation, implant size, approach, and screw trajectory can also be planned (▶Fig. 26.3).[2] It is important to obtain high-resolution, thin-slice, and contiguous axial and coronal scans that can be reformatted into long-axis sagittal and coronal views for operative planning. Finally, CT is considered the gold standard for assessment of healing, and can be used to quantify cortical bridging and provide guidelines for initiation of rehabilitation and return to activities.[12]

While CT scans can show the characteristic sclerosis, cysts, and fragmentation that are consistent with impaired vascularity, magnetic resonance imaging (MRI) is considered more informative in assessing fragment viability. MRI, however, is extremely operator dependent, and there is considerable controversy on the ideal sequencing algorithms and the role of contrast enhancement or perfusion studies.[13,14] MRI should be strongly considered in proximal third scaphoid nonunions. In one study, proximal fracture fragments with low T1 signal correlated with histologic evidence of osteonecrosis and poor uptake of tetracycline, whereas retention of proximal pole signal on T1 showed histologic viability. In this study, the investigators showed that nonunions with low signal on both T1- and T2-weighted sequences had the greatest compromise of vascularity and poor healing after nonvascularized bone grafting.[15] However, a more recent study demonstrated lack of correlation between MRI findings, presence or absence of intraoperative bleeding, histologic evidence of osteonecrosis, healing, or time to union.[16]

26.3 Treatment Options

26.3.1 Indications for Treatment

Fibrous Nonunion without Deformity

Scaphoid nonunions with delayed presentation (> 6 months) are unlikely to heal with casting alone, as the repair process has ceased. Electrical stimulation may be used as an adjunct to surgical intervention or casting.[17,18] In patients with delayed presentation, the success rate of

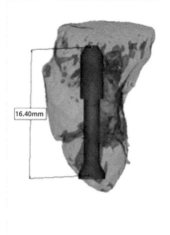
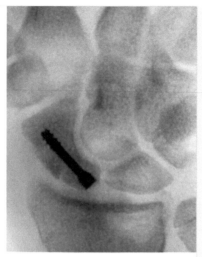
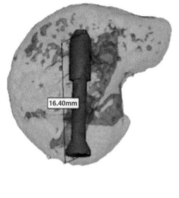
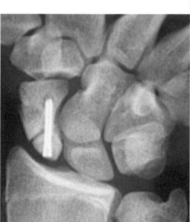

a   b

Fig. 26.3 (a) Three-dimensional CT surgical planning for optimal screw placement in a proximal pole fracture (Copyright © Joseph Lipman, PhD). (b) Intraoperative and postoperative imaging resulting from this preoperative plan (Copyright © Scott W. Wolfe, MD).

casting combined with electrical stimulation has been reported to be only 69%.[19] Therefore, rigid internal fixation with or without bone grafting is indicated for even nondisplaced scaphoid nonunions, unless medically contraindicated.

Historically, even in nondisplaced fractures, thorough debridement of the nonunion site was recommended prior to grafting and/or fixation. However, McInnes and Giuffre demonstrated that a more limited debridement (average 50%) achieved equivalent results, and therefore these authors concluded that full debridement is not necessary for healing.[20] Select stable scaphoid fractures without bone loss or deformity, an intact cartilaginous envelope, and with minimal sclerosis may be amenable to open, percutaneous, or arthroscopic-assisted screw fixation without need for autogenous graft.[21–23] Even in patients with significant bone resorption (> 2mm) but without humpback deformity, Mahmoud and Koptan reported 100% union with screw fixation without bone grafting after a mean of 11.6 weeks. The authors found time to union to be more related to delay in fixation rather than gap size.[24] However, controlled studies comparing stable fixation with more extensive debridement and grafting as compared to more limited techniques in stable nonunions have not yet been performed.

Scaphoid Waist Nonunion and Humpback Deformity

This is the most common type of nonunion faced by hand surgeons, with varying degrees of bone loss and deformity. Nonvascularized bone graft is most commonly indicated in cases with good vascularity of the proximal fragment. Graft can be obtained locally either from the distal radius or from the iliac crest. Matti originally described the process of removing all necrotic bone and fibrous tissue through a dorsal approach and packing the debrided nonunion site with a cancellous bone plugs.[25] Russe later described a method using a volar approach and two oblong corticocancellous grafts from the iliac crest as inlayed struts, in addition to packed cancellous graft (▶Fig. 26.4). This volar approach was believed to cause less damage to the dorsal blood supply.[26] Green later modified this procedure to use the volar aspect of the distal radius as the graft donor site.[27]

Fisk first proposed the technique of using a wedge graft taken from the distal radius to restore scaphoid length and simultaneously correct flexion deformity and DISI. However, his technique used a graft osteotomized from the styloid of the distal radius without internal fixation.[28] In 1984, Fernandez described use of a corticocancellous,

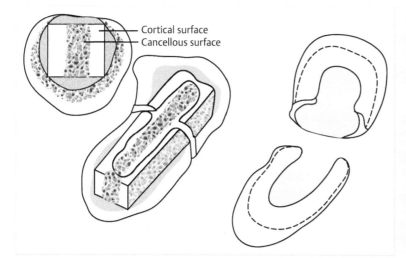

Cortical surface
Cancellous surface

Fig. 26.4 Russe's technique with two corticocancellous inlayed struts with cortical side facing out is used to restore height and correct flexion deformity.

trapezoidal wedge from the iliac crest through a volar approach with Kirschner's wire fixation.[29] Iliac crest graft was preferred to radial styloid graft as it was felt that the former resists compression forces better. Cohen et al reported treating scaphoid waist fractures with humpback deformity with purely cancellous bone graft and screw fixation. The authors proposed that screw fixation served as an internal strut without the need for corticocancellous interposition graft. However, this method is dependent on having proximal and distal fragments of sufficient size to support screw fixation, and the authors did not report the ability to correct DISI with this technique.[30]

26.3.2 Proximal Pole Nonunion

As long as the proximal fragment has good vascularity and size, surgical indications do not differ substantially for proximal pole fractures as compared to scaphoid waist fractures. Volar approaches for fixation result in less adequate reduction and union rates in both acute proximal pole fractures and nonunions.[31] Proximal pole fractures are most amenable to a dorsal approach, and in those with cavitation or cyst formation, cancellous bone graft from the dorsal distal radius or the iliac crest is generally recommended. Slade and Gillon recommended arthroscopically assisted percutaneous bone grafting from the distal radius, followed by rigid screw fixation for proximal pole nonunion, and his series demonstrated a 96% union rate by 9 months.[23]

Dysvascular Nonunions

Due to the tenuous retrograde blood supply of the scaphoid, proximal pole and even occasionally scaphoid waist nonunions may present with signs of poor vascularity either on preoperative imaging or with intraoperative inspection of punctate bleeding. Vascularized bone grafting has been recommended in the absence of punctate bleeding of the proximal pole. Initially described

techniques by Kuhlmann et al and others used vascularized pedicle grafts based on the pronator quadratus or the volar carpal artery.[32-35] The volar carpal artery pedicle lies between the palmar periosteum of the radius and the distal part of the superficial aponeurosis of the pronator quadratus and is harvested along with a 5-mm-wide strip of fascia and periosteum. In cases of humpback deformity, the harvested vascularized bone can be fashioned into a trapezoidal graft and wedged into the volar defect.[34]

However, many dysvascular nonunions involve the proximal pole, where a dorsal approach is preferred. In response to this, Zaidemberg et al[36] in 1991 described an anatomical and clinical study of a vascularized pedicle graft from the dorsal distal radius based on the 1,2 intercompartmental supraretinacular artery (1,2 ICSRA), a consistent branch of the radial artery.[37] In 2006, Sotereanos et al reported a dorsal capsular-based graft from the distal radius, which is supplied by the artery of the fourth extensor compartment and can be used as an inlay graft.[38] Criticism of dorsal vascularized grafts centers on their potential for disruption of the dorsal scaphoid blood supply. Bertelli et al described a thumb metacarpal graft based on the first dorsal metacarpal artery to be used as a volar interposition graft that does not require crossing the wrist joint.[39]

More recently, there has been enthusiasm for free vascularized grafts, particularly as there is concern that radial grafts are structurally inadequate for correction of humpback deformity. Sakai et al[40] first described the medial femoral condyle graft based on the articular branch of the descending genicular artery in 1991 and Gabl et al[41] described free iliac crest graft based on the deep circumflex iliac vascular pedicle in 1999. The medial femoral condyle graft technique has been further popularized by Bishop and Shin, and Jones et al reported superior results with free medial femoral condyle graft as compared to the 1,2 ICSRA graft.[42-44] Bürger et al[45] and Higgins and Bürger[46] demonstrated successful use of a free osteoarticular medial femoral trochlear graft to replace unsalvageable avascular and fragmented proximal poles. Disadvantages of free grafts include the potential for donor site morbidity. Current commonly used vascularized graft choices include 1,2 ICSRA pedicle, pedicled volar carpal artery, and free medial femoral condyle. Less commonly used options include dorsal capsular pedicle, thumb metacarpal graft, and free iliac crest or osteoarticular grafts.

As a sort of middle ground between nonvascularized and vascularized bone grafting, Hori et al originally described the transplantation of a vascular bundle in 1979. In this technique, a vascular pedicle (consisting of a peripheral artery, venae comitantes, and perivascular tissue) is transplanted and anchored directly into the nonviable bone fragment.[47] Fernandez and Eggli later described a similar procedure using a vascular pedicle from the second dorsal intermetacarpal artery with an iliac crest corticocancellous inlay graft. In this small series, 10 of the 11 healed at an average of 10 weeks, but further studies on this or similar techniques have not yet been performed.[48]

Considerable controversy remains as to the need for vascular grafting of dysvascular scaphoid nonunions, and the optimal means to determine the vascularity of the proximal pole. Neither MRI nor punctate bleeding has been validated as predictive of histologic trabecular viability, time to union, or union itself.[16] Robbins et al showed successful healing of scaphoid nonunions without punctate bleeding when treated with interposition iliac crest corticocancellous bone graft and rigid screw fixation, though the majority of cases in this study were waist or distal pole fractures.[49] A recent meta-analysis by Pinder et al on 1,602 patients in 48 publications demonstrated no benefit of vascular grafts over nonvascular grafts in the treatment of scaphoid nonunion.[50]

26.3.3 Surgical Techniques

Percutaneous Fixation and Bone Grafting

In select stable, nondisplaced scaphoid nonunions, a percutaneous approach may be appropriate, particularly in proximal pole fractures. Many surgeons prefer a mini-incision over the 3–4 portal to quickly expose the ideal screw starting point and avoid potential injury to the extensor tendons. For the mini-incision approach, the extensor pollicis longus (EPL) tendon is identified and retracted radially in order to make a small capsular incision to expose the proximal pole. If there is some displacement, 0.062-inch Kirschner's wires may be used as joysticks to aid in reduction prior to guide wire placement. The guide wire for the cannulated screw is passed from its starting point at the proximal pole, down the scaphoid axis, radially and distally, in line with the thumb under fluoroscopy. This is done with the wrist in slight flexion. Once reduction and wire placement are verified on fluoroscopy and the screw length is measured, the wire tip can be driven out through the volar skin and clamped. This is an important step, should the guide wire break during reaming or screw insertion. Reaming over the guide wire is then performed, being careful not to violate the most distal cortex. The volar aspect of the guide wire is then withdrawn into the distal fragment, and a curette is inserted through the dorsal

portal to debride the nonunion site. Care must be taken not to violate the outer fibrocartilaginous shell that maintains stability of the scaphoid. If the fragment is loose, a small cortical window is created just distal to the fracture site for cancellous grafting.

Bone graft may be obtained from the iliac crest or distal radius. For distal radius graft, a small incision and blunt dissection are used to expose the cortex over Lister's tubercle. For large amounts of graft, the tubercle is removed and abundant cancellous graft is harvested with curettes. Luchetti et al prefers to pack the graft in a small syringe, for ease of placement into the nonunion defect.[51] Alternatively, the cortex is opened and an 8-gauge bone biopsy cannula is inserted to obtain multiple cancellous bone plugs. Bone plugs are then passed into the nonunion site via the bone biopsy cannula, and packed into the nonunion defect with a trocar or curette. The scaphoid guide wire is then retrograde drilled back out the dorsal cortex. Prior to screw insertion, the hand reamer may be passed over the guide wire to gently pack the bone graft and advance it into the distal pole. The screw is inserted and final radiographs are obtained. The amount and type of postoperative immobilization varies in these cases, but nonetheless should be maintained until union is confirmed on CT scan.[52]

Surgical Fixation with Nonvascularized Bone Graft

Author's Favored Treatment Option: Local Bone Graft from Radius

The original Matti–Russe procedure with Green's modification utilized a volar approach to first excavate the nonunion site and remove all necrotic bone, cartilage, and fibrous tissues. This technique then includes inlay of two corticocancellous strut grafts from the distal radius with the cortical surfaces facing outward into the nonunion site to restore height and correct flexion deformity. The remaining cavity is then packed with cancellous bone graft. The author's preferred treatment is a further modification of this technique, or hybrid Russe, using a single cortical strut and cancellous graft packing in combination with rigid screw fixation.[53]

Under tourniquet control, a 4-cm volar incision is made along the flexor carpi radialis (FCR) tendon and extending another 2 cm along the glabrous border of the thenar eminence distally. After dividing its sheath, the FCR tendon is retracted ulnarly and the superficial branch of the radial artery is retracted radially or divided between sutures. The floor of the FCR tendon sheath is next incised longitudinally to expose extrinsic volar carpal ligaments. These capsular flaps should be carefully divided to expose the proximal and distal poles of the scaphoid, tagged, and preserved for later closure at the end of the case. The nonunion site is then wedged open using small osteotomes and the site is debrided using curettes to reach healthy bone with punctate bleeding. Small hooks or 0.062-inch Kirschner's wire joysticks can be used to keep the nonunion site open. Care is taken not to disrupt the dorsal cortex to maintain stability and preserve the blood supply.

Once the nonunion site is thoroughly debrided, the pronator quadratus is incised from its radial attachment to expose the radial metaphysis. A 20-mm-long by 8-mm-wide oval cortical window is marked out on the distal radial cortex (▶Fig. 26.5). A 0.045-inch Kirschner wire is used to make multiple holes along the marked line and the cortex is lifted using a small osteotome (▶Fig. 26.6). This cortical

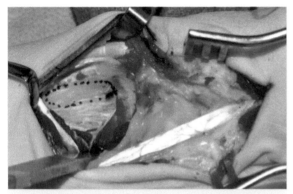

Fig. 26.5 An oval cortical window of 20 × 8 mm² is marked out on the distal radial cortex so that a 0.045-inch Kirschner wire can be used to make multiple holes along this line. (Copyright © Scott W. Wolfe, MD.)

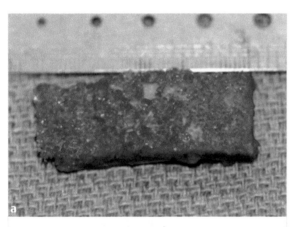

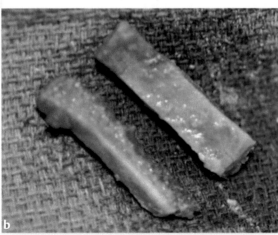

Fig. 26.7 (a, b) The cortical graft is sculpted using a rongeur to form a "matchstick" strut appropriately sized to the defect and deformity of the scaphoid. (Copyright © Scott W. Wolfe, MD.)

graft is sculpted using a rongeur to form a "matchstick" strut appropriately sized to the defect and deformity of the scaphoid (▶Fig. 26.7). Abundant cancellous bone graft is harvested using curettes. The defect is then packed with thrombin-soaked Gelfoam and the pronator quadratus is repaired over the defect.

Small hooks or joysticks are then used to extend the nonunion site for positioning of the cortical strut graft in an intramedullary fashion (▶Fig. 26.8). Alignment with the graft in place is verified on fluoroscopy. The remaining defect is then packed with abundant cancellous graft. Stable fixation is then obtained by placing an antegrade or retrograde headless cannulated screw. For proximal pole nonunions, a limited dorsal approach and antegrade screw fixation is recommended. The previously tagged volar ligaments and wrist capsule are then repaired to prevent graft extrusion, and the subcutaneous tissue and skin are then closed in layers. When severe humpback deformity and DISI are present, the proximal row is manually reduced using wrist flexion, while a percutaneous radiolunate 0.062-inch Kirschner wire is passed through the

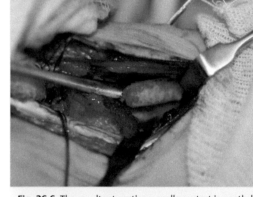

Fig. 26.6 The resultant corticocancellous strut is gently lifted out with a small elevator or osteotome. (Copyright © Scott W. Wolfe, MD.)

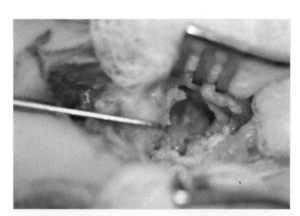

Fig. 26.8 Small hooks are used to open the thoroughly debrided nonunion site so that the strut graft can be inlayed in an intramedullary fashion. Cancellous graft is then packed into the remaining space around the strut. (Copyright © Scott W. Wolfe, MD.)

metaphyseal–diaphyseal junction of the radius into the lunate under fluoroscopy (▶Fig. 26.9).

A postoperative thumb spica splint is kept in place for 10 to 14 days. The patient is immobilized in a thumb spica cast for 6 to 8 additional weeks. Patients with a radiolunate pin require long-arm thumb spica immobilization for the first 4 weeks to protect the pin, at which time the pin is removed in the office under local anesthesia. After 8 weeks of casting, the patient is placed in a custom-molded orthosis until union is confirmed on CT scan.

Distant Bone Graft from Iliac Crest

When performing the Fernandez–Fisk wedge graft, preoperative planning based on comparative imaging of the opposite wrist is considered critical.[29,49] The goals are to analyze scaphoid length and angular deformity in order to plan resection of nonviable bone and design an appropriately sized graft. Preoperative PA, lateral, and ulnar deviation radiographs or CT scans in the longitudinal axis of the scaphoid of the injured and contralateral wrist are obtained. The surgeon must then measure the scapholunate and scaphocapitate angles, scaphoid

flexion deformity, and loss of height as compared to the uninjured side.

Under tourniquet control, a volar approach is made similar to that described earlier for the hybrid Russe technique. At the level of the volar capsule, this layer is incised obliquely from the distal radius to the scaphotrapezial joint. Resection of the sclerotic nonunion is then performed using an oscillating saw to obtain flat bony surfaces according to the preoperative plan. Depending on the degree of sclerosis or cavitation, additional curettage is performed and autogenous cancellous graft is utilized to fill voids. A bicortical or tricortical graft is then obtained from the iliac crest. The graft is then sculpted using a rongeur to fit the dimensions of the resection (▶Fig. 26.10). Osteotomes can be useful in measuring the trapezoidal defect.[49]

Lunate extension can be corrected with a radiolunate pin as previously described. The osteotomy site is then distracted using small hooks with the wrist in hyperextension. The wedge graft is impacted into the defect with the graft oriented such that the large cortical aspect faces palmarly. Any protruding bone is shaped flush with the proximal and distal fragments using a burr, and alignment of the graft is verified on fluoroscopy. While Fernandez's original technique used two or three Kirschner's wires for fixation, modern techniques utilize a cannulated headless compression screw.[49] The technique is exacting, and the tolerance for precise angular saw cuts is minimal. Careful closure of the

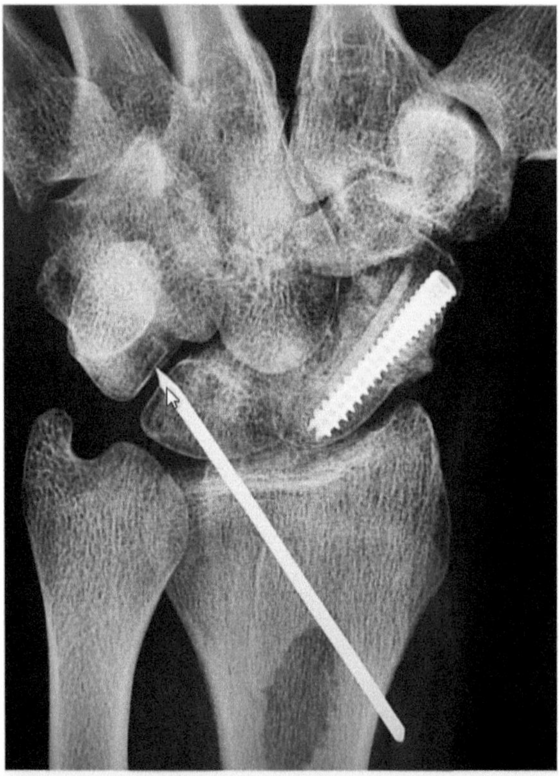

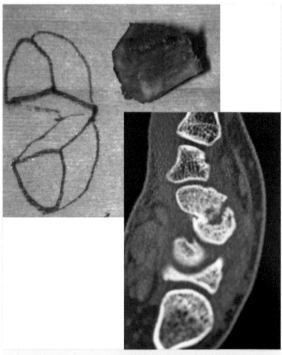

Fig. 26.9 Postoperative radiograph of a hybrid Russe technique. The cortical strut can be seen in line with the screw. A radiolunate pin was passed to correct DISI (dorsal intercalated segment instability) deformity. (Copyright © Scott W. Wolfe, MD)

Fig. 26.10 Corticocancellous bone graft is obtained from the iliac crest and shaped to fit into the trapezoidal defect created by the small oscillating saw. The resultant wedge is then impacted into the defect to correct scaphoid collapse and flexion deformity. (Copyright © Scott W. Wolfe, MD)

volar capsular flaps is then performed and the subcutaneous tissue and skin are then closed in layers.

A postoperative thumb spica splint is kept in place for 10 to 14 days and then converted to a short-arm thumb spica cast until radiographic union is confirmed. If present, a radiolunate pin is removed in the office at 4 to 6 weeks. Fernandez originally described criteria for healing based on absence of pain, bridging bony trabeculae on both sides of the graft, and disappearance of osteotomy lines on plain radiographs. However, modern treatment should include confirmation of healing on CT scan prior to initiating range of motion or return to activity.

Surgical Fixation with Vascularized Bone Graft

Pedicled Bone Graft

1,2 Intercompartmental Supraretinacular Artery Graft

Although the procedure is performed under tourniquet, it is recommended to elevate the extremity rather than exsanguinate using an esmarch to improve later visualization of small vessels. A dorsoradial, curved incision is made centered over the interval between the first and second dorsal compartments and the radiocarpal joint. The superficial radial nerve is then identified and preserved. Then, the 1,2 ICSRA can be located as it courses dorsally from the radial artery lying on the extensor retinaculum between the first and second dorsal compartments. An incision is then made at the bony attachments of the first and second compartments on either side of the artery to create a cuff of retinaculum. The 1,2 ICSRA pedicle is then carefully mobilized to the level of the radial artery in the anatomic snuff box. The nutrient vessels penetrate the dorsal radial cortex about 10 to 15 mm proximal to the joint line and care must be taken not to elevate past this point. It should be noted that the 1,2 ICSRA is a relatively short pedicle and the 2,3 ICSRA, which may provide more length, can be approached in an analogous fashion.

Once the pedicle is elevated, the scaphoid is exposed dorsally via a longitudinal or transverse incision in the capsule. The nonunion site is then thoroughly debrided using curettes. Attention is then turned back to the dorsal radial graft, which is centered at 15 mm from the joint line and elevated using small osteotomes. The graft may be fashioned to fit into the concavity of the two fragments in an inlay technique or may be used as a wedge graft. The 1,2 ICSRA is then ligated and divided proximal to the graft. The graft is then rotated and passed under the radial wrist extensors into the prepared scaphoid defect (▶Fig. 26.11). Once the graft is impacted into place, screw fixation is performed. If the fragments are grossly unstable screw fixation may be performed prior to grafting. Postoperative immobilization is achieved with a short- or long-arm cast for 6 weeks. Splinting should be continued until union is confirmed on imaging.[36]

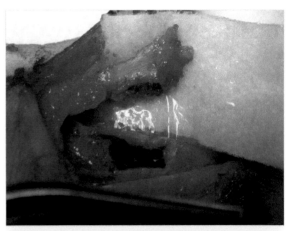

Fig. 26.11 The dorsal radial corticocancellous graft is rotated and passed under the radial wrist extensors into the prepared scaphoid defect. (Copyright © Scott W. Wolfe, MD)

Free Bone Graft

Medial Femoral Condyle Graft

A two-surgeon approach is often employed for scaphoid exposure and graft harvest, and the donor graft is usually obtained from the ipsilateral knee so that the appropriate hand can be used for a cane or crutch postoperatively. The patient is positioned supine with the hip and knee flexed and externally rotated. Under tourniquet, the previously described FCR approach is used to expose the nonunion site and if needed a radiolunate pin is placed. The nonunion site is prepared using an oscillating saw. However, if further necrosis is noted, the fragment can be excavated and packed with cancellous bone graft prior to placement of the vascularized graft.

Under tourniquet control, an incision is made positioned over the posterior border of the vastus medialis and extending from the articular aspect of the distal femur to around 20 cm proximal. The underlying fascia is longitudinally incised and the vastus medialis is elevated to expose the medial femoral condyle. The descending genicular vessels are identified and followed distally to their attachment to the medial femoral condyle. The presence and location of these vessels may be confirmed preoperatively using Doppler. Depending on the size of the descending genicular vessels (ideally >1 mm diameter), the superomedial vessels, muscular and osteoarticular branches, and saphenous branches are ligated. If the descending genicular vessels are insufficient, the superomedial vessels may be used. The graft is then harvested using a small oscillating saw and curved osteotomes being careful to retract the pedicle at the proximal border. A second 45-degree cut can be made distally and a triangle of bone removed to aid in removing the graft en bloc. The pedicle is then clipped and divided proximally at Hunter's canal.

The free graft is then sculpted to fit the trapezoidal osteotomy site in the scaphoid and gently tamped into place with the periosteum facing volar. A cannulated headless screw is then placed to secure the graft usually in a retrograde fashion. Next, the vascular pedicle is anastomosed to the radial artery (end to side) and its vena commitans (end to end). Although it is not routine, a monitoring skin paddle can be used. The volar radiocarpal ligaments are then repaired and the skin and subcutaneous tissue closed in layers. A long-arm thumb spica splint should be used and converted to a cast at 2 weeks. After 6 weeks, the patient may be switched to a short-arm cast until union is confirmed on imaging. The patient may weight bear immediately with a cane on the lower extremity.[42]

26.4 Evidence and Prognosis

Prognosis of surgically treated nonunions is primarily related to the time from injury and presence of avascular necrosis. A study by Shah and Jones looking at 50 cases of scaphoid nonunion treated with Herbert's screw fixation showed decreased union rates as time from injury increased. The authors also found avascular necrosis and history of previous surgery for nonunion to be determinants of adverse outcome.[21] Inoue et al performed a similar study reviewing 160 cases treated with Herbert's screw and bone grafting and found delay in treatment, avascular necrosis of the proximal fragment, instability, and fracture location to be associated with persistent nonunion.[54] A meta-analysis of the prevailing surgical techniques in 2002 showed that in stable nonunions screw fixation with grafting (94% union) as opposed to Kirschner's wire fixation with wedge grafting (74% union) yielded superior outcomes. This study also showed that in cases of proximal pole dysvascularity, union was achieved in 88% of those with vascularized graft as opposed to 47% with screw and nonvascularized corticocancellous graft.[55]

Controversy remains over whether deformity correction is essential to good outcomes. Amadio et al showed that scaphoid malunions of greater than 45 degrees had satisfactory clinical outcomes in only 27%, and posttraumatic arthritis later developed in 54%.[7] Other smaller studies have described improved pain and range of motion in patients with malunion after corrective osteotomy with anterior wedge grafting.[56,57] Jiranek et al found that malunited scaphoid fractures have a greater severity of arthritic changes irrespective of patient activity level. However, these same patients showed no significant differences in satisfaction or return to work or sport.[58] Inoue et al's study of outcomes with Herbert's screw fixation did not demonstrate a decrease in satisfactory outcomes with residual flexion deformity.[54] More recently, Forward et al showed that severity of malunion did not correlate to range-of-motion, grip strength, or subjective outcome scores.[59] Despite these conflicting data, the authors recommend attempting to correct malunion while surgically addressing nonunion.

Historically, there has been enthusiasm for vascularized bone grafting of scaphoid nonunions with concern for poor vascularity. However, in recent years reports of outcomes with vascularized grafts have been less optimistic. While some have reported healing rates as high as 100% using the 1,2 ICSRA graft, others have reported rates of 50 to 75% with similar techniques.[36,60–62] Historical reports of success with nonvascularized bone grafting in cases of poor vascularity were low. Green in 1985 reported poor results with nonvascularized bone grafting using the Russe technique in cases of complete avascularity of the proximal pole. In his series, 92% of patients with good vascularity went on to union, as compared to only 71% of patients with poor vascularity.[27] However, many of these historical techniques were performed using inadequate fixation by today's standards. It remains controversial as to whether thorough debridement, replacement with abundant nonvascularized bone graft and modern rigid screw fixation, or vascularized bone grafting with retention of necrotic bone is the preferred treatment for dysvascular nonunions. However, in the authors' experience, vascularized bone graft has rarely proved to be necessary.[16]

26.5 Salvage Procedures

Although good outcomes have been reported with the techniques described earlier, some fractures fail to heal. A number of "salvage" options exist for treatment of persistent, symptomatic nonunion of the scaphoid. Salvage treatments may be applicable to elderly or less active patients who initially chose to defer surgical treatment and subsequently become symptomatic. These techniques are generally performed in patients who present with advanced arthritic changes on preoperative imaging, because traditional scaphoid reconstruction is less likely to improve functional outcomes.

Radial styloidectomy has poor outcomes alone, but is indicated in stage I SNAC arthritis in conjunction with other procedures. The radial styloid may be approached through the anatomic snuff box or dorsally, and the procedure may be combined with partial denervation of the wrist. Removal of greater than 10 mm or more of volar bone may lead to instability from disruption of the volar radioscaphocapite (RSC) ligament attachment[63]; 6 mm is the current recommendation. We recommend that styloidectomy be considered an adjunct to operative treatment of SLAC I patients exclusively in mid and distal third nonunions.[64]

Distal scaphoid excision is also indicated for stage I SNAC wrist in which the distal pole has hypertrophic arthritic changes at the radioscaphoid articulation. This technique involves a dorsal approach with resection of the posterior interosseous nerve. The distal scaphoid fragment is excised using a key elevator in the scaphotrapeziotrapezoidal joint, while taking care not to disrupt the RSC ligament. After removal of the distal scaphoid fragment, stability of the distal row should be confirmed. If the capitate subluxates, conversion to scaphoid excision and four-bone fusion or proximal row carpectomy should be performed.[65] A 20-year study of outcomes with this procedure demonstrated significant improvement in pain relief, increased grip strength, and improved range of motion.[66]

In patients with more advanced arthritic changes (stage II SNAC wrist), whether noted on preoperative imaging or discovered intraoperatively, proximal row carpectomy and intercarpal fusion are the preferred options. Proximal row carpectomy is traditionally indicated in lower demand patients due to decreased grip strength, though more recent data have called this into question.[67] This procedure requires little immobilization and rehabilitation and affords excellent pain relief. This technique should not be used if there is exposed bone on the proximal capitate, as radiocapitate arthritis will progress prematurely. Despite long-term studies documenting a high percentage of radiocapitate arthritis, many patients describe little functional impact. Scaphoid excision with four-bone fusion addresses arthritis that has progressed to the radioscaphoid and midcarpal joints and is historically preferred in younger, higher demand patients or laborers.

References

[1]   Gelberman RH, Menon J. The vascularity of the scaphoid bone. J Hand Surg Am. 1980; 5(5):508–513

[2]   Bain GI. Clinical utilisation of computed tomography of the scaphoid. Hand Surg. 1999; 4(1):3–9

[3]   Doornberg JN, Buijze GA, Ham SJ, Ring D, Bhandari M, Poolman RW. Nonoperative treatment for acute scaphoid fractures: a systematic review and meta-analysis of randomized controlled trials. J Trauma. 2011; 71(4):1073–1081

[4]   Kim WC, Shaffer JW, Idzikowski C. Failure of treatment of ununited fractures of the carpal scaphoid. The role of non-compliance. J Bone Joint Surg Am. 1983; 65(7):985–991

[5]   Düppe H, Johnell O, Lundborg G, Karlsson M, Redlund-Johnell I. Long-term results of fracture of the scaphoid. A follow-up study of more than thirty years. J Bone Joint Surg Am. 1994; 76(2):249–252

[6]   Ruby LK, Stinson J, Belsky MR. The natural history of scaphoid non-union. A review of fifty-five cases. J Bone Joint Surg Am. 1985; 67(3):428–432

[7]   Amadio PC, Berquist TH, Smith DK, Ilstrup DM, Cooney WP, III, Linscheid RL. Scaphoid malunion. J Hand Surg Am. 1989; 14(4):679–687

[8]   Mack GR, Bosse MJ, Gelberman RH, Yu E. The natural history of scaphoid non-union. J Bone Joint Surg Am. 1984; 66(4):504–509

[9]   Vender MI, Watson HK, Wiener BD, Black DM. Degenerative change in symptomatic scaphoid nonunion. J Hand Surg Am. 1987; 12(4):514–519

[10] Herbert TJ, Fisher WE. Management of the fractured scaphoid using a new bone screw. J Bone Joint Surg Br. 1984; 66(1):114–123

[11] Slade JF, 3rd, Geissler WB, Gutow AP, Merrell GA. Percutaneous internal fixation of selected scaphoid nonunions with an arthroscopically assisted dorsal approach. J Bone Joint Surg Am. 2003; 85-A(Suppl 4):20–32

[12] Singh HP, Forward D, Davis TR, Dawson JS, Oni JA, Downing ND. Partial union of acute scaphoid fractures. J Hand Surg [Br]. 2005; 30(5):440–445

[13] Murthy NS. The role of magnetic resonance imaging in scaphoid fractures. J Hand Surg Am. 2013; 38(10):2047–2054

[14] Fox MG, Gaskin CM, Chhabra AB, Anderson MW. Assessment of scaphoid viability with MRI: a reassessment of findings on unenhanced MR images. AJR Am J Roentgenol. 2010; 195(4):W2 81:W286

[15] Trumble TE. Avascular necrosis after scaphoid fracture: a correlation of magnetic resonance imaging and histology. J Hand Surg Am. 1990; 15(4):557–564

[16] Rancy SK, Swanstrom MM, DiCarlo EF, Sneag DB, Lee SK, Wolfe SW; Scaphoid Nonunion Consortium. Success of scaphoid nonunion surgery is independent of proximal pole vascularity. J Hand Surg Eur Vol. 2018; 43(1):32–40

[17] Osterman AL, Bora FW, Jr. Electrical stimulation applied to bone and nerve injuries in the upper extremity. Orthop Clin North Am. 1986; 17(3):353–364

[18] Divelbiss BJ, Adams BD. Electrical and ultrasound stimulation for scaphoid fractures. Hand Clin. 2001; 17(4):697–701, x–xi

[19] Adams BD, Frykman GK, Taleisnik J. Treatment of scaphoid nonunion with casting and pulsed electromagnetic fields: a study continuation. J Hand Surg Am. 1992; 17(5):910–914

[20] McInnes CW, Giuffre JL. Fixation and grafting after limited debridement of scaphoid nonunions. J Hand Surg Am. 2015; 40(9):1791–1796

[21] Shah J, Jones WA. Factors affecting the outcome in 50 cases of scaphoid nonunion treated with Herbert screw fixation. J Hand Surg [Br]. 1998; 23(5):680–685

[22] Slade JF, III, Geissler WB, Gutow AP, Merrell GA. Percutaneous internal fixation of selected scaphoid nonunions with an arthroscopically assisted dorsal approach. J Bone Joint Surg Am. 2003; 85-A(Suppl 4):20–32

[23] Slade JF, III, Gillon T. Retrospective review of 234 scaphoid fractures and nonunions treated with arthroscopy for union and complications. Scand J Surg. 2008; 97(4):280–289

[24] Mahmoud M, Koptan W. Percutaneous screw fixation without bone grafting for established scaphoid nonunion with substantial bone loss. J Bone Joint Surg Br. 2011; 93(7):932–936

[25] Matti H. Uber die Behandlung der Naviculärefraktur und der refractura patellae durch plombierung mit spongiosa. Zentralbl Chir. 1937; 41:2353–2369

[26] Russe O. Fracture of the carpal navicular. Diagnosis, non-operative treatment, and operative treatment. J Bone Joint Surg Am. 1960; 42-A:759–768

[27] Green DP. The effect of avascular necrosis on Russe bone grafting for scaphoid nonunion. J Hand Surg Am. 1985; 10(5):597–605

[28] Fisk GR. An overview of injuries of the wrist. Clin Orthop Relat Res. 1980(149):137–144

[29] Fernandez DL. A technique for anterior wedge-shaped grafts for scaphoid nonunions with carpal instability. J Hand Surg Am. 1984; 9(5):733–737

[30] Cohen MS, Jupiter JB, Fallahi K, Shukla SK. Scaphoid waist nonunion with humpback deformity treated without structural bone graft. J Hand Surg Am. 2013; 38(4):701–705

[31] Slade JF, III, Jaskwhich D. Percutaneous fixation of scaphoid fractures. Hand Clin. 2001; 17(4):553–574

[32] Kawai H, Yamamoto K. Pronator quadratus pedicled bone graft for old scaphoid fractures. J Bone Joint Surg Br. 1988; 70(5):829–831

[33] Mathoulin C, Haerle M. Vascularized bone graft from the palmar carpal artery for treatment of scaphoid nonunion. J Hand Surg [Br]. 1998; 23(3):318–323

[34] Kuhlmann JN, Mimoun M, Boabighi A, Baux S. Vascularized bone graft pedicled on the volar carpal artery for non-union of the scaphoid. J Hand Surg [Br]. 1987; 12(2):203–210

[35] Braun RN. Pronator pedicle bone grafting in the forearm and proximal row. Orthop Trans.. 1983; 7:35

[36] Zaidemberg C, Siebert JW, Angrigiani C. A new vascularized bone graft for scaphoid nonunion. J Hand Surg Am. 1991; 16(3):474–478

[37] Sheetz KK, Bishop AT, Berger RA. The arterial blood supply of the distal radius and ulna and its potential use in vascularized pedicled bone grafts. J Hand Surg Am. 1995; 20(6):902–914

[38] Sotereanos DG, Darlis NA, Dailiana ZH, Sarris IK, Malizos KN. A capsular-based vascularized distal radius graft for proximal pole scaphoid pseudarthrosis. J Hand Surg Am. 2006; 31(4):580–587

[39] Bertelli JA, Peruchi FM, Rost JR, Tacca CP. Treatment of scaphoid non-unions by a palmar approach with vascularised bone graft harvested from the thumb. J Hand Surg Eur Vol. 2007; 32(2):217–223

[40] Sakai K, Doi K, Kawai S. Free vascularized thin corticoperiosteal graft. Plast Reconstr Surg. 1991; 87(2):290–298

[41] Gabl M, Reinhart C, Lutz M, et al. Vascularized bone graft from the iliac crest for the treatment of nonunion of the proximal part of the scaphoid with an avascular fragment. J Bone Joint Surg Am. 1999; 81(10):1414–1428

[42] Larson AN, Bishop AT, Shin AY. Free medial femoral condyle bone grafting for scaphoid nonunions with humpback deformity and proximal pole avascular necrosis. Tech Hand Up Extrem Surg. 2007; 11(4):246–258

[43] Jones DB, Jr, Moran SL, Bishop AT, Shin AY. Free-vascularized medial femoral condyle bone transfer in the treatment of scaphoid nonunions. Plast Reconstr Surg. 2010; 125(4):1176–1184

[44] Jones DB, Jr, Bürger H, Bishop AT, Shin AY. Treatment of scaphoid waist nonunions with an avascular proximal pole and carpal collapse. A comparison of two vascularized bone grafts. J Bone Joint Surg Am. 2008; 90(12):2616–2625

[45] Bürger HK, Windhofer C, Gaggl AJ, Higgins JP. Vascularized medial femoral trochlea osteocartilaginous flap reconstruction of proximal pole scaphoid nonunions. J Hand Surg Am. 2013; 38(4):690–700

[46] Higgins JP, Bürger HK. Medial Femoral Trochlea Osteochondral Flap: Applications for Scaphoid and Lunate Reconstruction. Clin Plast Surg. 2017; 44(2):257–265

[47] Hori Y, Tamai S, Okuda H, Sakamoto H, Takita T, Masuhara K. Blood vessel transplantation to bone. J Hand Surg Am. 1979; 4(1):23–33

[48] Fernandez DL, Eggli S. Non-union of the scaphoid. Revascularization of the proximal pole with implantation of a vascular bundle and bone-grafting. J Bone Joint Surg Am. 1995; 77(6):883–893

[49] Robbins RR, Ridge O, Carter PR. Iliac crest bone grafting and Herbert screw fixation of nonunions of the scaphoid with avascular proximal poles. J Hand Surg Am. 1995; 20(5):818–831

[50] Pinder RM, Brkljac M, Rix L, Muir L, Brewster M. Treatment of scaphoid nonunion: a systematic review of the existing evidence. J Hand Surg Am. 2015; 40(9):1797–1805.e3

[51] Luchetti TJ, Rao AJ, Fernandez JJ, Cohen MS, Wysocki RW. Fixation of proximal pole scaphoid nonunion with non-vascularized cancellous autograft. J Hand Surg Eur Vol. 2018; 43(1):66–72

[52] Slade JF, III, Dodds SD. Minimally invasive management of scaphoid nonunions. Clin Orthop Relat Res. 2006; 445(445):108–119

[53] Lee SK, Byun DJ, Roman-Deynes JL, Model Z, Wolfe SW. Hybrid Russe procedure for scaphoid waist fracture nonunion with deformity. J Hand Surg Am. 2015; 40(11):2198–2205

[54] Inoue G, Shionoya K, Kuwahata Y. Herbert screw fixation for scaphoid nonunions. An analysis of factors influencing outcome. Clin Orthop Relat Res. 1997(343):99–106

[55] Merrell GA, Wolfe SW, Slade JF, III. Treatment of scaphoid nonunions: quantitative meta-analysis of the literature. J Hand Surg Am. 2002; 27(4):685–691

[56] Nakamura P, Imaeda T, Miura T. Scaphoid malunion. J Bone Joint Surg Br. 1991; 73(1):134–137

[57] Lynch NM, Linscheid RL. Corrective osteotomy for scaphoid malunion: technique and long-term follow-up evaluation. J Hand Surg Am. 1997; 22(1):35–43

[58] Jiranek WA, Ruby LK, Millender LB, Bankoff MS, Newberg AH. Long-term results after Russe bone-grafting: the effect of malunion of the scaphoid. J Bone Joint Surg Am. 1992; 74(8):1217–1228

[59] Forward DP, Singh HP, Dawson S, Davis TR. The clinical outcome of scaphoid fracture malunion at 1 year. J Hand Surg Eur Vol. 2009; 34(1):40–46

[60] Steinmann SP, Bishop AT, Berger RA. Use of the 1,2 intercompartmental supraretinacular artery as a vascularized pedicle bone graft for difficult scaphoid nonunion. J Hand Surg Am. 2002; 27(3):391–401

[61] Hirche C, Heffinger C, Xiong L, et al. The 1,2-intercompartmental supraretinacular artery vascularized bone graft for scaphoid nonunion: management and clinical outcome. J Hand Surg Am. 2014; 39(3):423–429

[62] Chang MA, Bishop AT, Moran SL, Shin AY. The outcomes and complications of 1,2-intercompartmental supraretinacular artery pedicled vascularized bone grafting of scaphoid nonunions. J Hand Surg Am. 2006; 31(3):387–396

[63] Siegel DB, Gelberman RH. Radial styloidectomy: an anatomical study with special reference to radiocarpal intracapsular ligamentous morphology. J Hand Surg Am. 1991; 16(1):40–44

[64] Vutescu ES, Jethanandani R, Sneag DB, Wolfe SW, Lee SK. Radial styloidectomy for scaphoid nonunion advanced collapse - relevance of nonunion location. J Hand Surg Eur Vol. 2018; 43(1):80–83

[65] Malerich MM, Clifford J, Eaton B, Eaton R, Littler JW. Distal scaphoid resection arthroplasty for the treatment of degenerative arthritis secondary to scaphoid nonunion. J Hand Surg Am. 1999; 24(6):1196–1205

[66] Malerich MM, Catalano LW, III, Weidner ZD, Vance MC, Eden CM, Eaton RG. Distal scaphoid resection for degenerative arthritis secondary to scaphoid nonunion: a 20-year experience. J Hand Surg Am. 2014; 39(9):1669–1676

[67] Wagner ER, Werthel JD, Elhassan BT, Moran SL. Proximal row carpectomy and 4-corner arthrodesis in patients younger than age 45 years. J Hand Surg Am. 2017; 42(6):428–435

27 Other Carpal Fractures

Martin Richter

Abstract

Fractures of the carpals, which do not affect the scaphoid, are less common fractures. The most common is the dorsal chip fracture of the triquetrum, which can usually be treated conservatively. In carpal body fractures, on one hand, the possibility of a complex injury with carpal instability is to be considered, on the other hand, the exact restoration of height and joint surfaces is required to avoid carpal malalignment and secondary osteoarthritis. When diagnosing, it should be noted that the fractures are often difficult to detect on the plain X-rays. At the slightest suspicion, therefore, a CT-scan should be made, which usually shows the diagnosis clearly. This is the only way to ensure timely treatment, which can safely avoid the long-term consequences of overlooked fractures, which often cannot be corrected later.

Keywords: carpal fracture, trapezium, triquetrum, pisiform, Lunate, hamate, treatment options, making diagnosis

27.1 General Considerations

In the region of the carpus, the scaphoid fracture is the most common fracture by far. Their frequency is given according to literature with up to 60 to 85%.[1,2] In this light, the fractures of the other carpal bones seem to play only a minor role, since its frequency is only about 20% of carpal fractures in the literature. Considering that this number is distributed even on the remaining seven carpal bones, we find for the other carpal bones even only frequency rates in the single-digit range, sometimes by 1% or less depending on which carpal bones it is calculated and which literature is cited (▶Fig. 27.1). It should be noted, however, that it is precisely the rare occurrence of a fracture that often leads to uncertainty in the treatment, as in the daily routine not always immediately available knowledge of comparable cases is available to the hand surgeon. Also in this respect, it is interesting to deal with these fractures.

Regarding the trauma mechanism, the most common mechanism is certainly the fall on the hand. However, in rare cases of carpal fractures, bruising and axial forces can lead to individual trauma. Open fractures in complex hand injuries can cause unusual fracture patterns (▶Fig. 27.2). Basically, three types of carpal fractures can be distinguished from the severity of the acting force. In the case of very severe trauma forces, dislocation fractures can occur which, in addition to the fracture, also lead to instability in the area of the carpus and are therefore originally classified as carpal instabilities. Typical are the perilunate fracture dislocations, which not necessarily have to affect the scaphoid, as in De Quervain's dislocation fracture, but can also involve other carpal bones such as the triquetrum. These fracture dislocations can be classified in the instabilities in the so-called greater arc injuries.[3] The treatment of the carpal fractures itself, however, usually follows the guidelines of the care of the isolated carpal fracture. The second group of fractures

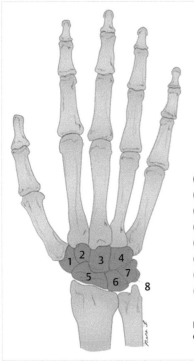

Fig. 27.1 Carpal bones. (This illustration is provided courtesy of Dr. Nasa Fujihara.)

(1) Trapezium (3-5%)
(2) Trapezoid (<1%)
(3) Capitate (1-2%)
(4) Hamate 2%
(5) Scaphoid (58-66%)
(6) Lunate (0.5-4%)
(7) Triquetrum (3-5%/15-18%)
(8) Pisiform (1-2%)

Percentage indicate published fracture rate of each bone in regard to all carpal bones

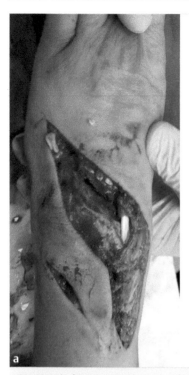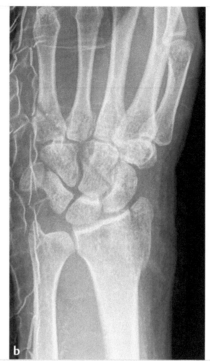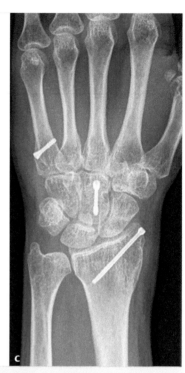

Fig. 27.2 (a, b) Open complex injury of the dorsal wrist by a cutting machine with involvement of tendons and bones. (c) After open reduction and internal fixation with different cannulated headless screws.

represents the fracture of the remaining carpals, which runs through the carpal bones themselves and thus represents a classic dislocated or nondislocated fracture. The slightest severity of injury is the bony avulsion. This is not rare at the carpal bones where many intrinsic and extrinsic ligaments attach. The most common and universally known is the dorsal triquetrum chip fracture.

With regard to the diagnosis, it can generally be said that localized pain and swelling follow the anatomical localization of the affected carpal. Corresponding anatomical knowledge of the landmarks of the carpus are required here. The X-ray image of the wrist in two planes, possibly with oblique views, is certainly the basic diagnosics for the carpal fractures. In all unclear or confusing situations, the application of computed tomography (CT) scan should be generous, as in the simple X-ray images, just in the area of the carpus and carpometacarpal (CMC) joints, overlappings often occur which do not clearly indicate fractures. Also, wrist arthroscopy can be helpful in making or confirming the diagnosis and can be used as assistance for closed reduction and fixation (see also Chapter 8).

With regard to the treatment of other carpal fractures, it can generally be said that reduction and fixation in dislocated fractures is usually either closed or open. As osteosynthesis material are primarily Kirschner's wires, mini screws or headless screws of the Herbert screw type used. For nondislocated fractures or undisplaced bony avulsions, conservative treatment is also possible. This conservative treatment usually consists in a 4-week immobilization of the wrists, leaving the finger joints and the thumb free.

27.2 Fracture of Triquetrum

27.2.1 Trauma Mechanism

The triquetral fracture is the most common carpal fracture after the scaphoid fracture with a range of 3 to 5% of carpal fractures. The most common trauma mechanism is the fall on the extended hand and wrist. Hyperflexion is also blamed for some avulsions at the dorsal side of triquetrum. In the dorsal, cortical chip fracture of the triquetrum, the ulnar styloid shall act as a chisel to shear off the dorsal, cortical surface in hyperextension and ulnar inclination of the wrist.[4]

27.2.2 Classification

Triquetrum fractures are classified generally in three different types. The majority of fractures is the small cortical fracture on the dorsal aspect of the triquetrum which is with 93% the most frequent triquetrum fracture.[4] The second type is the body fracture of the triquetrum. Body fractures can be classified by the course of the fracture line in the sagittal or horizontal or oblique plane. The rarest condition is the palmar avulsion fracture which is probably a bony avulsion of the strong palmar lunotriquetral (LT) ligament.

27.2.3 Clinical Signs and Tests

In triquetrum fractures, the pain is typically located over the dorsal ulnar aspect of the wrist. Using the landmarks

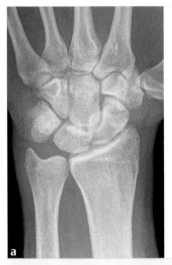
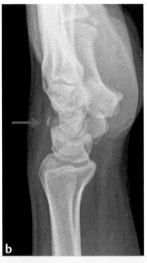
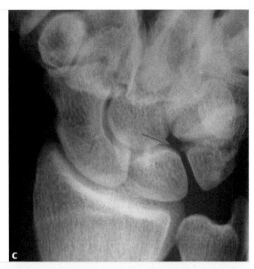

Fig. 27.3 (a) Dorsal chip fractures of the triquetrum are usually not visible on AP view, (b) but they are easy to detect on lateral X-rays of the wrist. (c) Body fractures are also visible on AP view.

of pisiform bone and ulnar styloid, it is easy to locate the precise spot of the triquetrum.

27.2.4 Investigatory Examinations

Basic imaging is X-ray of the wrist in anteroposterior (AP) and true lateral view. X-rays in AP view are often not helpful because the most frequent dorsal cortical fracture is usually hidden behind the bony structure of the carpal bones. For the easy dorsal cortical fracture, true lateral X-ray is usually sufficient to make definitely the diagnosis of this fracture (▶ Fig. 27.3). In cases of the body fracture, it is recommendable to have a CT scan to be sure that the fracture is not dislocated and that there is a normal alignment of the carpus.

27.2.5 Possible Concurrent Lesions

Dorsal cortical fractures usually show no additional lesions. When diagnosing a body fracture, one should be aware of an additional fracture in the carpus or a malalignment due to a greater arc injury with carpal instability.

27.2.6 Evidence

No randomized controlled studies exist.

27.2.7 Author's Favored Treatment Option

The majority of the triquetrum fractures are the dorsal cortical chip fractures and nondisplaced body fracture. I usually treat the dorsal chip fractures conservatively with a forearm splint or cast. It should not include metacarpophalangeal (MCP) joints and the thumb, so that early

active motion of the fingers is possible. For chip fractures, the period of immobilization is 3 weeks. After the immobilization, there will be a longer period with tenderness in the area of the chip fracture. Sometimes, for some weeks there is no bony union of the chip fragment. Sometimes, it remains a nonunion, but usually pain and tenderness disappears after 3 to 6 months. If pain persists over 6 months or longer, treatment of choice is the excision of the pseudarthrotic fragment. However, this is really a rare condition. Only very large dorsal fragments can be fixed with a small screw if they have a significant amount of join surface.

In nondisplaced body fracture, I immobilize the wrist for 4 weeks in the same type of splint or cast. Afterward mobilization of the wrist begins with loading of the wrist only 2 months after injury. The wrist can be loaded gradually to full activity after 3 months.

In displaced body fractures, I treat with open reduction and internal fixation to ensure that the joint surfaces are really congruent. The material for fixation depends on the type of fracture. In these rare conditions, I have used wires, and small headless compression screws and mini screws (▶ Fig. 27.4). If K-wires have been used, they should be removed after 4 to 8 weeks depending on the X-rays. Depending on the function after immobilization, physiotherapy could be recommendable.

27.2.8 Alternative Treatment Options

Concerning the small fragments some, authors recommend 4 weeks immobilization.

Dislocated body fractures of the triquetrum can also be reduced in a closed manner with percutaneous fixation. For the internal fixation in open reductions also mini plates and staples can be used.

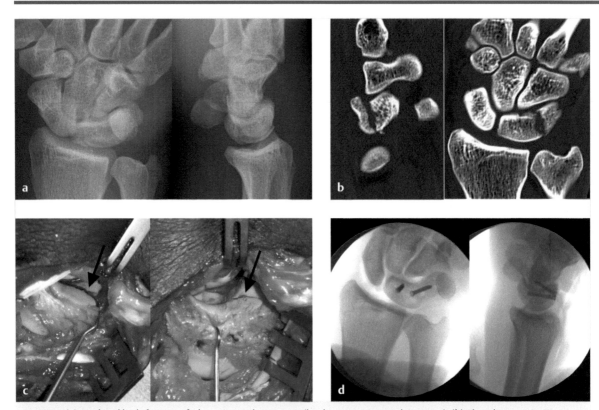

Fig. 27.4 (a) Displaced body fracture of a lunotriquetral synoytosis (hard to recognize on plain X-rays). (b) Clear diagnosis in CT scan. (c) Open reduction and screw fixation (*arrows* show fracture line before and after reduction). (d) X-ray after surgery.

27.2.9 Prognosis

The prognosis of the cortical dorsal chip fractures is good. Höcker and Menschik[5] published a series of 65 patients where conservative treatment with immobilization for 3 weeks was successful after a mean period of 47 months.

For the body fractures, due to the small number of cases, exist no reliable data. If joined surface is restored smoothly, prognosis will be good as well.

In fracture dislocations of the carpus, prognosis is determinated less by the fracture then by the carpal ligament injury.

27.3 Fracture of the Pisiform

27.3.1 Trauma Mechanism

Pisiform fractures are rare fractures with a frequency of about 2% of carpal fractures. Most of them caused by a direct blow or a fall on the outstretched hand.[6] The pisiform is a special carpal bone because it is the only one which is not integrated in the carpus and actually a sesamoid bone of the flexor carpi ulnaris (FCU) tendon. So, fracture can occur either due to direct force to the bone or due to traction of the FCU tendon while the pisiform bone is compressed against the triquetrum during the fall on the outstretched hand.

27.3.2 Classification

Four different types of pisiform fractures were distinguished. First is the transverse fracture of the pisiform; second is the parasagittal fracture line; third is the comminuted fracture; and the 4th is the impression fracture of the pisiform into the triquetrum.

27.3.3 Clinical Signs and Tests

The pisiform bone can easily be palpated on the palmar surface of the wrist close to the ulnar side of the distal flexion crease of the wrist and in the course of the FCU tendon. Pressure on the palmar surface leads to pain. Also pushing the pisiform from ulnar to radial while shifting it over the triquetrum courses usually pain.

27.3.4 Investigatory Examinations

Standard X-ray of the wrist in two planes are usually not appropriate to detect the pisiform fracture. The typical clinic in pain should directly trigger the special view 40 degrees supination compared to the true lateral view (▶Fig. 27.5). In X-ray view, the pisiform bone is free from overlapping of other bones and the diagnosis can usually be made without further investigations. Only in the rare case of an unclear situation, a CT scan can be performed.

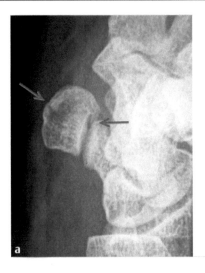
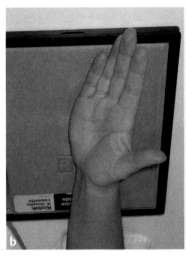

Fig. 27.5 Pisiform fractures can best be diagnosed by an oblique X-ray in 40-degree supination. (a) X-ray with fracture (red arrows). (b) Position of the hand for X-ray of the pisiform.

27.3.5 Possible Concurrent Lesions

Potentially, there can be a rupture of the FCU tendon, but this is really a rare condition.

27.3.6 Evidence

There are only about 200 pisiform fractures, which are published in the literature, so we cannot find reliable evidence.

27.3.7 Author's Favored Treatment Option

In nondisplaced fracture, I treat with a forearm cast with free MCP joints and thumb for 4 weeks. After removal of the cast and X-ray, control gradually loading is usually possible even if there is some tenderness projection of the passive form during the following weeks. In these cases, physiotherapy is usually not required.

In displaced fractures, and fractures with comminution of the joint surface, I excise the pisiform. I use an angular incision over the palmar aspect of the pisiform. After neurolysis and protection of the ulnar nerve, the FCU tendon is longitudinally split and the pisiform is removed in the subperiosteal layer. The longitudinal split of FCU tendon is sutured with an absorbable running suture. The wrist is immobilized for 3 weeks.

27.3.8 Alternative Treatment Options

In nondisplaced fracture, there is no alternative to immobilization of the wrist.

In simple fractures, open reduction end fixation of bone could be an option.

27.3.9 Prognosis

The results after conservative treatment end usually in bony union and are usually good.

In cases of pisiform excision, Carroll and Coyle[7] reported about good outcome with free function regarding the FCU tendon as well.

27.4 Fracture of the Lunate

27.4.1 Trauma Mechanism

Lunate fractures are really a very rare condition and are responsible for not more than 1% of the carpal fractures.[8] If we see a fracture of the lunate, we should always be aware that most of the fractures of the lunate are caused by the Kienböck's disease (▶ Fig. 27.6). Another condition, which is not really a lunate fracture, is the bony avulsion of the dorsal scapholunate (SL) ligament, which looks like a small fracture, but indeed is the SL rupture which leads to malalignment of the carpus with dorsal intercalated segmental instability (DISI) deformity. Because of this fact and the classification of five different acute fracture types, there is no typical trauma mechanism defined. So, there can be shear, compression, and hyperextension forces.

27.4.2 Classification

According to Teisen and Hjarbaek,[8] there exists a classification of five types of lunate fractures:
  Type I: palmar pole fracture
  Type II: osteochondral chip fracture
  Type III: dorsal pole fracture
  Type IV: sagittal fracture
  Type V: transverse fracture

27.4.3 Clinical Signs and Tests

Pain over the the middle part of the wrist especially on the dorsal side with increase while moving or loading.

27.4.4 Investigatory Examinations

Standard X-rays of the wrist in AP and true lateral view are the basic instruments of diagnosis. If there is suspicion

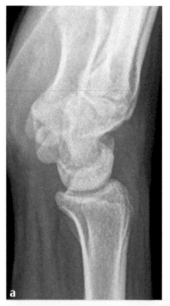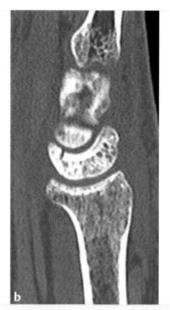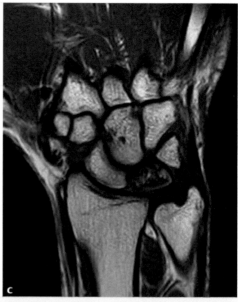

Fig. 27.6 Lunate fractures must not be mixed up with Kienböck's disease. **(a)** X-ray **(b)** CT scan, and **(c)** MRI help making the diagnosis.

of lunate fracture, CT scan and magnetic resonance imaging (MRI) should both be performed to rule out a Kienböck disease or carpal instability.

27.4.5 Possible Concurrent Lesions

Acute fractures should not be mixed up with bony SL lesions or Kienböck's disease.

27.4.6 Evidence

Because of the small number of fractures, we have no evidence about different treatment options.

27.4.7 Author's Favored Treatment Option

First of all, I would like to emphasize again the importance of excluding Kienköck's disease and SL instability, because in these cases we have to follow the guidelines which are valid for these conditions.

In nondisplaced fractures, nonoperative treatment with casting for 4 to 6 weeks in a forearm cast is my preferred treatment. In these nondisplaced fractures, physiotherapy is only prescribed if rehabilitation can't be accomplished by the patient himself in a successful manner.

In dislocated fractures of the lunate, open reduction and internal fixation is necessary depending on the type of fracture. You can use a dorsal approach between third and fourth external compartment or in the palmar pole fracture an extended approach to the carpal tunnel which gives direct access to the volar pole of the lunate. For fixation, I use mini screws or small headless screws (▶Fig. 27.7).

Also, in surgically stabilized fractures, I apply a cast for 4 weeks after surgery to ensure that patients will not load the wrist too early.

27.4.8 Alternative Treatment Options

Concerning the fixation of the fragments, small K-wires can also be used.

Earlier mobilization after internal fixation is generally possible. However, care must be taken that patients don't load their wrists too early and develop nonunions in the critical perfused carpal bone.

27.4.9 Prognosis

Potential complications are nonunion, osteonecrosis, and osteoarthritis.

Because of the limited number of cases, there exist no reliable data about the prognosis. However, if the diagnosis is made correctly and the fracture is treated in the proposed way, usually bone healing can be expected.

27.5 Fracture of the Trapezium

27.5.1 Trauma Mechanism

The frequency of the trapezium fracture is 1 to 5% of all carpal fractures. Located between the first metacarpal and the carpus, the trapezium is generally well protected. So, usually only major indirect forces lead to a fracture of this bone. In these cases, the main forces are external compression forces and shear forces of the thumb. Depending on this, forces of different fracture types can occur.

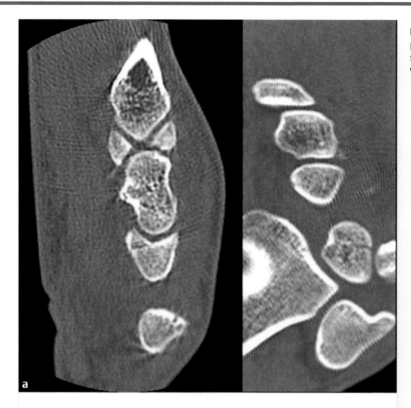

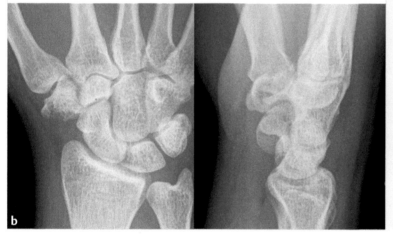

Fig. 27.7 Combined fracture of palmar pole of the lunate and scaphoid **(a)** in CT scan. **(b)** X-ray after fixation from palmar with headless screws.

27.5.2 Classification

Classification by Walker and colleagues[9]:

Type 1: vertical transarticular fractures
Type 2: horizontal fractures
Type 3: fractures of the dorsal radial tuberosity
Type 4: fractures of the medial ridge
Type 5: comminuted fractures

The most frequent type is the vertical transarticular fracture pattern.

27.5.3 Clinical Signs and Tests

We find swelling and hematoma over the CMC 1 joint with pain when this joint is moved. The pinch grip is painful and the power for this grip is reduced.

27.5.4 Investigatory Examinations

The base of diagnostics is the AP and lateral X-ray view of the wrist. Like in Bennett's fractures, a pronated AP view gives a good insight into the joint space. If there is any doubt, CT scan is recommended. Even if we detect the fracture in the plain X-rays, only CT scan gives us an impression of the 3D situation of the fracture at trapezium (▶Fig. 27.8). This is also very helpful for planning the surgery.

27.5.5 Possible Concurrent Lesions

Trapezium fractures are rare. Mostly they are combined with other fractures, in the majority with distal radius or metacarpal fractures and especially together with the Bennett fracture.

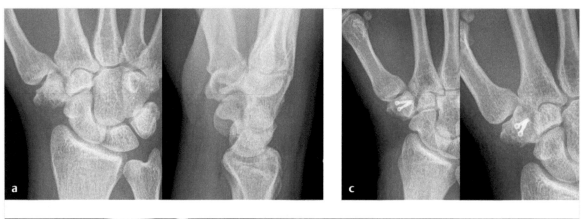

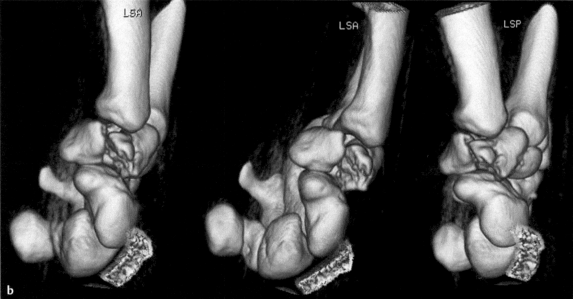

Fig. 27.8 (a) On plain X-rays, the amount of displacement is not clear. (b) On CT 3D reconstruction, the real severe displacement of the intra-articular trapezium fracture is visible. (c) After open reduction and screw fixation.

27.5.6 Evidence

There are no studies comparing different treatment options, probably because of the rarity of the fractures.

27.5.7 Author's Favored Treatment Option

Nondisplaced fractures can be treated in a cast including the thumb up to the interphalangeal (IP) joint like the typical scaphoid forearm cast. However, most of the trapezium fractures are dislocated. I prefer open reduction and internal fixation with screws or K-wires. I only use close reduction and can wire fixation in cases of easy fractures if I can be sure that the joint surface is definitely congruent after reduction.

However, in the majority of trapezium fractures, I use an open approach from palmar to address the fracture.

The incision is longitudinal to the first metacarpal and at the proximal thenar, the incision runs in 90 degrees in palmar direction in projection of the CMC 1 joint. After elevating, the skin care must be taken not to damage sensory nerves. Afterward, the thenar muscle is elevated from proximally to distally and the trapezium with the CMC 1 joint is exposed. From this approach, reduction with the safe reconstruction of the joint surface of CMC 1 joint is possible. For fixation, I use small screws in the case of two main fragments or K-wires in more comminuted situations with multiple fragments (▶ Fig. 27.9). In comminuted trapezium fractures, I also like to drill a K-wire as transfixation through the base of the first metacarpal and the second one. Transfixation remains for 4 weeks and ensures absolute immobilization and unloading of CMC 1 joint. Immobilization of the fracture depends on the stability of the fixation and ends usually between 4 and 6 weeks after surgery.

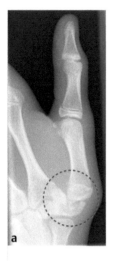
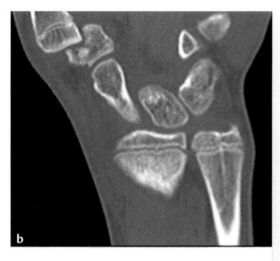

Fig. 27.9 (a) Trapezium impression fracture (b) confirmed in CT. (c) After open reduction and interal fixation with K-wires and transfixation. (d) Reconstructed trapezium and joint after K-wire removal.

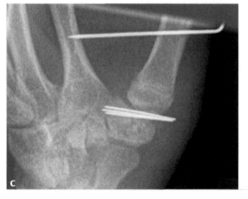
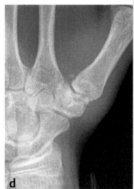

27.5.8 Alternative Treatment Options

Some authors prefer close reduction and K-wire fixation and others prefer more open reduction and screw fixation.

Excision of small fragments, especially if they were not united, is possible.

27.5.9 Prognosis

Most of the series which are published are small or case reports. The reports of nondisplaced or well-reduced trapezium fractures (open or closed) show a good prognosis. McGuigan and Culp reported about a case series of 11 patients with an articular displacement over 2 mm which had a good clinical outcome. However, 5 of 11 patients show secondary osteoarthritis in the CMC 1 joint 47 months after trauma.[10] So, even if we have no evidence in these special subgroup of carpal bones, it seems to be advisable to restore the articular surface like in other joints as good as possible.

27.6 Fracture of Capitate

27.6.1 Trauma Mechanism

Fractures of the capitate accounts for approximately 1 to 2% of carpal bone fractures.[11] The rarity of this fracture is most probably related to its protected position in the center of the carpus. Different trauma mechanisms are possible and can lead to different fracture types. Hyperextension of the carpus can lead to not only transverse body fractures but also fractures due to distal pressure of the third metacarpal or a direct blow occurs as well.

During a forced hyperextension, the capitate may strike against the dorsal edge of the radius, and further bending forces may then result in a transverse fracture with separation of the proximal pole. The distal fragment of the capitate dislocates posteriorly and during retraction to palmar, it can rotate the broken proximal capitate pole 180 degrees. This results in a typical malposition of the proximal pole, which points with the fracture surface to the lunate and with the articular surface distally (▶ Fig. 27.10).[12]

Another manifestation of capitate fracture is the combination of a capitate fracture with a scaphoid fracture as the transscaphoid transcapitate perilunate fracture dislocation.[13] This is usually caused by a high-energy trauma. These injuries are primary carpal instabilities classified according to the Mayo Classification as carpal instability complex (CIC).

27.6.2 Classification

Capitate fractures can be classified as follows:
• Transverse fracture of the body.
• Transverse fracture of the proximal pole.

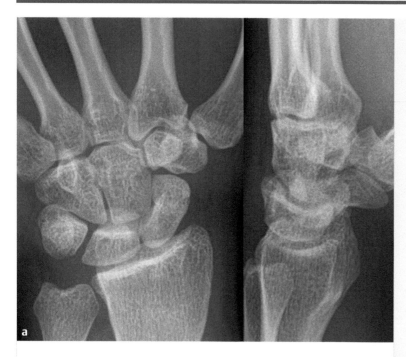

Fig. 27.10 Proximal pole fracture of the capitate with displacement and rotation of the proximal pole fragment. **(a)** No evidence in the X-rays. **(b)** Diagnosis with CT scan. **(c, d)** Fixation with screws in CT scan and X-ray after surgery.

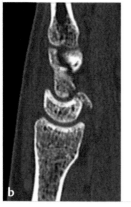
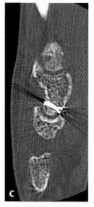
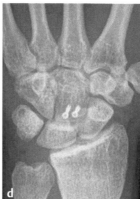

- Coronal oblique fracture.
- Parasagittal fracture.

27.6.3 Clinical Signs and Tests

There are no special signs or clinical tests for capitate fractures. They usually show pain and swelling and inability of motion or restricted range of motion of the wrist. In nondisplaced fractures, sometimes mild pain in the center of the wrist is the only clinical finding.

27.6.4 Investigatory Examinations

X-rays of the wrist in AP, lateral, and oblique view are the first step in making the diagnosis. If there is the suspicion of capitate fracture, next diagnostic tool to be used is the CT scan. Nondisplaced capitate fractures with mild symptoms which cannot be seen in plain X-rays are sometimes incidental findings in MRI (▶ Fig. 27.11).

27.6.5 Possible Concurrent Lesions

Capitate fractures, can occur with the scaphoid fracture, has transscaphoid transcapitate perlunate dislocations.[13]

27.6.6 Evidence

Because of the small number of cases, we don't have any evidence for treatment options.

27.6.7 Author's Favored Treatment Option

I usually treat nondisplaced capitate fractures nonoperatively, with a forearm cast with free MP joints and free thumb for 4 weeks. Before conservative treatment, I usually perform a CT scan to be sure that the fracture is nondisplaced.

I operate displaced fractures with open reduction and internal fixation. From a dorsal approach, it is easily

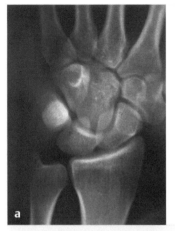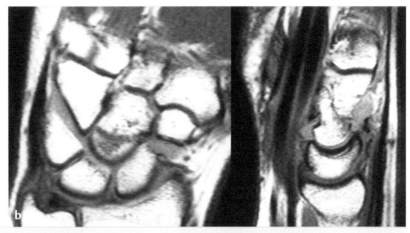

Fig. 27.11 Nondisplaced coronal oblique fracture of capitate as incidental finding in MRI. **(a)** X-ray. **(b)** Only MRI confirms a fracture.

accessible. If possible, I use headless bone screws like the Herbert screw. An urgent indication for surgery is the dislocated transverse proximal pole fracture, because it can end up in an avascular necrosis of the proximal capitate pole.

27.6.8 Alternative Treatment Options

Depending on the size of the fragments also, wires or mini screws can be used for fixation. Disadvantage of the K-wires is that they have to be removed, but the cost of the implant is lower.

In greater arc injuries, closed reduction and arthroscopically assisted percutaneous screw fixation is another option.

27.6.9 Prognosis

Most of the capitate fractures heal uneventfully, especially the nondisplaced fractures.

Care must be taken regarding the transverse proximal pole fractures. The proximal pole is nearly completely covered with cartilage. A dislocation of this pole leads to minor blood supply or nonperfusion of the fractured pole similarly as in scaphoid fractures. So, in these cases, risk of nonunion is higher and should be checked by X-ray examination during follow-up. Also, osteonecrosis of the proximal pole is possible.

27.7 Fracture of Hamate
27.7.1 Trauma Mechanism

In the literature, the hamate fracture is described only with a frequency of 2%. In comparison to the other carpal fractures, this seems to me to be a relatively minor amount. Maybe these figures do not cover all the hamate fractures that occur together with CMC dislocations. The

two main mechanisms of injury are once for the body fracture of the hamate the axial force through the fourth and fifth metacarpal base and on the other hand for the hook of hamate the direct blow against the proximal palmar palm of the hand. The hook of hamate is relatively prominent to the palmar side of the hand and is at risk when falling on the outstretched hand. Athletes who swing a racket, club, or bat (tennis, golf, baseball) have a greater risk of hook of hamate fracture. In these cases, repeated trauma is a potential cause. In our Hand Surgery department, the hamate fractures occur most frequently as additional injury in CMC dislocations of the fourth and fifth meatacarpal (▶ Fig. 27.12).

27.7.2 Classification

The two main categories of the hamate fractures are the body fracture and the fracture of the hook of hamate.

The fractures of the hook of hamate are subdivided into fractures of the of the tip, the waist, and the base of the hook.[14]

The fractures of the body have four types: There is the dorsal coronal fracture which usually appears with the 4, 5 CMC fracture dislocation. Furthermore, there are fractures of the proximal pole, medial tuberosity, and sagittal oblique fractures.

27.7.3 Clinical Signs and Tests

In fractures of the hook of hamate, you usually find the local pain and a tender spot exactly over the tip of the hook of hamate on the palmar side of the hand. Since the flexor tendons use the hook of hamate as a pulley, forceful finger flexion against resistance in an ulnar deviated wrist position usually increases pain. The clinical findings show in series of Kadar et al,[15] a higher sensitivity than the carpal tunnel view X-ray.

Regarding the body fractures, pain and swelling is located dorsally over the hamate, which can easily be found by localizing the CMC 5 joint by gentle passive

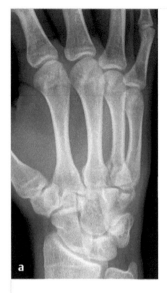
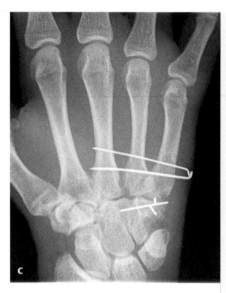
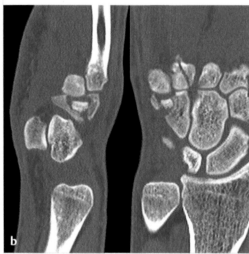

Fig. 27.12 Impression fracture of the hamate in combination with fracture dislocation of carpal base 4/5. **(a)** Oblique X-ray shows fracture of fourth metacarpal and impression of hamate. **(b)** CT scan reveals the severity of the injury. **(c)** After open reduction and transfixation of the metacarpals.

motion of the fifth metacarpal from palmar to dorsal. In cases which are combined with CMC 4 and 5 dislocations, the clinical aspect is determined by the dislocation or fracture dislocation.

27.7.4 Investigatory Examinations

For hook of hamate fractures, X-rays of the wrist are of low significance.[16] Usually, the hook of hamate can be seen as an elliptically contour in AP view of the wrist. If it is not detectable, it could be suspicious of a fracture. Carpal tunnel views were the main diagnostic tool in the pre-CT era. However, today the CT scan is the best imaging technique to make the diagnosis of a hook of hamate fracture.

The body fractures can often be found already in the X-ray AP view of the wrist. X-rays in AP view, lateral and oblique view should be the first diagnostic measures. To confirm the suspicion of a fracture and to get an accurate idea of the fracture, also with regard to surgery, CT is the best further investigation. MRI is usually not necessary.

27.7.5 Possible Concurrent Lesions

Because dorsal coronal fractures of the hamate almost always occur along with CMC 4/5 dislocation, one should always be aware of these dislocation in that fracture type.

The motor branch of the ulnar nerve and the concomitant deep branch of the ulnar artery are in very close vicinity of the base of the hook and the palmar surface of the body of the hamate. So, both can be at risk if the hamate is injured or the whole hook is excised as well.

Body fractures can be associated with a perilunate greater arc lesion.

27.7.6 Evidence

Regarding hook of hamate fractures, Kadar et al[15] reviewed 51 patients where the diagnosis was made with advanced imaging within 27 days. The group with nonoperative treatment developed a nonunion in 24%, while in the operative group no nonunions occured. However, concerning the clinical results there was no significant difference.

If the hook of hamate is resected in symptomatic non-unions, most series has published more than 90% good results.[17,18] However, arguments for preserving the hook of hamate also exist. The hook acts as a pulley at the ulnar border of the carpal tunnel that directs the flexor tendons of fifth and fourth finger from the palm to the forearm, especially in ulnar inclination of the wrist. So, after resection, maximum power could be reduced.[18] If a nonunion exists at the base of the hook of hamate, the flexor tendons 4 and 5 can rupture in the long term due to a chronic attrition at the sharp edges of the nonunion.

27.7.7 Author's Favored Treatment Option

For nondisplaced fractures of the hook of hamate and body fractures of the hamate as well, I prefer a nonoperatively treatment with a forearm cast for 4 weeks.

In displaced fractures of the hamate, I tend to open reduction and internal fixation with the cannulated Herbert screw if the base is involved. I prefer especially in younger patients to maintain maximum power and avoid flexor tendon rupture, which I have already seen in two of these patients with nonunion at the base. With the advanced image technique, it is possible today to make the diagnosis in due time and perform primary stabilization of these fractures, which is not a very difficult operation. Via a carpal tunnel incision, the tip of the hook of hamate at the border of the carpal tunnel can be easily accessible and through carpal tunnel, the reduction of the base of the hook can be easily controlled. Thanks to cannulated headless screw technique, also internal fixation is uncomplicated.

In displaced fractures, only of the tip of the hook, I also prefer nonoperative treatment, because later excision of the tip of the hamate, if necessary, has no biomechanical influence to the power grip.

In displaced body fractures, I use an open dorsal approach with opening of the distal fifth extensor compartment. Because usually the distal joint surface is involved, I open the fourth and/or fifth CMC joint to control proper reduction. Depending on the fracture, it could also be necessary to check the midcarpal joint surface of the hamate (▶Fig. 27.13). In coronal fractures, I

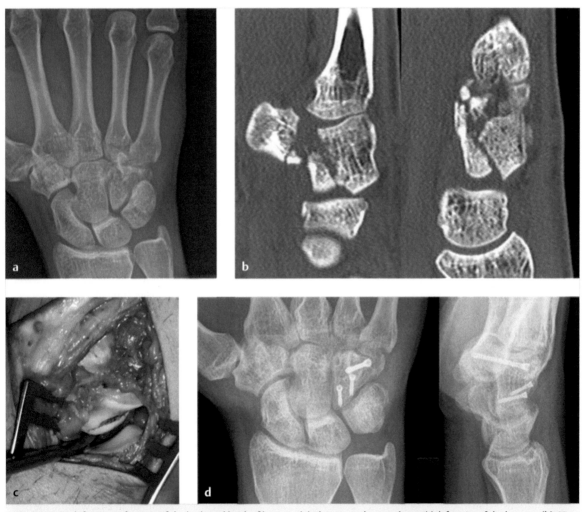

Fig. 27.13 Multifragment fracture of the body and hook of hamate. **(a)** Plain X-ray shows only a mild deformity of the hamate. **(b)** CT scan reveals the severe fracture type. **(c)** Reduced hamate joint surface from dorsal **(d)** postoperative X-rays.

use mini screws and cannulated mini headless screws for fixation. In small fragments, K-wires are an alternative. If the situation especially close to the CMC joint is rather comminuted, I secure the bone fixation with a transfixation of the fifth and fourth metacarpal horizontally then the third metacarpal. Thus, the pressure on the hamate is reduced. I leave the transfixation for 4 to 6 weeks.

27.7.8 Alternative Treatment Options

Closed reduction and percutaneous K-wire fixation is an alternative. I use this technique only in CMC dislocations with small dorsal shear fractures which is reduced properly with the CMC joint under fluoroscopy.

Some authors recommend the excision of the hook of hamate in any case independent from the location of the fracture, that means, even if the fracture is located at the base as well and report about good results.[19]

27.7.9 Prognosis

Prognosis of fractures of the hook and body of hamate is good if not displaced.

Displaced fractures of the hook have shown in different case series good clinical results even if there is a remarkable number of nonunions after nonoperative treatment.[15,19,20]

The prognosis depends on the diagnosis in due time and correct restoration of height and articular surfaces of the hamate.

References

[1] Dunn AW. Fractures and dislocations of the carpus. Surg Clin North Am. 1972; 52(6):1513–1538
[2] Auffray Y. [Fractures of the pyramidal bone. Study of 72 cases] Acta Orthop Belg. 1970; 36(3):313–345
[3] Garcia-Elias M. Carpal instability. In: Wolfe SW, Hotchkiss RN, Pederson PC, Kozin SH, eds. Green's Operative Hand Surgery. 6th ed. Philadelphia, PA: Elsevier Churchill Livingstone; 2011:465–522
[4] Levy M, Fischel RE, Stern GM, Goldberg I. Chip fractures of the os triquetrum: the mechanism of injury. J Bone Joint Surg Br. 1979; 61-B(3):355–357
[5] Höcker K, Menschik A. Chip fractures of the triquetrum. Mechanism, classification and results. J Hand Surg [Br]. 1994; 19(5):584–588
[6] McCarty V, Farber H. Isolated fracture of the pisiform bone. J Bone Joint Surg Am. 1946; 28:390
[7] Carroll RE, Coyle MP, Jr. Dysfunction of the pisotriquetral joint: treatment by excision of the pisiform. J Hand Surg Am. 1985; 10(5):703–707
[8] Teisen H, Hjarbaek J. Classification of fresh fractures of the lunate. J Hand Surg [Br]. 1988; 13(4):458–462
[9] Walker JL, Greene TL, Lunseth PA. Fractures of the body of the trapezium. J Orthop Trauma. 1988; 2(1):22–28
[10] McGuigan FX, Culp RW. Surgical treatment of intra-articular fractures of the trapezium. J Hand Surg Am. 2002; 27(4):697–703
[11] Adler JB, Shaftan GW. Fractures of the capitate. J Bone Joint Surg Am. 1962; 44-A:1537–1547
[12] Stein F, Siegel MW. Naviculocapitate fracture syndrome. A case report: new thoughts on the mechanism of injury. J Bone Joint Surg Am. 1969; 51(2):391–395
[13] Fenton RL. The naviculo-capitate fracture syndrome. J Bone Joint Surg Am. 1956; 38-A(3):681–684
[14] Milch H. Fracture of the hamate bone. J Bone Joint Surg Am. 1934; 16:459–462
[15] Kadar A, Bishop AT, Suchyta MA, Moran SL. Diagnosis and management of hook of hamate fractures. J Hand Surg Eur Vol. 2017:1753193417729603
[16] Carroll RE, Lakin JF. Fracture of the hook of the hamate: radiographic visualization. Iowa Orthop J. 1993; 13:178–182
[17] Stark HH, Chao EK, Zemel NP, Rickard TA, Ashworth CR. Fracture of the hook of the hamate. J Bone Joint Surg Am. 1989; 71(8):1202–1207
[18] Watson HK, Rogers WD. Nonunion of the hook of the hamate: an argument for bone grafting the nonunion. J Hand Surg Am. 1989; 14(3):486–490
[19] Aldridge JM, III, Mallon WJ. Hook of the hamate fractures in competitive golfers: results of treatment by excision of the fractured hook of the hamate. Orthopedics. 2003; 26(7):717–719
[20] Smith P, III, Wright TW, Wallace PF, Dell PC. Excision of the hook of the hamate: a retrospective survey and review of the literature. J Hand Surg Am. 1988; 13(4):612–615

Index

Note: Page numbers set **bold** or *italic* indicate headings or figures, respectively.

A

Anterolateral thigh flap (ALT), in compound hand injuries 87, *88*
Arthroscopic surgery
- in metacarpal fractures 209
- in scaphoid fractures **75**, *76, 77, 78, 79, 80*
- in scapholunate injuries 119
Athletes
- capitate fractures in **117**
- carpal fractures in **113**
- hamate fractures in **115**
- lunate fractures in **117**
- metacarpal fractures in **112**, *113*
- phalangeal fractures in
-- intra-articular **109**, *110*, *111*
-- shaft **110**
- pisiform fractures in **116**
- scaphoid fractures in **113**, *114*, *115*
- scapholunate injuries in **118**, *119*
- trapezium fractures in **116**
- trapezoid fractures in **117**
- triquetral fractures in **116**

B

Bagpipes *129*
Bennett's fracture 5, *6*
- K-wire fixation in **34**, *35*
- osteosynthesis in 209
- reduction in 208
- subluxations, nonoperative treatment of **24**, *25*
Biomechanical results, in evidence-based medicine **13**
Bone necrosis
- as complication **140**
- causes **140**
- surgical indications **140**
- surgical treatment **140**
Bones
- carpal *8*
- metacarpal *4*
- phalangeal *5*
Bone tie 182
Botulinum toxin, paralytic extremity fractures and **103**
Boutonniere fractures 189
Brachial plexus palsy, obstetric, paralytic extremity fractures and **103**
Brass instruments *125*, *126*, *127*
Buddy taping *92*

C

Capitate *8*
Capitate fractures
- classification of **269**
- clinical signs **270**
- concurrent lesions with **270**
- in athletes **117**
- incidence **8**
- investigatory examinations in **270**, *271*
- prognosis **271**
- tests **270**
- trauma mechanism in **269**, *270*
- treatment of **270**
Carpal bones *8*, 261
Carpal fractures 259
  See also Capitate fractures;Hamate fractures;Lunate fractures;Pisiform fractures;Trapezium fractures;Trapezoid fractures

- arthroscopic surgery in **75**, *76, 77, 78, 79, 80*
- diagnosis of 262
- gender in 6
- general considerations with **261**
- in athletes **113**
- incidence **6**, *7*
- in musicians 132, *133*
- K-wire fixation in **34**, *35*
- pediatric **97**
- plate and screw fixation in **51**, *59, 61, 62*
- trauma mechanism in 261, *262*
Carpometacarpal joint (CMC) arthritis, as complication **141**
Casting
- in pediatric hand fractures *92*
Cello *125*
Cembalo *126*
Cerclage wires 259
  See also Intraosseous wiring
- in fracture dislocation around joints **30**, *31*
- in metacarpal fractures **29**
- in phalangeal fractures **29**, *167, 169*
Cerebral palsy, paralytic extremity fractures and **103**
Charcot-Marie-Tooth (CMT) disease **103**
Clarinet *129*
Complications
- bone necrosis as **140**
- infections as **135**
- in intra-articular fractures **141**
- in intramedullary screw placement **46**
- in K-wire fixation **38**, *39*
- in plate and screw fixation **61**
- malunion as **136**
- nonunion as **139**
Compound hand injuries
- bone fixation in **83**, *84, 85, 86*
- classification of **82**
- clinical examination in **81**, *82*
- debridement in **83**
- extensor tendon reconstruction in **86**
- flexor tendon reconstruction in **84**
- imaging in **81**
- nerve reconstruction in **86**
- patient expectation in **81**
- revascularization in **83**
- skin coverage in **87**, *88*
- surgery for **83**
- surgical steps **83**
- timing of treatment of **82**
Conservative treatment **12**, 259
  See also Nonoperative treatment
- in metacarpal fractures, intra-articular, at base of 2 to 5 **197**
- in metacarpal neck fractures **226**, *227*, *228*
- in wrist rehabilitation *153*

D

Debridement, in compound hand injuries **83**
Distal interphalangeal joint (DIP)
- in bony mallet injuries 18, *20*
- in musicians 124, *125*, *126*
- intraosseous wiring in **29**, *93*
Dynamic compression plate (DCP) *48*, 259
  See also Plate and screw fixation

E

Evidence-based medicine (EBM)
- biomechanical results in **13**
- conservative treatment in **12**
- grafts in **13**
- hamate fractures in **272**
- in metacarpal malunion **233**
- in phalangeal malunion **233**
- metacarpal fractures in **11**, **206**
- operative treatment in **12**, **13**
- phalangeal fractures in **11**, **160**, **165**
- recommendations from **12**
- scaphoid fractures in **12**
- scaphoid nonunion in **258**
Extension sleeve, in rehabilitation **150**
Extensor avulsion fractures
- in boutonniere fractures **189**
- in mallet injury **185**, *186*, *187*, *188*, *189*, *190*
Extensor carpi radialis longus avulsion fractures **189**, *190*
Extensor tendon reconstruction, in compound hand injuries **86**
External minifixation
- history of 65
- in comminuted articular fractures 68
- in corrective osteotomies 68
- indications for 65, 66, 67, **68**
- in finger lengthening 68, *69*
- in metacarpal fractures 66, *67*, *68*
- results with **69**
- surgical technique 55, **65**

F

Finger lengthening, external minifixation in 68, *69*
Fixation
- external minifixation
-- history of 65
-- in comminuted articular fractures 68
-- in corrective osteotomies 68
-- indications for 65, 66, 67, **68**
-- in finger lengthening 68, *69*
-- in metacarpal fractures 66, *67*, *68*
-- results with **69**
-- surgical technique 55, **65**
- in compound hand injuries **83**, *84, 85, 86*
- open reduction and internal
-- in base of proximal phalanx **160**, *161*
-- in lunate fractures 266, *267*
-- in metacarpal fractures 200, *201*, *202*, 209, **218**, *219*, *220*, *229*, *230*
-- in musicians 128, *130*
-- in triquetral fractures 263, *264*
Flexor digitorum profundis (FDP) avulsion fractures
- classification of **190**, *191*
- intraosseous wiring in *31*
- prognosis **192**
- surgical options **191**
- trauma mechanism in **190**
Flexor tendon avulsion fracture
- in extensor carpi radialis longus avulsion fractures **189**, *190*
- intraosseous wiring in *31*
Flexor tendon reconstruction, in compound hand injuries **84**

Flossing **148**, *149*
Flute *126*

G

Gender
- in carpal fractures 6
- in metacarpal fractures 3
Grafts
- in evidence-based medicine **13**
- in scaphoid nonunion **254**, *255, 256*, **257**
- nonvascularized vs. vascularized **13**
Guitar *125*, *129*

H

Hamate *8*
Hamate fractures
- classification of **271**
- clinical signs in **271**
- concurrent lesions with **272**
- in athletes **115**
- in evidence-based medicine **272**
- investigatory examinations in **272**
- prognosis **274**
- tests in **271**
- trauma mechanism in **271**, *272*
- treatment of **273**
Home exercises, in rehabilitation **151**, *153*
Horn *125*

I

Imaging
- in capitate fractures **270**, *271*
- in compound hand injuries **81**
- in diaphyseal metacarpal fractures 213
- in hamate fractures **272**
- in intra-articular metacarpal fractures *197*, *198*, **206**, *207*
- in lunate fracture 265
- in metacarpal neck fractures **225**
- in phalangeal base fractures **160**
- in phalangeal extra-articular fractures **164**
- in pisiform fractures **264**, *265*
- in proximal interphalangeal joint fractures *175*, *176*
- in scaphoid fractures 252
- in scaphoid nonunion 251
- in trapezium fractures **267**, *268*
- in triquetral fractures 263
Incidence **3**
- in musicians 123
- of capitate fractures 8
- of carpal fractures **6**, *7*
- of lunate fractures 8
- of metacarpal fractures 3, *4*
-- neck 3
- of phalangeal fractures 3, *4*, *5*
- of pisiform fractures 8
- of scaphoid fractures 7
- of thumb fractures 5
- of trapezium fractures 7
- of trapezoid fractures 8
- of triquetral fractures 7
Infection
- as complication **135**
- causes of **135**

– in K-wire fixation 38
– surgical indications for **135**
– surgical methods with **136**
Intra-articular fractures 259
 See also Bennett's fracture
– complications with **141**
– distal metacarpal 58
– intramedullary screw fixation
 in *42*
– K-wires in 32
– metacarpal
– – at base of 2 to 5
– – – anatomy in **195**
– – – classification of **195**
– – – clinical signs in **196**
– – – investigatory examinations in
 197, *198*
– – – K-wire fixation in **200**, 202
– – – nonoperative treatment of
 197, *198*, *199*
– – – open reduction and internal
 fixation in 200, *201*, *202*
– – – operative treatment of **197**,
 200
– – – tests in **196**
– – – trauma mechanism in **195**,
 196
– – – treatment of **197**, *198*, *199*,
 200
– – at base of first metacarpal
– – – arthroscopic surgery in 209
– – – classification of **205**
– – – clinical signs in 206
– – – in evidence-based medicine
 206
– – – investigatory examinations in
 206, *207*
– – – K-wire fixation in **206**, *208*
– – – open reduction and internal
 fixation in 209
– – – prognosis in **210**
– – – trauma mechanism in **205**
– – proximal **56**, *57*
– – phalangeal
– – in athletes **109**, *110*
– – in musicians *131*
– – in proximal interphalangeal
 joint
– – – bone tie in 182
– – – classification of **175**
– – – clinical signs in **175**
– – – condylar **176**, *177*, *178*, *179*,
 180, *181*, **182**
– – – dorsal lip **177**
– – – external fixation in **182**, *183*
– – – grafting in 183
– – – investigatory examinations in
 175, *176*
– – – K-wire fixation in **181**
– – – lag screws in **180**, *181*
– – – middle phalangeal base **177**,
 179, **180**, *181*, **182**
– – – palmar lip **177**, *179*, **180**
– – – pilon *179*, **180**, *181*, **182**, *183*
– – – prognosis in **183**
– – – tests in **175**
– – – trauma mechanism in **175**,
 176
– – plate and screw fixation in
 52, *55*
Intramedullary nails, in diaphyseal
 metacarpal fractures **216**, *218*
Intramedullary screws
– complications with **46**
– history of **41**
– in diaphyseal metacarpal
 fractures **216**
– indications for **42**
– in distal phalanx **43**
– in metacarpals **44**, *45*
– in middle phalanx **43**
– in proximal phalanx **44**
– intra-articular approach
 for *44*
– postoperative treatment
 with **45**
– surgical technique **42**

– transmetacarpal approach
 for **44**
Intraosseous wiring
– in flexor digitorum profundus
 avulsion 31
– in fracture dislocation around
 joints **30**
– in metacarpal fractures **29**
– in phalangeal fractures **29**
– surgical technique **31**
– theta loop in 29

J

Jamar dynamometer **146**, *147*

K

K-wire fixation
– complications with **38**, *39*
– history of **31**
– in Bennett's fracture **34**, *35*
– in carpal fractures **34**, *35*
– indications for 36
– infection and 38
– in hamate fracture 273
– in mallet fracture **36**, *38*
– in metacarpal fractures 200,
 202, **206**, *208*
– – neck **36**, *37*
– – shaft **36**
– in musicians 129, *131*
– in phalangeal fractures **36**, *37*,
 161, *162*, **166**, *167*, *168*
– in proximal interphalangeal
 joint fracture dislocation **36**,
 38, *181*
– in trapezium fractures **268**,
 269
– technique **32**, *33*
– trocar tip in 31, *32*
– wire design in **31**, *32*

L

Lag screws
– in extra-articular phalangeal
 fracture **167**, *168*
– in intra-articular proximal
 interphalangeal joint fracture
 180, *181*
Lunate 8
Lunate fractures
– classification of **265**
– clinical signs in **265**
– in athletes 117
– incidence 8
– investigatory examinations
 in **265**
– open reduction and internal
 fixation of 266, *267*
– prognosis in **266**
– trauma mechanism in **265**,
 266
– treatment of **266**
Lymphatic drainage, in rehabilitation **148**, *149*, *150*, 153

M

Mallet injuries
– classification of **185**, *186*
– clinical signs in **185**
– flexion vs. hyperextension
 186
– investigations in **185**
– K-wire fixation in **36**, *38*
– nonoperative treatment of **18**,
 19, *20*, *21*, *23*
– prognosis in **189**
– tests in **185**
– trauma mechanism in **185**
– treatment options **186**, *187*,
 188, *189*, *190*

Mallet injury
– extensor avulsion fractures
 in **185**
Malunion
– as complication **136**
– causes of **136**
– in metacarpal fractures
– – acceptable levels of 17, *137*
– – classification of **233**
– – clinical signs in **233**
– – in evidence-based medicine
 233
– – surgical technique in **234**,
 235, *236*
– – surgical timing in **233**
– – tests in **233**
– – trauma mechanism in **233**
– in phalangeal fractures
– – classification of **233**
– – clinical signs in **233**
– – in evidence-based medicine
 233
– – surgical technique in **234**,
 235, *236*
– – surgical timing in **233**
– – tests in **233**
– – trauma mechanism in **233**
– surgical indications for **136**
– surgical methods with **138**,
 139
Metacarpal bones **4**
Metacarpal fractures
– diaphyseal
– – anatomy in **214**
– – classification of **205**
– – clinical signs in **205**
– – concurrent lesions in **214**
– – external fixation of **217**, *219*
– – intramedullary approaches for
 216, *218*
– – intramedullary nails in **216**,
 218
– – intramedullary screws in
 216, *218*
– – investigatory examination
 in **213**
– – long oblique 215
– – nonsurgical treatment of **215**,
 216, *217*
– – open reduction and internal
 fixation of **218**, *219*, *220*
– – pinning in 216
– – prognosis in **220**
– – short oblique 215
– – surgical indications in **214**,
 218
– – surgical treatment of **216**
– – transverse 215
– – trauma mechanism in **213**
– external minifixation in *66*,
 67, *68*
– gender in 3
– in athletes **112**, *113*
– incidence 3, *4*
– in evidence-based medicine
 11
– intra-articular
– – at base of 2 to 5
– – – anatomy in **195**
– – – classification of **195**
– – – clinical signs in **196**
– – – investigatory examinations in
 197, *198*
– – – K-wire fixation in **200**, 202
– – – nonoperative treatment of
 197, *198*, *199*
– – – open reduction and internal
 fixation in 200, *201*, *202*
– – – operative treatment of **197**,
 200
– – – tests in **196**
– – – trauma mechanism in **195**,
 196
– – – treatment of **197**, *198*, *199*,
 200
– – at base of first metacarpal
– – – arthroscopic surgery in 209
– – – classification of **205**

– – – clinical signs in **206**
– – – in evidence-based medicine
 206
– – – investigatory examinations in
 206, *207*
– – – K-wire fixation in **206**, *208*
– – – open reduction and internal
 fixation in 209
– – – prognosis in **210**
– – – trauma mechanism in **205**
– – intramedullary screws in 42,
 44, *45*
– – intraosseous wiring in **29**
– malunion in
– – acceptable levels of 17, *137*
– – classification of **233**
– – clinical signs in **233**
– – in evidence-based medicine
 233
– – limits in 17, *137*
– – surgical technique in **234**,
 235, *236*
– – surgical timing in **233**
– – tests in **233**
– – trauma mechanism in **233**
– neck
– – angulation measurement
 in **225**
– – bouquet pinning in 229
– – classification of **223**, *224*
– – clinical signs in **223**, *224*
– – concurrent lesions in
 226
– – conservative treatment of
 226, *227*, *228*
– – incidence 3
– – K-wire fixation in **36**, *37*
– – open reduction and internal
 fixation of **229**, *230*
– – operative treatment of **227**,
 228, *229*
– – prognosis in **230**
– – radiography in **225**
– – reduction in 228
– – shortening measurement
 in **225**
– – tests in **223**
– – trauma mechanism in
 223
– nonoperative treatment of
– – finger transverse **16**, *17*
– – long oblique **15**, *17*
– – spiral **15**, *16*, *17*
– pediatric **96**
– plate and screw fixation in
 51, **56**
– – in comminuted fractures **56**
– – in distal intra-articular metacarpal fracture **58**
– – in first metacarpal fractures
 58, *59*, *60*
– – in long oblique fractures **56**
– – in proximal intra-articular
 fractures **56**, *57*
– – in short oblique fractures
 56, *57*
– – in subcapital fractures **58**
– – in transverse fractures **56**
– – rehabilitation in **154**, *155*
– – shaft, K-wire fixation in **36**
– – spiral
– – intraosseous wiring in 30
– – nonoperative treatment of
 15, *16*, *17*
Metacarpophalangeal joint (MP)
– in musicians 124, *125*, *126*
– thumb, avulsion fractures of
 22, *24*
Mirror therapy **149**, *150*
Musicians
– emotional consequences of
 hand injury in 124
– general principles with **128**
– incidence of hand fractures
 in 123
– instruments used by **124**
– surgical planning with 128,
 129

N

Nerve reconstruction, in compound hand injuries **86**
Nonoperative treatment
- in evidence-based medicine **12**
- of Bennett's fracture subluxation **24**, *25*
- of bony mallet injuries **18**, *19, 20, 21, 23*
- of metacarpal fractures
-- finger transverse **16**, *17*
-- long oblique **15**, *17*
-- spiral **15**, *16, 17*
- of phalangeal fractures
-- collateral ligament avulsion **18**, *19*
-- in base of middle phalanx **21**, *22*
- of thumb fractures
-- metacarpophalangeal avulsion **22**
-- radial collateral ligament injuries in **24**
-- ulnar collateral ligament injuries in **22**, *23*
Nonunion
- arthroscopy in **73**, *76*
- as complication **139**
- capitate **117**
- carpal, in musicians *132*
- causes **139**
- external minifixation in **68**
- plate and screw fixation in **48**, *50*
- scaphoid
-- classification of **250**
-- clinical signs in **251**
-- dysvascular **253**
-- fibrous, without deformity **251**
-- fixation and grafting in **254**, *255, 256*
-- iliac crest graft in **256**
-- imaging in **251**, *252*
-- in athletes **113**
-- in evidence-based medicine **258**
-- medial femoral condyle graft in *257*
-- natural history of **249**, *250*
-- pedicled graft in *257*
-- percutaneous fixation and grafting in **254**
-- prognosis in **258**
-- proximal pole **253**
-- salvage procedures in **258**
-- surgical techniques for **254**
-- tests in **251**
-- trauma mechanism in **249**
-- treatment indications **251**
-- waist, and humpback deformity **252**, *253*
- scaphoid, in musicians *133*
- surgical indications for **139**
- surgical treatment of **139**
- trapezium **117**
- triquetral, in athletes **116**

O

Oboe *126, 127, 129*
Obstetrical brachial plexus palsy, paralytic extremity fractures and **103**
Open reduction and internal fixation (ORIF)
- in base of proximal phalanx **160**, *161*
- in lunate fractures *266, 267*
- in metacarpal fractures *200, 201, 202, 209*, **218**, *219, 220*, **229**, *230*
- in musicians *128, 130*

-- in triquetral fractures *263, 264*
Operative treatment, in evidence-based medicine **12**, *13*
Osteomyelitis *259*
See also Infection
Osteoporosis, paralytic extremity injury and *102*, **104**

P

Paralytic extremity fractures
- and bone changes in paralysis **101**
- basic science of **101**
- botulinum toxin and **103**
- calcium homeostasis and *102*
- cerebral palsy and **103**
- Charcot-Marie-Tooth disease and **103**
- diagnosis of **105**
- epidemiology of **104**
- lower motor neuron lesions and **103**
- management of **105**
- obstetrical brachial plexus palsy and **103**
- osteoporosis and *102*
- prevention of **104**
- spinal cord injury and **101**
- stroke and **103**
Pediatric hand fractures
- age in *91*
- buddy taping in *92*
- carpal *97*
- casting in *92*
- diagnosis of *92*
- frequency of *91*
- metacarpal *96*
- phalangeal
-- neck **94**, *95, 96*
-- proximal **95**, *97*
- physes in *91*
- scaphoid *97, 98*
- Seymour's fracture in *92, 93, 94*
- tuft fractures in *94*
Percussion instruments *126, 127, 129*
Phalangeal bones *5*
Phalangeal fractures
- at base of proximal
-- classification of **159**
-- clinical signs in **159**
-- comminuted *160*
-- concurrent lesions in *160*
-- displaced *160*
-- in evidence-based medicine **160**
-- investigatory examinations in **160**
-- K-wire fixation in *161, 162*
-- metaphyseal *160*
-- open reduction and internal fixation of *160, 161*
-- prognosis in **161**
-- tests in **159**
-- trauma mechanism in **159**
- extra-articular
-- cerclage wire in **167**, *169*
-- classification of **163**
-- clinical signs in **164**
-- comminuted **170**, *171*
-- concurrent lesions in **164**
-- conservative treatment of *165*
-- distal **171**
-- in evidence-based medicine **165**
-- investigatory examinations in **164**
-- K-wire fixation in **166**, *167, 168*
-- lag screws in **167**, *168*
-- malrotated **171**, *172*
-- metaphyseal **170**, *171*
-- plates in **167**
-- prognosis **173**

-- proximal **169**
-- shaft **171**
-- spiral **169**, *170*
-- tests in **164**
-- transverse **170**
-- trauma mechanism in **163**, *166*
-- tuft **171**
-- undisplaced **169**
- in athletes
-- intra-articular **109**, *110, 111*
-- shaft **110**, *111, 112*
- incidence *3, 4, 5*
- in evidence-based medicine **11**
-- intraosseous wiring in **29**
- K-wire fixation in **36**, *37*
- malunion in
-- classification of **233**
-- clinical signs in **233**
-- in evidence-based medicine **233**
-- surgical technique in **234**, *235, 236*
-- surgical timing in **233**
-- tests in **233**
-- trauma mechanism in **233**
- nonoperative treatment of
-- collateral ligament avulsion **18**, *19*
-- in base of middle phalanx **21**, *22*
- pediatric
-- in neck **94**, *95, 96*
-- proximal **95**, *97*
- plate and screw fixation in *50, 51*, **52**
-- in bony avulsions *55*
-- in comminuted diaphyseal fractures **53**
-- in condylar fractures **54**
-- in distal phalanx **52**
-- in dorsal avulsion fractures *55*
-- in long oblique fractures *52*
-- in middle phalanx **52**
-- in proximal phalanx **52**
-- in short oblique fracture **52**, *53*
-- in transverse fracture **52**
-- in volar fractures *55*
- rehabilitation of **154**, *155, 156*
Pisiform *8*
Pisiform fractures
- classification of **264**
- clinical signs in **264**
- concurrent lesions in **265**
- in athletes **116**
- incidence *8*
- investigatory examinations in **264**, *265*
- prognosis in **265**
- tests in **264**
- trauma mechanism in **264**
- treatment of **265**
Plate and screw fixation
- complications in **61**
- history of **47**
- implants in **47**
- in bony avulsions *55*
- in carpal fractures *51*, **59**, *61, 62*
- in comminuted diaphyseal fractures **53**
- in condylar fractures **54**
- indications for **51**
- in distal phalanx **52**
- in dorsal avulsion fractures *55*
- in long oblique fractures *52*
- in metacarpal fractures *51*, **56**
- in comminuted fractures **56**
- in distal intra-articular metacarpal fracture **58**
-- in first metacarpal fractures **58**, *59, 60*
-- in long oblique fractures **56**

-- in proximal intra-articular fractures **56**, *57*
-- in short oblique fractures **56**, *57*
-- in subcapital fractures **58**
-- in transverse fractures **56**
- in metacarpal malunion **234**, *235, 236*
- in middle phalanx **52**
- in phalangeal fractures *50, 51*, **52**, *167*
- in phalangeal malunion **234**, *235, 236*
- in proximal phalanx **52**
- in short oblique fracture **52**, *53*
- in transverse fracture **52**
- in volar fractures *55*
- plates in **47**, *48, 49*
- screws in **48**, *49, 50*
- technical principles in **47**, *48, 49*
Postoperative treatment
- in evidence-based medicine **13**
- in intramedullary screw placement **45**
Proximal interphalangeal joint (PIP)
- fracture dislocation, K-wire fixation in **36**, *38*
- fracture subluxation *21*
- in musicians *124, 125, 126, 128*

R

Radial collateral ligament injury, nonoperative treatment of **24**
Rehabilitation
- challenges in **145**
- circumference measurement in **146**, *147*
- extension in **150**
- extension sleeve in **150**
- flossing in **148**, *149*
- force measurement in **146**, *147*
- hand span distance in **146**
- home exercises in **151**, *153*
- incomplete fist closure in **146**
- in metacarpal fractures **154**, *155*
- lymphatic drainage in **148**, *149, 150, 153*
- manual therapy in **146**, *148, 153*
- measurement tools in **145**, *146*
- mirror therapy in **149**, *150*
- neurological evaluation in **146**, *147*
- of phalangeal fractures **154**, *155, 156*
- patient evaluation in **145**
- scar treatment in **150**, *151, 152*
- sensibility training in **150**, *151*
- splints in **151**, *152*
- techniques **146**
- traction in **150**
- volume measurement in *147*
- wrist *153*
Revascularization, in compound hand injuries **83**

S

Salter-Harris classification *4, 6, 91*
Salter II fractures, locations of *4*
Saxophone *126, 127*
Scaphoid fractures
- arthroscopic surgery in **75**, *76, 77, 78, 79, 80*
- conservative treatment of *73*

- diagnosis of **75**
- in athletes **113**, *114, 115*
- incidence **7**
- indications for surgical treatment of **73**, *74*
- in evidence-based medicine **12**
- in musicians **132**, *133*
- nonunion
-- classification of **250**
-- clinical signs in **251**
-- dysvascular **253**
-- fibrous, without deformity **251**
-- fixation and grafting in **254**, *255, 256*
-- iliac crest graft in **256**
-- imaging in **251**, *252*
-- in athletes 113
-- in evidence-based medicine **258**
-- medial femoral condyle graft in 257
-- natural history of **249**, *250*
-- pedicled graft in 257
-- percutaneous fixation and grafting in **254**
-- prognosis in **258**
-- proximal pole **253**
-- salvage procedures in **258**
-- surgical techniques for **254**
-- tests in **251**
-- treatment indications **251**
-- waist, and humpback deformity **252**, *253*

- nonunion in
-- trauma mechanism in **249**
-- pediatric 97, *98*
-- plate and screw fixation in *50*
Scaphoid nonunion advanced collapse (SNAC) 51, 113
Scapholunate injuries, in athletes **118**, *119*
Scar treatment, in rehabilitation **150**, *151, 152*
Screw fixation 259
  See also Intramedullary screws; Plate and screw fixation
- in intra-articular proximal interphalangeal joint fracture **180**, *181*
- in phalangeal extra-articular fractures **167**, *168*
Sensibility training, in rehabilitation **150**, *151*
Seymour's fracture **92**, *93, 94*
Skin coverage, in compound hand injuries **87**, *88*
Spinal cord injury, paralytic extremity fractures and **101**
Splints, in rehabilitation **151**, *152*
Sports 259
  See also Athletes
String instruments **124**, *125, 126, 129*
Stroke, paralytic extremity fractures and **103**

T

Theta loop 29
Thumb fractures 259
  See also Bennett's fracture
- incidence **5**
- nonoperative treatment of
-- metacarpophalangeal joint avulsion **22**
-- with radial collateral ligament injury **24**
-- with ulnar collateral ligament injury **22**, *23*
Tinel's sign *147*
Trapezium *8*
Trapezium fractures
- classification of **267**
- clinical signs in **267**
- concurrent lesions in **267**
- in athletes **116**
- incidence of **7**
- investigatory examinations **267**, *268*
- plate and screw fixation in *50*
- tests **267**
- trauma mechanism in **266**
- treatment of **268**, *269*
Trapezoid *8*
Trapezoid fractures
- in athletes **117**
- incidence **8**
Triquetral fractures
- classification of **262**
- clinical signs in **262**

- concurrent lesions with **263**
- in athletes **116**
- incidence **7**
- investigatory examinations in **263**
- open reduction and internal fixation of 263, *264*
- prognosis in **264**
- test in **262**
- trauma mechanism in **262**
- treatment of **263**, *264*
Triquetrum *8*
Trombone 125
Trumpet 125
Tuba 126
Tuft fractures **94**, **171**

U

Ulnar collateral ligament injury, nonoperative treatment of **22**, *23*

V

Viola 124
Violin 124

W

Woodwind instruments **126**, *129*
Wrist rehabilitation **153**, *154, 155*